THE VENEREAL DISEASES;

THEIR

PATHOLOGICAL NATURE, CORRECT DIAGNOSIS,

AND

HOMŒOPATHIC TREATMENT.

PREPARED IN ACCORDANCE WITH THE AUTHOR'S OWN, AS WELL AS WITH THE EXPERIENCE OF OTHER PHYSICIANS, AND ACCOMPANIED WITH CRITICAL DISCUSSIONS,

BY G. H. G. JAHR, M.D.

TRANSLATED, WITH NUMEROUS AND IMPORTANT ADDITIONS FROM THE WORKS OF OTHER AUTHORS, AND FROM HIS OWN EXPERIENCE,

BY CHARLES J. HEMPEL, M.D.

NEW YORK:
PUBLISHED BY WM. RADDE, 550 PEARL STREET.
PHILADELPHIA: F. E. BOERICKE, 635 ARCH STREET.
Boston: OTIS CLAPP. St. Louis: H. C. G. LUYTIES. Cincinnati: SMITH & WORTHINGTON.
Pittsburg: J. G. BACKOFEN & SON. Cleveland: BECKWITH & CO. Detroit: E. A. LODGE.
Chicago: KEEN & CO., and C. S. HALSEY.
LONDON: H. TURNER & CO., and JAMES EPPS.
1868.

THE TROW & SMITH
BOOK MANUFACTURING COMPANY,
46, 48, 50 Greene Street, N. Y.

TRANSLATOR'S PREFACE.

Of the different works on venereal diseases that have been given to the profession, we consider this the best. It not only presents the subject of which it treats in the accredited forms of science, but it likewise shows, most conclusively, that there can be no truly scientific treatment of syphilis, or of disease generally, without a thorough knowledge of its pathological nature. Following the impulse of his naturally investigating mind, Jahr has in this work, more than in any other of his publications, been led beyond the boundaries of a barren treatment by mere symptoms, and has boldly and manfully proclaimed the doctrine which all progressive and philosophical physicians of our School have advocated long ago, that disease is not a mere string of symptoms, but an internal state of the organism deviating more or less from its normal condition, and that the phenomena amenable to sensual observation indicate the character and extent of this deviation. An analysis and accurate perception of these phenomena very properly belong to the province of the understanding; but an appreciative comprehension of the meaning and value of these phenomena, and their connection and relation in one or more broad generalizations, is the business of another equally legitimate faculty of the mind, whose claims, in the department of Medicine, have been denied by many of the older adherents of Hahnemann, and are still denied by a few modern falsifiers of Homœopathy: the Scientific Reason. We confess it has afforded us a genuine pleasure to be the instrument of enabling such of our physicians as are not conversant with the author's own language, to render themselves familiar with the highly instructive, practical, and philosophical teachings of this volume.

We cannot be sufficiently grateful to Jahr for the efforts he has been making for a period of forty years in behalf of the spread and popularity of Homœopathy. His "French Manual" first placed the subject of Homœopathy fairly before the profession in France. Hering's excellent translation of Jahr's original work introduced the subject to the progressive inquirer of our own country. Since that time Jahr's numerous works, some of which, like his "Symptomen-codex," and "Repertory," are of large size, have been continually adding to our stock of knowledge and to our means of usefulness. We cannot sufficiently honor a man for having worked so zealously in a cause involving the dearest interests of humanity.

In perfecting the translation of this work, we desire to tender to our friend and colleague, Doctor Lilienthal of New York, our thanks for having aided us with his valuable suggestions and efficient coöperation in accomplishing a task, the difficulties of which those who are acquainted with Jahr's peculiar, interminable, and fatiguing phraseology will be best able to appreciate. The sense, and even the text of the original work, had to be faithfully rendered in a language, the laws and precise brevity of which are utterly at variance with the heavy and entangled periods of our friend, the Author.

We have taken the liberty of rendering the term "*Syphiliden,*" which is frequently made use of by German authors, by the corresponding term "*Syphilidæ;*" and to some of the intermediate forms of syphilis we have applied the term "*syphiloid.*"

In conclusion, we beg leave to direct the reader's attention to numerous additions with which the original work has been interspersed. Every useful suggestion and observation, concerning the employment of new remedies and the value of different modes of treatment, which are recorded in our periodicals, as well as in our larger publications, has been carefully weighed and appropriated for the benefit of the professional reader.

In return for the good which this volume will undoubtedly accomplish, we bespeak for it a liberal and generous reception.

CHARLES J. HEMPEL, M.D.

GRAND RAPIDS, MICH.,
January, 1868.

TABLE OF CONTENTS.

FIRST DIVISION.

THE PRIMARY FORMS OF THE VENEREAL DISEASES.

FIRST CHAPTER.

OF THE VENEREAL PHENOMENA GENERALLY.

SECOND CHAPTER.

THE DIFFERENT FORMS OF GONORRHŒA.

THIRD CHAPTER.

THE VARIOUS FORMS OF CHANCRE.

FOURTH CHAPTER.

OTHER PRIMARY FORMS OF SYPHILIS.

SECOND DIVISION.

THE SECONDARY FORMS OF SYPHILIS.

FIRST CHAPTER.

OF SECONDARY SYPHILIS GENERALLY.

SECOND CHAPTER.

SYPHILITIC CUTANEOUS AFFECTIONS.

THIRD CHAPTER.

INTERMEDIATE FORMS OF SECONDARY SYPHILIS.

THIRD DIVISION.

GENERAL PATHOLOGICAL OBSERVATIONS ON SYPHILIS AND ITS COURSE GENERALLY.

FIRST CHAPTER.

PATHOLOGICAL NATURE AND ORIGIN OF SYPHILIS.

SECOND CHAPTER.

OF VENEREAL CONTAGIA.

THIRD CHAPTER.

GENERAL DEVELOPMENT, COURSE, AND TERMINATION OF SYPHILIS.

FOURTH DIVISION.

GENERAL THERAPEUTIC OBSERVATIONS ON THE TREATMENT OF SYPHILIS.

FIRST CHAPTER.

GENERAL DIAGNOSTIC REMARKS.

SECOND CHAPTER.

GENERAL THERAPEUTIC OBSERVATIONS.

THIRD CHAPTER.

PHARMACO-DYNAMIC OBSERVATIONS.

ADDENDA.

ALPHABETICAL INDEX

OF THE

DIFFERENT SUBJECTS TREATED OF IN THIS VOLUME.

PREFACE.

It is now more than twenty years since the study of the "*Cutaneous Syphilitic Affections*," by Doctor Cazenave, of Paris, whose labors in this department of medical knowledge occupy such a deservedly eminent rank, induced me to devote particular attention to the multifarious and frequently misjudged forms of secondary and constitutional syphilis, and to observe the character and general development of this disease, among a number of individuals of both sexes and varied ages, temperaments, and constitutions, from the first origin of the malady to its return to masked forms of existence. The greater, however, my opportunities, by pursuing this course, of becoming acquainted, by personal experience, with every known form of this disease, and of comparing my own observations with those of the different writers on syphilis, and with the statements of other physicians generally, the more I became convinced that, with the single exception of special treatises on syphilis by ancient and modern writers, most pathological and therapeutic manuals, especially when arranged by authors who only knew syphilis from books, are filled with the most fanciful hypotheses as irrefutable articles of faith, and that even among our own number, many practitioners are still far removed from a lucid and positive knowledge of syphilis, of the true nature of its primary and secondary products, of the different forms in which they manifest themselves as specific pathological alterations, or are frequently found concealed under the mask of other apparently different diseases. For this reason I have frequently been tempted to treat various points of this disease and its treatment, in our homœopathic periodicals; but, being satisfied that a few isolated compositions on this subject would do little good in the absence of a work which would present the most important and best-substantiated observations of our specific writers on syphilis, not, after the fashion of our present manuals, in a series of dogmatic assertions, but likewise *with critical acumen*, I have deemed it preferable to condense in one volume all the noteworthy facts concerning syphilis which I have been able to gather during the last twenty years both in my own private practice and from the study of a variety of the most reputable works. In offering this volume, my special aim has been to furnish the busy practitioner of our school, who has not the time to verify, in such cases as may fall under his notice, the correctness of the observations contained in our manuals by comparing them with upwards of a hundred original works, a treatise where he finds condensed and critically considered, in as brief a space as possible, every thing noteworthy that the authors of those works have written on the pathological nature, diagnosis, and course of venereal diseases, but where the cures of these diseases, reported by our own authors, are likewise subjected to a careful review and analysis. In one word, what I designed to accomplish in arranging this work, was to place the practitioner in possession of a guide both intelligible and trustworthy, that should lead him, without much useless trouble, through the still comparatively unknown domain of chronic syphilis, and render a knowledge of this disease, even under its most hidden forms, as easy as that of primary gonorrhœa, chancre, bubo, and sycosic condylomata.

Had the *founder of our school*, instead of sojourning in a small city of Germany, resided in Paris or London, and only seen the tenth part of the venereal diseases which any physician in those cities, who devotes a more or less exclusive attention to the study and treatment of syphilis, has occasion to observe in the course of several years of practice, in all its varied forms among men, women, and *children*, he would most likely have treated of these diseases as fully as of his so-called *psora*, and, with his habitual acumen and in his masterly manner, would have diagnosed and delineated the varied forms of *chronic*, *secondary*, or constitutional syphilis. For be it ever so much insisted upon that Hahnemann was a declared enemy of *diagnosis* and *names of diseases*, and that, from principle, he would never have consented, even if he had been able, to fill this great gap in his system; such an opinion is either derived from an entire ignorance of the *true spirit* of his doctrine, or else is based upon an intentionally *malicious interpretation* of all his pathological and diagnostic tendencies and endeavors. What he rejected, and was absolutely unwilling to regard as scientific, was, that certain names, such as *dropsy, jaundice, cough, nervous debility*, etc., whose symptomatic manifestations may be peculiar to pathological conditions of the most different natures, should be described as idiopathic diseases. What he, on the contrary, admitted and even demanded, was an exact knowledge and correctly discriminating appreciation of the pathognomonic characteristics of all diseases which nature herself has distinguished from each other, and which depend upon some *permanent, unchanging, specific cause*, such as scarlatina, purpura miliaris, measles, whooping-cough, croup, cholera, etc. If he had taught his *psora doctrine* at the commencement of his homœopathic career, we have no reason to doubt that, at a later period, his innate energy of mind, which had become somewhat weakened in after-years, would have led him to delineate separate forms of scrofulosis, tuberculosis, and such like diatheses, and even to describe characteristically distinct forms of psora, as he had formerly described gonorrhœa, syphilis, and *sycosis*, as distinct diseases. Be this, however, as it may, even if Hahnemann has left us no definite theoretical opinions on these subjects, the necessity of investigating all *idiopathic, specific* diseases results from his teachings *implicitly*, just as much as the investigation of specific drug-effects is *explicitly* taught by him. As long, therefore, as the so-called *physiological* school has not succeeded in prevailing upon us to regard the doctrine of idiopathic diseases, after its founder, Broussais, as an absurdity, so long it is not only the right, but it becomes the duty of *our* school, provided it means to progress in the true spirit of its founder, to enrich the science of medicine both by an exact investigation of all *specific diseases*, and their *fixed forms of manifestation*, as well as by the study of specific *drug-effects*. This cannot be denied by any body whom the doctrines of our master have inspired with their true spirit, and with a clear perception of the task and destiny of our school.

It is strange, indeed, that Hahnemann should never have seemed able to attain to a sufficiently lucid knowledge of the essential differences between different diseases, which must, however, have presented themselves to his mind in his own practice, to embody them in some positive doctrine, and thus to prevent the one-sided doctrines of the *specific school* as well as the errors of the *physiologists.* I mean the difference between *specific pathological* and more or less purely *physiological* disturbances of health. Both exist. The physiologists err in rejecting all idiopathic diseases, and the adherents of the specific school in regarding all, even purely accidental disturbances of an organ, as *absolute pathological* forms of disease which require to be controlled by definite specifics, thus rejecting a consideration of the *individual symptoms* as mere Hahnemannism, even in cases where the *physiological* phenomena are alone capable of pointing out the true remedy. Among the so-called *physiological* forms of disease, we number without exception all the more or less unimportant or extensive *functional disturbances* which originate in some transitory and frequently trifling cause of disease, such as violent emotions, a cold, derangement of the stomach, excessive bodily or mental exertions, or other trifling causes. Although we are in possession of remedial agents which are more specially related to these causes as well as to the affected organ, yet we should commit a great mistake, if, in such cases, we were to select a remedy, not as Hahnemann teaches, almost exclusively in accordance with the symptoms characterizing the individual case, but, as is demanded by the *specific school,* in accordance with the *name* of the disease or with one of its leading forms. The case is different with *specific pathological* diseases depending upon some specific cause, of which Hahnemann, in his "*Medicine of Experience*" teaches that a *specific* remedy, if known, will always cure them provided they are "*uncomplicated.*" To this class belong all the *miasmatic,* and likewise all clearly marked *drug-diseases.* If we extend the limits of Hahnemann's categories so far as to admit these *pathological* disturbances not only *in the gross,* but likewise class them with reference to their *special forms* in so far as they can be regarded as *fixed* and strictly *pathognomonic,* without being obscured or modified by *extraneous* or *individualizing* influences, we must concede it as a fact that in these diseases, if not absolutely in all cases, at least in most of them, it is the *pathological form* which determines the remedy, in the same way as, in all other not *idiopathic* diseases, the choice of the remedy must always depend upon the *individual physiological symptoms.* To be neither a *one-sided* adherent of the specific school, nor a one-sided *physiologist*, but to act in the one case as a *pathological specificist*, and in the other case as a *physiological symptomist*, and to be guided in either case by the law "*similia similibus*," is the task of every physician who means to practice our art not merely according to the *letter*, but likewise according to the *spirit* of its author; in other words, in accordance with the fundamental ideas to which he has given utterance with more or less scientific fulness and precision.

As regards the classification and correct delineation of the *acknowledged fixed* forms of primary and secondary syphilis, I believe I have accomplished all that I was able to do at the present period, in accordance with the facts which I have gathered in my own practice as well as from other sources, although I feel very sensibly that a great deal yet remains to be done to complete a knowledge of their remedial agents, and the mode of applying them, agreeably to the nature of each particular case. Yet even in this respect I have frequently indicated certain general rules which beginning practitioners may avail themselves of, to great advantage, in the treatment of certain definitive forms belonging to the same class of syphilitic diseases. A single physician, however, cannot be expected to meet a sufficient number of cases of syphilis to enable him to draw positive conclusions regarding the most appropriate remedies in the different forms of this disease. Nevertheless, if we mean to obtain truly useful results by co-operation, we should never content ourselves with mentioning mere *names* in reporting our cases of cure, but we should likewise furnish an exact *symptomatic* description of every case, in order that the reader may be enabled to judge for himself whether the pretended simple gonorrhœa, the regular, raised, *phagedenic* or *Hunterian* chancre, was indeed a gonorrhœa simplex, an *ulcus regulare, elevatum, phagedænicum* or *induratum*, or not; a subject which will remain of the highest importance as long as many a physician is still disposed to talk about figwarts or even chancres which he professes to have cured with this or that remedy; whereas it appears from all his statements that the case in point was one of *mucous tubercles.* These remarks apply still more forcibly to the different forms of secondary syphilis, where we are frequently plunged into doubt by the advice of those who recommend to us remedies for tertiary or quaternary forms of this disease without informing us, in spite of the notorious indefiniteness of these disorders, *what* forms, in their opinion, belong to one or the other class; or in spite of the fact that the *gummatose swellings* which are seated in the cellular tissue are located among the osseous affections by some, or mercurial ulcers are confounded with secondary chancres by others. Pathological *names* for *fixed* pathological forms of *idiopathic* diseases do very well, provided the forms which are designated by these names, are fixed and clearly defined, and the reporter does not err in his diagnosis. But should the least doubt prevail regarding the correctness of the diagnosis, names may do a great deal of mischief, more particularly since the homœopathic law may lead us to decide *à priori* in favor of more than one remedial agent as adapted to a given case, one or more of which will undoubtedly prove curative; however, their truly specific character as curative agents, and their scientifically specific relation to the case in hand, will have to be determined by their practical application.

For the reasons here stated, I have not deemed it advisable to follow the example of Attomyr and of several other homœopaths, to recommend, as *probably useful*, in accordance with mere provings, agents that had not yet been tested in practice, or to suggest, as adapted to similarly named *syphilitic* affections, in accordance with mere external *analogies*, drugs that had been found curative in cases of *common warts*, *scrofulous glandular swellings*, or *rhachitic affections.* He who approves of such therapeutic conclusions is at liberty to consult general repertories for the similarly-named symptoms of such drugs in non-syphilitic diseases, and to apply them upon his own responsibility, *by way of experiment;* if they help, in such a case we shall have enlarged the boundaries of our practical experience; if they do not help, the practitioner has to accuse himself alone for his erroneous conclusions. It is indeed *possible* that one or the other remedy which produces *similar anatomical changes,* may likewise prove curative against *syphilitic alterations of tissue;* but we can only depend with certainty for curative results upon remedies which, like *Mercurius, Nitri acidum, Thuja, Cinnabris, Lycopodium* and the like, not only cover with their symptoms the functional derangements of single organs, but correspond to the totality of the syphilitic process; and, since this correspondence of their total characteristics to the totality of the syphilitic process is very frequently difficult to determine *a priori,* we feel bound to advise beginners to depend upon *well-tried* remedies, before they undertake to use drugs that only enjoy a theoretic recommendation; or, guided by a few more or less hazardous therapeutic conclusions, to look for other remedial agents in some general repertory. Thus, for instance, whatever may have been said in favor of *Sulphur* or *Lachesis* in consequence of their induration-symptoms, neither of these remedies is as efficient against the Hunterian chancre as *Mercurius,* which, indeed, has not the induration-symptom, but otherwise corresponds to the totality of the peculiar characteristics of the syphilitic process; and if, in this case, which is reported by its author for the purpose of backing up his theory, the patient had not already been drugged by his allopathic physician with large doses of Mercury, every practitioner will admit that the use of *Sulphur* and *Lachesis* would have been a loss of time. Otherwise, as regards the *characteristic induration of the Hunterian chancre,* which some regard as the genuinely pathognomonic sign of the true *gummatose* or *cellular syphilis* first described by Professor Virchow of Berlin, I am likewise of opinion, as may be seen in the third division of this work (§§ 152–166), that the indurated ulcer constitutes the true type of the chancre-syphilis; nevertheless I cannot agree with recent syphilographs of Lyon, who traces the soft, elevated, phagedenic, gangrenous chancre to some *other virus;* but I am to this day of opinion, with Ricord of Paris, that this form of ulcer is simply a mismanaged or degenerated Hunterian chancre. However, since the facts which both parties have adduced in support of their respective theories are still very contradictory, and my own observations are still too imperfect to furnish me with irrefutable arguments on this subject, I have deemed it preferable *not to institute any further* inquiry into a question of this kind, and to postpone a discussion of this point as well as of Virchow's still problematical observations concerning gummata in the lungs, heart, liver, etc., until more satisfactory observations shall have been accumulated by the Profession. I am all the more persuaded to pursue this course since the diagnosis of all these gummata of *internal* organs is still enveloped in great obscurity, and all that can as yet be said on this subject with any thing like certainty, is confined to the swellings described in the subsequent paragraphs, §§ 147–149.

These are the leading ideas which I have sought to embody in this work with as much logical correctness as possible, and which have guided me in perfecting as lucid and comprehensible an arrangement of the different forms of venereal diseases as can be obtained in the present state of medical science. Having explained the purpose and plan of my work thus far, I might perhaps be allowed to conclude this preface, if it were not for some other matter which has weighed heavily upon my mind even while I was writing this work, and which I feel bound to touch upon before I lay down my pen. This is the unfortunate *systematic-anti-Hahnemannism* which, since the first appearance of the great specificist *Rau* and his followers, has unhappily taken possession of the minds of some of our recent homœopaths, and which, as I have learned to my great grief from various oral discussions, is pushed so far in many quarters, out of a pure *spirit of opposition*, as not only to reject the *dynamic* effect of our attenuations, but every action of any morbific agent that is not *demonstrable by chemical tests*, and thus to stifle all belief in a concealed syphilis which may still exist in certain cases in spite of the absence of all perceptible symptoms; yea, to reject even the dangerous character of cauterizations of chancres as mere *Hahnemannism*, and to silence those who differ from them in opinion, by reproaching them with a brainless desire to imitate the master. More than once, when thinking of these quarrelsome disturbers and of their malicious criticism, I was on the point of destroying my manuscript; not because I fear them *personally* (for it will be seen in the course of this work that I know how to answer them); oh, no! simply because I did not wish to furnish an opportunity of seeing truths that have been recognised as such by the greatest physicians, repudiated in the style and after the fashion of the former Carlsruhe clique, for no better reason than because their defence emanated from the pen of one of Hahnemann's partisans. Fortunately this systematic opposition-party does not constitute a majority in our School, which still numbers among its adherents *competent* men; if only one of these competent and serious men, a V. Meyer, Clotar Müller, Vehsemeyer, or any one of the present *Leipsic*, *Berlin*, or *Vienna* School should be pleased to read this book without prejudice, and to subject the views therein expressed to further scientific discussions, such treatment would compensate me more than any thing else for the time and labor which I have devoted to this work. For, even if I differ in my understanding of this or that point of Hahnemann's doctrine from the opinions entertained by these honorable men, on the other hand I have profited too much by their teachings, not to accept every suggestion that is offered to me from that quarter, so much the more gratefully as I have constantly entertained the highest respect for the serious, truth-seeking and truth-loving minds of the above-mentioned practitioners, and have frequently desired that some of them might attack others who differ from them in opinion, a little more *sine ira et studio.* Whatever reception this book may meet with, it will have to be admitted that I have considered every fact which has been made public on this subject, down to the most recent period; that I have condensed with logical brevity all the facts which experience has confirmed and demonstrated; that I have added my own observations to every statement which I had verified in my own practice; and that I have not mentioned a single *questionable* point without examining it on all sides as fully as possible. In conclusion I beg the reader to accept this book in the spirit in which it is offered: as a proof of the author's desire not to remain behind with his contributions in building up an edifice for which a sufficient number of workmen are still wanting to furnish the material.

Paris, December 24th, 1866.

The Author.

THE

VENEREAL DISEASES.

THEIR

PATHOLOGICAL NATURE, CORRECT DIAGNOSIS, AND HOMŒOPATHIC TREATMENT.

INTRODUCTION.

Among all the diseases that weigh upon suffering humanity, there are probably none which are more extensively discussed by physicians, more dreaded by some, more frivolously regarded by others, and at the same time less definitely determined, with regard to their course and the boundaries of their various forms, than the diseases designated as *venereal.* According to *Fallopius*, *Girtanner*, *Astruc*, *Hunter*, *Van Swieten*, etc., among the older, or *Carmichael*, *Bell*, *Cazenave*, *Biett*, *Baumès*, and others, among recent physicians, there exists nothing more fearful and insidious in the world than these diseases. Fostered in the fatal bosom of a degrading passion, and conceived at a moment of burning lust, they scatter, according to some, silently and mysteriously their poisonous seed whose offspring, which, at its first appearance, is but lightly regarded and extirpated from the sphere of observation as speedily as possible by the criminal hand of indiscreet or ignorant physicians, nevertheless continues silently to unfold its manifold germs in the organism, until they break forth anew in a variety of different forms and thus announce to every eye the presence of the still raging malady. Again repressed by external means and again sprouting forth in other parts, they penetrate, according to the assertions of observers, all the tissues of the patient, who, far from suspecting the enemy that is gnawing at his vital forces, very frequently sees one organ after the other invaded and destroyed, his face disfigured in the most horrible manner, his muscles and bones perforated, and his frame generally overwhelmed by the most horrid tortures without knowing how his distress can be alleviated were it only in a trifling degree. Whatever revolting and horrifying diseases are met with in large cities, in the huts of misery and in the gloomy abodes of vice: all those wretches who are covered with ugly scars and horrid ulcers; whose *faces* are disfigured by pustules and suppurating blotches; who are not unfrequently deprived of their noses and even eyes; who are emaciated to skeletons; whose livid and shrivelled skin is dangling around their fleshless bones; and who, spreading a pestilential fetor all around, wander about like half-rotten cadavers from the tombs, or who, removed from human society and avoided even by their own friends, are stretched upon the torture-bed of despair, praying for death as their greatest blessing: all these unfortunates, according to the common opinion of the greatest physicians, owe the whole sum of their sufferings to no other cause than to venereal infection, which, having been contracted in an unguarded moment, had been neglected, disregarded and afterwards mismanaged throughout. Yea, if these physicians are to be believed, a whole number of the most chronic and most incurable organic affections of various kinds, with which inhabitants of large cities are afflicted, emanate from this cause as their true fountain-head; their true character, unless they had reached the previously described fearful height, being almost always misapprehended, so that they are confounded with other less dangerous diseases, and the poison, even if, favored by peculiar circumstances, it should not break forth in actual disease in all cases, is transmitted to the children and entails upon them the distressing and irresistible processes of destruction from which the parents had luckily escaped. It is the opinion of the above-named physicians that these diseases contain a *virus* which, if once introduced into the organism, germinates unless previously neutralized by its *specific antidote*, and sprouts in the organism, after the fashion of parasitical growths, at the expense of its vital essence and strength, and continues to sprout until the body perishes by the poison. Where, according to the testimony of these physicians, nothing is done against these diseases than merely to obliterate their sprouting growths, the root remains in the organic tissues and may sprout forth again any time until life is annihilated by this murderous destroyer.

On the other hand, these physicians are opposed by others, more particularly by the adherents of the Physiological School founded by Broussais. Starting from the view, which may not be erroneous of itself, that all *pathological* processes are, primarily, deviations from the normal physiological form, they not only reject all belief in some peculiar *contagium* or *virus*, but likewise repudiate the doctrine of *idiopathic* diseases, tracing, as they do, the first cause of all imaginable diseases to a simple inflammation which may have been caused by some mechanical or chemical irritation, and whose ulterior course and form depend exclusively upon the character of the invaded organ, upon the physiological temperament of the individual, and upon the accidental supervention of external, either ameliorating or deteriorating influences. This school, which, in the department of venereal diseases, may be said to be represented by *Jourdan*, *Devergie*, and *Desruelles*, does not deny the existence of the disorders which the opponents of Broussais describe as the products of the syphilitic virus; but it maintains that it is wrong to attribute them to impure coition or, still worse, to some *specific contagium*, contending as they do that the so-called venereal disease owes its origin to nothing else than a *simple inflammation* caused by acrid menstrual blood, an acrid hemorrhoidal discharge, or some other acrid humor, and that this inflammation, like any other that had been caused by purely chemical agents, such as lunar caustic, etc., only becomes worse in case the affected individual either has constitutionally bad humors, or had been abusively treated with Mercury or some other irritating agents. In corroboration of this view, the Physiological School partly refers to the total ignorance which prevailed among the ancients, of *particular*, so-called *venereal ulcers* or venereal affections generally as a special class, and partly to the proportionally small number of cases where accidental discharges or ulcers, that had been occasioned by an *inflammatory* or *irritating* coït, were succeeded by derangements of a different kind. By thus attributing a large portion of the disorders that other physicians traced to the *venereal virus*, exclusively to individual disposition or to the action of irritating drugs, the Physiological School at the same time holds that what are falsely called venereal diseases have no existence in fact, nor would these supposed venereal diseases ever have existed if we had always taken the precaution of combating, at the outset, the inflammation that might have resulted from an inflammatory or irritating coït, by such *antiphlogistic* means as leeches, cups, bleeding, etc. Between the physiological physicians —who not only deny the existence of a specific virus, but the pathognomonic character of all venereal diseases—and their above-named opponents, there are many physicians who occupy an intermediate position, in so far as they not only accept the essential nature of these diseases, but likewise admit the existence of a specific virus as indispensably necessary to cause venereal infection; but, on the other hand, neither recognize all the phenomena of syphilitic poisoning described by their opponents as such, nor admit the absolute danger which the artificial extirpation, cauterization or suppression of supervening discharges, ulcers, etc., is said to involve. Some English physicians, for instance, ascribe, if not all the phenomena which are generally supposed to constitute *secondary syphilis*, at least the *affections of the bony system*, and a variety of *cutaneous diseases* which others regard as venereal, to the abuse of mercury; and other practitioners want to know, with *Girtanner*, *Hecker* and *Ricord*, whether the internal administration of some *specific* antidote is at all necessary, and whether it is not sufficient to suppress the incipient products of the contagion as speedily as they appear upon the skin, and to prevent them, as they imagine, in this manner from becoming rooted in the organism.

But even among those who believe in the existence of a specific virus as well as in the necessity of annihilating it in the interior of the organism by some specific antidote, the views concerning the *pathological* nature of syphilitic diseases and the specific poison which produces them, differ a good deal.

It is well known that several physicians, more especially *Bell*, *Carmichael*, and others, as well as *Hahnemann*, whose views, as expressed in the year 1788, had undergone a radical change in the year 1816, held that there are three different kinds of virus leading to three different classes of syphilitic diseases, which have to be combated by three corresponding specific antidotes: 1. *syphilis* or *chancre;* 2. *sycosis* or *figwart-diseases;* and 3. the common or *idiopathic gonorrhœa.* Any one who is acquainted with modern syphilography, must know that, even among the greatest physicians of France, the dispute concerning the homogeneousness or heterogeneousness of *chancre, mucous condylomata* and *gonorrhœa,* is not yet ended even at this late period. It is indeed true that more recently the essential oneness of the different forms of syphilis has been advocated by *Davasse* of Paris, *Lancelot* of Lyons, and generally by the physicians of this last-named city. They base this advocacy upon the assertion that they had never yet seen in hospitals *mucous tubercles* that had not been demonstrably preceded by chancre; in opposition to which Parisian physicians continue to assert that these mucous tubercles may be generated *protopathically* by direct infection, without any previous chancre. We have, moreover, to consider that the advocates of the homogeneous oneness of syphilis, nothwithstanding they derive mucous tubercles from the Hunterian chancre, which they regard as the the only true *ulcus regulare,* on the other hand attribute to the elevated, soft, phagedænic, and other chancre forms, the property to propagate their *own specific forms* by infection without engendering *constitutional syphilis* as in the case of the regular chancre—a distinction which we cannot receive from a pathological stand-point without being logically led to the doctrine of essential differences in the nature of the *contagium.* In our own school, where it seemed to be the chief endeavor of some, at a previous period, to differ from Hahnemann, short work has been made of this subject. Without even instituting the least inquiry into this subject, Hartmann's system of therapeutics, for instance, teaches the doctrine of a homogeneous *lues venerea,* of which chancre, as well as gonorrhœa, are products of equal import and character; whereas, beside *Hahnemann,* several of the greatest physicians of England and France, such as *Baumès, Bell, Bafour, Duncan, Hernandez,* even *Ricord,* contend for the non-malignant character of a simple, *idiopathic gonorrhœa* as a non-syphilitic disease. These physicians are indeed opposed by others, like *Hunter, Lagneau,*

Ritter, *Cazenave*, *Castelnau*, and others, who not only consider gonorrhœa a syphilitic disease, but attribute to the gonorrhœal virus the power, unless previously eradicated by specific anti-syphilitic antidotes, to produce the same *secondary* and *constitutional phenomena* as *chancre*. Now, inasmuch as, according to the universally received doctrines of our school, so far, at least, *mercury* continues to be regarded as the sovereign specific against *primary* as well as *secondary syphilis*, how can we account for the fact that Hartmann, as well as all those who believe in the homogeneous oneness of the different forms of syphilis, can be content with curing a case of gonorrhœa with *cannabis*, which is no remedy for syphilis, without feeling uneasy regarding ulterior pernicious results of the syphilitic virus? It is plain enough that Hahnemann, who fancied he had discovered three distinct syphilitic miasms and three corresponding antidotes, had a perfect right to imagine that these antidotes would radically annihilate the virus; but if it was proper to upset his theory, what right had one to continue his practice, which was based upon this very theory? And if his practice was correct, with what right was his theory abandoned?

It is an easy thing to oppose Hahnemann's views and the opinions of those who agree with him, with all sorts of bold assertions of a contrary character, especially if one does not take the trouble to show the scientific correctness of antagonistic arguments. As for ourselves, we frankly confess that we are far from accepting unconditionally every thing that this excellent observer has taught on the subject of venereal diseases; but have those who make it their business to contradict him in every thing without rhyme or reason, ever considered why syphilis, if it is indeed a disease *one* and *indivisible*, manifests itself under various forms, both protopathically and deuteropathically, each form being endowed with a capacity of reproducing itself *specifically* by contagion? Have they a more palpable hypothesis in the place of Hahnemann's, which accounts for all contradictions between theory and practice, as well as all apparently contradictory facts, in a most natural and comprehensible manner, and explains the most opposite statements to the satisfaction of every body, in such an easy and unaffected manner that each separate fact in the series seems authorized to claim its place as equally possible and legitimate? More than one, who knows how to accuse others of a deficient knowledge of pathology, brags of *tertiary* and *quarternary* syphilis; but are these gentlemen prepared to show the characteristic differences even between primary and secondary syphilis, and to explain why the same remedies that will remove the primary disease, have to be exchanged for others in combating the secondary form? Are they able to say where the primary form ends, and the truly secondary symptoms commence, and what *fixed* symptoms always characterize the former, and can never, nor ever ought to, characterize the latter? Whence do we at all know, provided we do not blindly follow some pathological manual, that there exists a *secondary* syphilis, and that every morbid manifestation which we consider as a secondary symptom of this disease is not, as some of us indeed believe, if not of a *mercurial*, at least of an herpetic, scrofulous, or *psoric* origin? And if the latter should not be the case; if there are phenomena that owe their origin to the mismanagement of some primary form of the disease, what primary form, among those which constitute this category, is it that serves in every case as an undoubted basis to the former? As we said before, many authors regard the external suppression of the Hunterian chancre, which they would like to preserve as an everlasting scourge at the spot where it first made its appearance, as the sole cause of all the mischief, whereas they dry up a *gonorrhœa* as a most innocent precursor of syphilis, or even as a non-syphilitic disease, and cut away figwarts with a pair of scissors as a *purely local excrescence* of the chancrous disease; others, again, suspect a character of malignancy in either of these two categories of phenomena as much as in chancre itself, and trace every morbid symptom, of whatever name, which is occasioned by an impure coït, to the action of a virus which, unless neutralized by its specific antidote, must and always will produce the same ravages of disease. We know what Hahnemann thought of the evil consequences that might result from an unnatural suppression of gonorrhœa and of a chancre or figwarts; but who is able, even in this respect, to show by irrefutable testimony where the truth is to be found, in Hahnemann, who met with the most determined opposition even in his own ranks, or in the writings of his opponents? And, finally, if there are morbid phenomena that owe their origin to the action of some specific contagium, what are the phenomena to which this fact applies with axiomatic certainty, and what scientific reason is there, that might justify a belief in the emanation, from a similar origin, of a variety of other phenomena which often do not show themselves until years after the infection had taken place, and which we nevertheless seek to combat in accordance with such a supposition?

It will be seen that, the more earnestly we seek to solve the questions which present themselves for our consideration in the domain of diseases that, for a period of over four centuries, have been attributed to the action of a specific venereal virus, not every thing, or indeed scarcely any thing that is to be found on this subject in pathological manuals, is perfectly positive and certain, and that the different opinions which prevail among authors, even on the most important points of doctrine, are sufficiently founded in fact to divest the perception of truth, at first sight, of all difficulty. Nevertheless, if we mean to practise our art with intelligence and a thorough knowledge of the subject, and do not wish to imitate the crude empiric who employs his remedies for no better reason than because they had helped in other similar cases, we should not content ourselves with individual *opinions*, nor with the *dicta* of *authority* or general *articles of faith*, but we should strive, by a thorough examination of the most essential points, to attain to independent, positive, and lucid views concerning the true nature of the cases occurring in this particular branch of medicine. And even if we should not find it possible to solve the questions that have presented themselves, and may still present themselves, as satisfactorily as possible, we certainly agree on one point, which is, whether our therapeutic means are properly chosen; whether, if it be true that all venereal phenomena depend upon a virus that never becomes extinct of itself, spontaneously, we may be sure of its utter annihilation without saturating the organism with mercury, not to salivation, as used to be the method in former times, at least to the extent which Hahnemann recommended as late as the year 1788, until a mercurial fever has become developed; or whether we are privileged not only to limit the use of this metal as much as possible, but to substitute in its place other remedial agents whenever the case may seem to demand it. If our present methods of treatment seem to bring about a *radical* cure of our patients, this does not show that, sooner or later, even after the lapse of years, the marked signs of the syphilitic disease may not break forth, unless we are in possession of *some diagnostic signs* by which a *radical cure* may be ascertained with infallible certainty, and unless we are likewise enabled to show that the remedial agents which we are in the habit of employing are capable of fulfilling *these indications*. It is the object of this work to furnish contributions to the solution of these all-important questions. Even if it should be found insufficient to solve these questions, yet it may point out the road that may lead to their solution, and may show with sufficient clearness the points that should form the chief object of our inquiries. If we do not mean, in these inquiries, to go astray at the very first step, it is evident that we should not, after the fashion of pathological manuals, begin with the building up of *general hypotheses* concerning *the nature of syphilis* generally, but, *vice versâ*, pursue an *opposite course*, passing from particular and *concrete facts* to general *abstractions*, and well considering that we should not hazard general conclusions regarding the *specific nature* of syphilis until we have considered all the special forms resulting from syphilitic infection, either *mediately* or *immediately*, in all their pathological and therapeutic relations, with such completeness and so much accuracy that all further conclusions and deductions result as a matter of course. This course is indicated by Nature herself, in so far as she first displays single forms of the disease which she continues to develop until finally the whole image of the disease is presented to our view. Let us pursue this road, which is the only safe one, and let us consider in the following *four divisions* of this work:

I. Under the designation of *primary forms*, the *indisputable*, *immediate* products of venereal infection.

II. Under the designation of *secondary forms* that category of phenomena which always make their appearance as the *more remote* consequences of the syphilitic infection, to which they have necessarily to be attributed; and let us afterwards determine,

III. What *general pathological conclusions regarding syphilis* are suggested by a consideration of these different forms of this disease; as well as,

IV. What *diagnostic, therapeutic* and *pharmaco-dynamic maxims* we may derive from these considerations for the practical treatment of syphilis.

In order to enable the reader to study the original works which we have consulted in the composition of this volume, we here subjoin as complete as possible a list of these works, most of which deserve the most *attentive perusal* with reference to any particular theory or set of opinions.

LITERATURE

OF THE

VENEREAL DISEASES.

I. German and More Ancient Latin and Italian Works.

Albers, Joh. Fr. Ueber die Erkenntniss und Kur der syphilitischen Hautkrankheiten. Bonn, 1832.

Albrecht, Lehrbuch zur sichern Heilung der venerischen Krankheiten. 2. Auflage von Fr. Stehmann. Quedlinburg, 1844.

Aronssohn, Tac. Ez., Vollständige Abhandlung aller venerischen Krankheiten, mit Vorrede und Anmerkungen vom Fr. W. Wolf. Berlin, 1808.

Baerensprung, von, Die hereditäre Syphilis, Berlin, 1864.

Behrend, Syphilidologie, oder die neuesten Erfahrungen, etc. Leipzig, 1838–1845.

Bergman, G. A., Anweisung, die veralteten und vom Missbrauch des Quecksilber's entstandenen Krankheiten gründlich zu heilen Leipzig, 1825.

Boerhaave, Herm., Academische Vorlesungen oder medicinish-praktische Abhandlungen von der Venusseuche. Aus dem Lateinischen von Burghardt. Breslau, 1753.

Bolschwing, Theod v., Ueber Syphilis und Aussatz. Dorpat, 1839.

Bonorden, Herm. Friedr., Die Syphilis, pathologisch, diagnostisch und therapeutisch dargestellt. Berlin, 1834.

Clossius, C. Friedr., Ueber die Lustseuche. Tubingen, 1799.

Dieterich, G. Ludw., Die Krankheitsfamilie Syphilis. Landshut, 1842.

—— Die Merkurial-krankheit in allen ihren Formen, etc. Leipzig, 1837.

Dollmayr, Joh., Praktische Anleitung, die örtlichen, primären und secundären syphilitischen Krankheitsformen richtich zu beurtheilen und gründlich zu heilen. Wien, 1839.

ESSIG, Pracktische Anleitung zur gründlichen Kur aller nur möglichen venerischen Krankheiten, Augsburg, 1787.

EYEREL, Darstellung der neuesten Theorieen über syphilitische Krankheiten. Wien, 1802.

FALLOPII, Gabrielis, Mutensis, de morbo gallico liber absolutissimus. Venetiis, 1574.

FRACASTORIUS, de contagiorum morborum cura. Venetiis, 1584.

FRANKKEN, Anweisung alle venerischen Krankheiten gründlich und schnell zu heilen etc. Quedlinburg, 1812.

FRITZ, Joh. Frieder. Handbuch der venerischen Krankheiten. Leipzig, 1797.

GIRTANNER, Abhandlung über die venerischen Krankheiten. 3 Bdl. Göttingen, 1788–1789.

GRÜNBECK, venera. magist. de Burkhausen, Tractatus de pestilentia, scorra, sive malo de Frantzos. 1496 (in the library of the "Institute de France" at Paris).

HACKER, H. Aug., Literatur der syphilitischen Krankheiten, als Fortsetzung zu Girtanner's Literatur, etc. Leipzig, 1830.

—— Neueste Literatur der syphilitischen Krankheiten, nebst Nachträgen zu früheven Jahren. Leipzig, 1839.

—— Praktisches Handbuch der syphilitischen Krankheiten. Leipzig, 1847.

HAGER, Die Entzündungen (und die Merkurialkrankheit). Wien, 1835.

HAHNEMANN, S., Unterricht für Wundärzte über die venerischen Krankheiten, etc. Leipzig, 1789.

HANDEL, Kenntniss und Kur der venerischen Kranhheiten. Weilburg, 1801.

HANDSCHUCH, G. Fr., Die syphilitischen Krankheitsformen und ihre Heilung, mit steter Rücksicht auf die Beobachtungen und Erfahrungen der neuesten Zeit. Stuttgart, 1831.

HECKER, Aug. Friedr., Anweisung, die venerischen Krankheiten genau zu erkennen und zu behandeln, 3. Ausgabe von Walch. Erfurt, 1791–1815.

HEIM, Inaugural Abhandlung über die Merkurial-krankheiten. Erlangen, 1835.

HERGT, F. Carl, Geschichte, Erkenntniss und Heilung der Lustseuche, Hadamar, 1826.

HERMANN, Ueber die Merkurial-krankheiten, die nach lange fortgesetz tem Gebrauche des Quecksilbers in venerischen Krankheiten entstehen. Leipzig, 1835.

Hock, Joh. Dan., Von der Kenntniss und den vorzüglichsten Heilungsmitteln aller Arten venerischer Zufälle. Leipzig, 1792.

Hoffmann, Fr. (II)., Dass der bösartige Tripper wirklich venerish sei. Frankfurt *a* M., 1778.

—— Über den Tripper und Tod. Koppenhagen, 1781.

Huber, Ueber die Geschichte und die Behandlung der venerischen Krankheiten. Stuttgart, 1825.

Ingarden, Syphilidologie nach geläuterten hämatopathologischen Ansichten, etc. Wien, 1845.

Kuber, Kurze Beschreibung einer besonderen Art der Syphilis und des Mercurialismus. Leipzig, 1845.

Lahner, Das Wesen der Lustseuche, die Natur und Eigenschaften derselben, der Ursprung, etc. Pressburg, 1818.

Lippert, Heinr., Die Pathologie und Therapie der venerischen Krankheiten nach Ricord's neuesten Vorträgen. Hamburg, 1846.

Ludolph, Beweis, dass die heftigsten Zeichen der Lues keine venerischen, sondern mercurielle Zeichen sind. Erfurt, 1750.

Luisini, Collectio scriptorum de morbo gallico. Venetiis, 1566.

Martens, Friedr. Heinr., Handbuch zur Kenntniss und Kur der venerischen Krankheiten. 2. Thle. Jena, 1805.

Monteggia, Abhandlung über die venerischen Krankheiten und ihre Heilart. Translated from the Italian by Schlessing. Wien, 1804.

Müller, Taschenbuch sämmtlicher syphilitischen Krankheitsformen nach den neuesten Entdeckungen, nebst Angabe der verschiedenen Behandlungsweisen. Ludwigsburg, 1841.

Müller, J. V., Der Arzt für venerische verlarvte Krankheiten. Frankfurt *a* M., 1808.

—— Gründliche Anleitung alle Arten der venerischen Krankheiten richtig zu erkennen und gründlich zu behandeln. 2 Bde. Bremen, 1796, 1797.

Parenotti, de Cigliano, von der Lustseuche. From the Italian by Sprengel. Leipzig, 1791.

Plenck, Lehre von den venerischen Krankheiten. Wien, 1793.

Ritter, Darstellung der scheinbaren Aehnlichkeit und wesentlichen Verschiedenheit, welche zwischen der Schanker und Tripperseuche wahrgenommen wird. Leipzig, 1819.

Rosenbaum, Die Geschichte der Lustseuche im Alterthum, für Ärzte, Philologen, etc., etc. Halle, 1839.

Schaarschmidt, Sam., Abhandlung von venerischen Krankheiten. Berlin, 1759.

Schmidt, I. Adam, Beiträge zu den Resultaten der Versuche mit der Salpetersäure bei syphilitischen Krankheitsformen. Wien, 1802.

SCHMIDT, I. Adam, Lehrbuch der Syphilidoklinik. Wien, 1810.
—— Vorlesung über die syphilitische Krankheit und ihre Gestalten. Wien, 1812.
SCHREIBER, J. C., Theoretische und praktische Betrachtungen über alle Arten der syphilitischen Krankheiten. Berlin, 1775.
SIMON, F. A., Über die Zeichen der venerischen Krankheit und deren Bedeutung. Leipzig, 1725.
SWIETEN, von, von den venerischen Krankheiten und ihrer Heilart, nebst Boerhave's Vorrede. From the Latin. Cœthen, 1777.
TILING, Uber Syphilis und Syphiloiden. Mitan, 1833.
ULRICI de Hutten, de guajaci medicina et morbo gallico liber unus. Moguntiæ, 1519.
VIRCHOW, die constitutionelle Syphilis. Berlin, 1859.
WALCH, Fr. Aug., Ausführliche Darstellung des Ursprunges, der Erkenntniss, Heilung und Vorbauung der venerischen Krankheiten. Jena, 1711.
WEDEKIND, Fragmente über die Erkenntniss venerischer Kraukheiten. Hanover, 1790.
WENDT, Joh., Die Lustseuche in allen ihren Richtungen und allen ihren Gestalten, zum Behufe akademischer Vorlesungen. Breslau, 1816.
WETZEL, Wie kann man sich von dem im Körper befindlichen venerischen und Merkurial-gifte befreien. Pilna, 1809.

II. WORKS OF ENGLISH AND FRENCH AUTHORS.

a. English Authors.

ANDREE, Bemerkung über die Theorie und die Heilung der venerischen Krankheiten. Leipzig, 1781. (Theory and treatment of venereal diseases.)
BACOT, A treatise on Syphilis. London, 1829.
BELL, Benj., Abhandlungen über den bösartigen Tripper und die venerischen Krankheiten. 2. Theile, mit einem Kupfer. Leipzig, 1794. (Essays on Gonorrhœa and the Venereal diseases, 2 parts).
BLAIR, W. M., Versuche über die venerischen Krankheiten und die sie begleitenden Zufälle, erläutert durch Krankheits-geschichten. 2 Theile, Altenburg und Görlitz, 1799. (The Venereal diseases and their complications, illustrated by cases.)
CARMICHAEL, Rich., Beobachtungen über die Zufälle und specifischen Unterschiede der venerischen Krankheiten. Translated by C. G. Kühn. With one illum. plate. Leipzig, 1819. (Observations on the complications and specific differences of the venereal diseases.)

Carmichael Rich., Klinische Vorlesungen über die syphilitischen Krankheiten. Mit color. Abbildungen. Leipzig, 1843. (Clinical lectures on Syphilis.)

—— Bemerkungen über die Zeichen und besondere Unterscheidung der venerischen und Merkurial-Krankheiten. Translated by Kühn. Leipzig, 1819. (Observations on the symptoms and specific distinctions between the venereal and mercurial diseases.)

Colles A., Practical Observations on the use of Mercury. London, 1836.

Deacon, Anweisung zur Kenntniss und Heilung venerischer Krankheiten. Translated by Spohr. Stendal, 1791. (Diagnosis and treatment of venereal diseases.)

Dease, Heilart der Lustseuche und der damit vergesellschafteten Zufälle. Translated by Michaëlis. With one plate. Zittau, 1778. (Treatment of Syphilis and its complications.)

Falk, A Treatise on the Venereal Diseases. Translated by Möller. Hamburg and Kiel, 1775.

Foot, Abhandlungen über die Lustseuche und Urinverhaltungen. Translated by C. G. Reich. 2. Bde. Leipzig, 1793. (A Treatise on Syphilis and retention of urine.)

Fordyce, Genaue Untersuchung der venerischen Krankheiten. Altenburg, 1769. (Critical examinations of the venereal diseases.)

Hunter, Treatise on the Venereal Diseases. With three plates.

—— The same work, with notes by Ricord, Babington and Behrend.

Judd, A Practical Treatise on Urethritis and Syphilis. London, 1836.

Mayo, A Treatise on Syphilis.

Murphy, Practical Observations, showing that Mercury is the sole cause of what is termed Secondary Syphilis. London, 1839.

Nisbett, Theoretical and Practical Treatise on Syphilis. Translated by Michaëlis with notes. Leipzig, 1789.

Rose, Observations on the Treatment of Syphilis, etc.

Thomson, Observations on the Treatment of Syphilis with Mercury. Edinburgh, 1817.

Tilley, Maddon, a Practical Treatise on Diseases of the Genitals of the male. London, 1829.

Turner, Practical Treatise on Syphilis, with a number of cases. 1754.

Wallace, Will., A Treatise on the Course and Treatment of the Primary and Constitutional Venereal Disease and its Varieties. Translated into German under the supervision of Fr. Behring. Leipzig, 1842.

b. French authors.

Astruc, Joach., Abhandlung und Cur aller Venus-Krankheiten. Translated from the Latin by Heisse. Francfort on the Main. (Exceedingly interesting.)

Baumès, Précis historique et pratique sur les maladies vénériennes. Paris et Lyon, 1840.

Bertin, Traité de la maladie vénérienne, chez les nouveaux-nés, les femmes enceintes et les nourices. Paris, 1810.

Botten, Alex., Sur la nature et le traitement des maladies syphilitiques. Traduit en allemand, avec un postcript par Aug. Droste. Osnabruck, 1834.

Bouchut, Traité des maladies des nouveaux-nés. Paris, 1855.

Boyer, Traité pratique de la syphilis. Paris, 1836.

Calderon (Luna), Démonstration pratique de la prophylaxie syphilitique, etc. Paris, 1815.

Capuron, Aphrodisiographie, ou Tableau des maladies vénériennes. Paris, 1807.

Castelnau, Annales des maladies de la peau et de la syphilis. Paris, 1840.

Cazenave, Les syphilides ou maladies vénériennes de la peau. Translated into German by W. Walther and C. Streubel. With 12 plates. Leipzig, 1844.

Cirillo, Traité complet et observations sur la maladie vénérienne. Paris, 1803.

Cullerier, Traité sur la gonorrhée primaire et secondaire, sur les bubos et le chancre. With additions, by J. Renard. Mentz, 1815.

—— Sur la syphilis, ses complications et rémèdes. With additions by J. Renard, and 2 lithog. tables. Mentz, 1822.

—— Sur le Mercure, et son emploi contre les maladies syphilitiques. With additions by J. Renard. Perth, 1822.

Davasse, la syphilis, sa forme et son unité. Paris, 1865.

Desruelles, Lettres sur les maladies vénériennes et leur traitement. Translated into German by Frank and Hain. Leipzig, 1848.

Devergie, Clinique de la maladie syphilitique. Avec 126 planches. Paris, 1833.

Diday, Exposition critique et pratique des nouvelles doctrines de la syphilis. Paris, 1854.

—— Syphilis des nouveaux-nés. Paris, 1858.

Dubled, Exposition de la nouvelle doctrine de la syphilis, 1830.

Faber, Traité de la diagnose et du traitement des maladies vénériennes. Translated into German by Schrœder, with annotations by Tode. 2 parts. Copenhague, 1777.

FOURNIER, M. L., Traité de la syphilis, avec des planches. Translated by Wendt. Leipzig, 1820.

GIBERT, Manuel pratique des maladies vénériennes. Paris, 1837.

HERNANDEZ, Essai analytique sur la non-identité du virus gonorrhéique. Toulon, 1812.

JOURDAN, Traité complet de la maladie vénérienne. Paris, 1836.

LACOSTA, de, Traité de la vérole et de toutes les maladies vénériennes. Berlin, 1769.

LAGNEAN, L' art de reconnaitre toutes les formes de la syphilis, de les guérir et de s'en préserver. Translated into German. 4th edition. Gotha, 1815.

PLISSON, Monographe sur la syphilis, ses diverses formes, etc. Translated by Fitzler. Jlmenan, 1827.

REYNARD, Traité des maladies vénériennes. Paris, 1840.

RICORD, Observations sur la syphilis et la gonorrhée. Translated, with notes, by Eisenmann. With one plate. Edangen, 1836.

—— Examen de la méthode de l'inoculation. Translated into German. Reutlingen, 1838.

—— Traité pratique des maladies vénériennes. Translated into German by Herm. Müller. Leipzig, 1838.

—— Tableaux cliniques de l'hôpital des maladies vénériennes à Paris. In German by Gottschalk. With 15 colored plates. Dusseldorf, 1842–1844.

—— Doctrine de la syphilis. In German by L. Türck. Vienna, 1846.

—— Cours récent sur la syphilis et les blennorrhées vénériennes. In German by Gerhardt. Berlin, 1848.

SWEDIAUR, sur la syphilis. Translated into German by Kleffel. With a preface and notes by Sprengel. 2 vols. Berlin, 1803.

—— Exposition des théories modernes sur la syphilis. Translated by Egerel. Vienna, 1802.

—— Traité des symptomes, des effets et du traitement des maladies syphilitiques. Leipzig, 1799.

YVAREN, Des métamorphoses de la syphilis. Paris, 1854.

III. HOMŒOPATHIC LITERATURE.

This is only practical, with very few pathological or diagnostic notes, but replete with therapeutic observations. The most important publications are:

ATTOMYR, Die venerischen Krankheiten. Leipzig, 1836.

—— Rhapsodien über latente syphilis in Stapf's Archiv. Leipzig.

BICKING, das Hervortreten latenter syphilis. All. hom. zeit., Band 15 and 19.

BUCHNER, Notizen über Syphilis. Hygea, Bd. 13.

GASPARY, Über die homöopathische Behandlung der Bubonen. Vehsemeyer's Jahrbücher, Band 4.

HAHNEMANN, S., Die chronischen Krankheiten. Dresden, Arnold'sche Buchhandlung, 1837.

—— Belehrung über die venerische Krankheit und deren gewöhnlich unrichtige Behandlung Hahnemann's kleine med. Schriften, Band 2.

HOFRICHTER, Einige syphilitische Krankheitsformen und ihre homöopathische Behandlung. Allg. hom. Zeitung. Band 35.

KOPP, Denkwürdigkeiten, Band 2. Über Hahnemann's Lehre der Behandlung der Syphilis.

LIEDBECK, Praktische Mittheilungen über Syphilis, Tripper, etc. Hygea, Band 4.

MÜLLER, Clotar, Bericht über die Leipziger Polyklinik und die homœopathische Behandlung der venerischen Krankheiten. Erster Bericht, in der All. hom. Zeitung, Band 34. Zweiter Bericht, ebend. Band 37.

ROSENBERG, Rhapsodische Beiträge zur Syphilidologie. All. hom. Zeitung, Bd. 32, 35, 36, 37.

RÜCKERT, Klinische Erfahrungen in der Homœopathie, Eine vollständige Sammlung aller in der homöopathischen Literatur niedergelegten Heilungen, Band 2. Seite 66–207. Die syphilitischen Krankheiten. Denan, 1855.

RUMMEL, Über Trippercontagium und Sycosis. Stapf's Archiv, Band 8, Heft 1.

—— Beiträge zur Syphilidoklinik. All. hom. Zeitung, Bd. 18.

SOMMER, über den Gebrauch des Cinnabaris bei Behandlung des primären Schankers. All. hom. Zeitung, Bd. 38.

STARKE, Bemerkungen über Vehsemeyer's Beitrag zur Behandlung der syphilitischen Krankheiten. All. hom. Zeit. Bd. 20.

THORER, Syphilis und Sycosis. Stapf's Archiv, Band 19, Heft 3.

TRINKS, Kurze, Abhandlung der Feigwarzenkrankheit und ihrer Heilung. Annalen von Trinks und Hartlaub, Band 1.

—— Marginalien zu Rau's Organon der homœopathischen Heilkunst. Allg. hom. Zeitung, Band 15.

VEHSEMEYER, Beitrag zur Behandlung der syphilitischen Krankheiten. Vehsemeyer's Jahrbücher, Bd. 3.

WISLICENUS, über zweckmäszige Anwendung des Quecksilbers in der syphilitischen Krankheit, Stapf's Archiv, Band 2, Heft 3.

WOLF (in Dresden), Praktische Andeutungen, Stapf's Archiv, Band 11, Heft 1.

Besides these publications we have articles by the following writers:

a. On the Treatment of Gonorrhœa.

Argenti, Bernstein, Ehrhardt, Fielitz, Goullon, Gross, Hartlaub, Hanbold, Hering, Hirsch, Kämmerer, Knorre, Kreussler, Lingen, Lobethal, Müller, Noack, Nunez, Ohlhaut, Pleyl, Schelling, Schréter, Seidel, Tietze, Wahle, Weber, Wurda.

b. On the Treatment of Chancre and its Consequences.

Aegidi, Altmüller, Baudis, Bernstein, Bigel, Fielitz, Ganzke, Glaser, Goullon, Hartlaub, Hartmann, Hermann, Horner, Knorre, Kramer, Kreussler, Kratzenstein, Kurz, Laughammer, Lingen, Lobethal, Mayrhofer, Nithack, Ohlhaut, Schwab, Schelling, Schréter, Schrœn, Schindler, Segin, Seidel, Simon, Schulz, Stapf, Tietze, Wahle, Wesselhœft, Wurda, whose contributions may be found in the following publications:

ALLGEMEINE homœopathische Zeitung. Leipzig, 1833–66.

ANNALEN für homœopathische Heilkunst, von Hartlaub und Trinks. Leipzig, 4 Bände.

ARCHIV für homœopathische Heilkunst von Stapf's. Leipzig, Band 1–23.

BERNSTEIN, Mosaik, Leipzig, Shumann; Griesselich, Hygea, Zeitschrift für Homöopathie. Carlsruhe, Band 1–24.

HARTMANN, homöopathische Therapie der acuten und chronischen Krankheiten. Leipzig, 1854.

OESTERREICHISCHE Zeitschrift für Homœopathie, Wien, 4 Bände.

THORER, Praktische Beiträge im Gebiete der Homöopathie. Leipzig, 4 Bände.

FIRST DIVISION.

THE PRIMARY FORMS

OF THE

VENEREAL DISEASES.

FIRST CHAPTER.

OF VENEREAL PHENOMENA GENERALLY.

I. DEFINITIONS OF THE VENEREAL DISEASES.

Section 1.—Various Definitions.

EVERY BODY knows that, when speaking of *venereal diseases*, we mean *gonorrhœa*, *chancre*, *buboes*, *figwarts*, and other affections occasioned by an *impure coït;* but if we refer to what authors understand by this term, we shall meet such a great diversity of opinions, or even such a radical *confusion of ideas*, that it almost becomes impossible to comprehend all the different views in one universal definition of the phenomena that belong to this category. Even if we were to confine the meaning of this term to the simplest limits, and simply understand by it the diseases that had been contracted by an impure coït, or *in usu veneris*, we should satisfy neither party, inasmuch as such a definition would be too comprehensive for some, and not sufficiently comprehensive for others; according as they regard most of these diseases as depending upon a *specific virus* which may be transmitted without the act of coïtion, by simply being brought in contact with susceptible parts of the organism; or according as they hold with the *Physiological School* that these diseases constitute nothing but *simple inflammations*, the particular form of which is supposed to be determined by individual or other accidental influences. For whereas the former exclude from the class of syphilitic products as *non-venereal*, all those that are incapable, by the transmission of their secretions, of developing like phenomena in healthy persons, and, on the other hand, comprehend under the term of *venereal* phenomena even those that had been caused by contact with the infectious virus *between* the acts of coïtion; the latter, on the contrary, apply the term *venereal* even to the most innocent discharges and ulcerations caused, during the act of coït, by a want of cleanliness, acrid menstrual blood, or a corrosive leucorrhœa, and absolutely unable to transmit a like infection; yet, not recognizing idiopathic diseases, they refuse to recognize as venereal a whole category of products which are considered as absolutely *venereal* by the former, even though it may not be possible to show a direct transmission through an impure coït. A similar confusion of ideas prevails among those who believe in a specific virus as the generator of certain venereal products; some referring the term *venereal* exclusively to chancre and the phenomena that can be traced to it as their producing cause, thus regarding even *infectious* gonorrhœa as a *non-venereal* product; others, on the contrary, who distinguish several varieties of venereal affections, designating the phenomena that owe their development to chancre as *syphilitic*, the phenomena that constitute the category of figwarts as *sycosic*, and the phenomena that belong to the class of *common gonorrhœa* as *simply venereal*. In addition to this, others again, not content with the already excessive confusion of ideas, apply the term *syphilitic*, which properly belongs only to a *subdivision* of this class of diseases, indiscriminately with that of *venereal*, to all kinds of products of an impure coït, speaking for instance of syphilitic orchitis, phimosis, strictures of the urethra, affections of the prostate, etc., whereas such affections really only accompany or result from a simple venereal gonorrhœa; so that, if we read of *non-syphilitic* or *non-venereal gonorrhœas* or other products, we have first to ask ourselves whether the reporter only meant affections that were not caused by a chancre, or such as cannot be numbered among the products of an *infectious coït*. The same difficulty prevails in regard to special names of venereal products, such as *gonorrhœa*, *chancre*, *inguinal swellings*, etc., by which some understand exclusively the *venereal contagious* discharges, ulcers and buboes; whereas other physicians, especially the French adherents of the *Physiological School*, call every non-contagious ulcer on the genital organs a *chancre*, every discharge from these organs a *gonorrhœa*, and every scrofulous or other inguinal swelling a *bubo;* deducing from these similarly named products whose homogeneousness is only predicated upon their anatomical locality, but which differ essentially in regard to their *pathological* character, therapeutic propositions (such as the *spontaneous* cure of some *chancres*) that might lead any one who is not acquainted with their *mode of expressing themselves*, and imagines they mean *specific* chancres, gonorrhœas or buboes, into the gravest errors.

Sec. 2.—Precise Definitions.

It is easily seen to what misunderstandings and errors in science such a babylonic confusion of terms must and will lead, if the reader, guided by his own customary technical terms, should understand perhaps the opposite of what the author intended to convey by his own language; and it is morally certain that so many endless disputes concerning the nature and treatment of venereal diseases would never have taken place, if the disputants had, in the first place, endeavored to attach the same meaning to the terms which they respectively made use of. In the course of this work we shall touch upon several of these points, and, for the present, confine ourselves to the statement, that, *for ourselves*, we do not by any means understand by the term *venereal diseases* all those that may have been *occasioned by sexual excesses*, but only a category of phenomena which, having arisen from this source, may, by transmitting the virus to susceptible parts of a healthy organism, *reproduce a like series of phenomena*, endowed with a like power of reproducing the original malady. In thus stating our general definition we do not yet concern ourselves with the inquiry whether the venereal phenomena spring from a *simple* or *compound* virus; our general definition not only comprehends all the products of an infectious coït, hence, likewise, a simple but *contagious gonorrhœa*, but likewise that further series of products which may result from the former products being brought in contact with susceptible parts in any other manner than by sexual intercourse. Inasmuch as, however, even if all these phenomena should be caused by a single contagium, *gonorrhœa*, *chancre*, and *figwarts* have been described by several authors as so many distinct forms of venereal disease; and inasmuch as we shall be obliged, in discussing their different theories, to adopt particular terms, in order to avoid one set of definitions being confounded with another; we shall distinguish, for the purpose of proceeding in a more systematic manner: *a*) *syphilitic*-venereal, or simply *syphilitic* phenomena, that is to say, those that can be traced to *chancre; b*) *sycosic*-venereal, or simply *sycosic*, that is to say, all the phenomena which belong to the domain of *condylomata;* and *c*) *simply* venereal phenomena, or all such as do not seem to refer to either of the above-mentioned categories. This shows that we do not, like other physicians, regard the terms *syphilitic* and *venereal*, as *synonymous*, but as *strictly distinct.* If we use the term *venereal*, we mean to include all the phenomena of this class, even *syphilis*, *sycosis* and *simple* lues, opposing this whole series to the *non-venereal*, *non-contagious* products of sexual intercourse as excluded from it. In order to illustrate, we hold that any, ever so simple form of gonorrhœa, which had resulted from an infectious coït, is not, on that account, to be considered of a *syphilitic* or *sycosic* nature, unless we are certain that it owes its origin to *chancre* or *sycosis*. By *non-venereal* gonorrhœa we mean a gonorrhœa that has nothing in common with the products of *infectious coït*, but is the result of irritating *scrofulous* humors, *hæmorrhoids* or other similar causes. And, in order to avoid even in this respect all confusion of ideas, we do not, like other authors, first speak of non-venereal gonorrhœa, chancre and bubo, but understand by these terms in every case all such *venereal products* as have emanated from an impure coït, and are, in their turn, capable of *transmitting the infection.* Further on, we shall see by what diagnostic signs a venereal gonorrhœa, chancre or bubo is distinguished from a non-venereal discharge, ulcer or inguinal swelling; previously, however, we will cast a glance at the *general forms* under which the venereal diseases may appear.

II. FORMS UNDER WHICH VENEREAL DISEASES MANIFEST THEMSELVES.

Sec. 3.—Essential Distinctions.

On surveying the totality of the phenomena of venereal origin, which authors have described either as venereal or as syphilitic, we cannot fail to perceive at first sight, that they constitute two *essentially distinct classes*, namely:

a) Those which, like *gonorrhœa* and *chancre*, generally make their appearance soon after an impure coït, or which, even if, like *buboes* and *figwarts*, they break out at a somewhat later period, still are so closely connected with the first-mentioned phenomena that their origin from an impure venereal source cannot be doubted; and

b) Those which, like *affections of the skin, mucous membranes and bones*, frequently do not make their appearance until long after the first-named symptoms had disappeared, so that their probable *derivation from a similar source* can only be accounted for by the absence of any other cause, or by the resemblance existing between their course and character and that of the first-named phenomena.

The phenomena of this second class, which never appear as the *primary symptoms* of a direct infection, but always follow such an infection at an earlier or later period, have, on that account, been designated by many authors as *secondary symptoms*, or, inasmuch as they are principally traceable to a chancre, as *secondary syphilis*, whereas the phenomena constituting the first class have been comprehended under the general name of *lues venerea primaria*, or the *primary forms* of venereal disease. On the other hand, there are physicians who would not even recognize those *secondary symptoms* as *venereal*, and even go so far as to deny the existence of secondary syphilis, for the reason that the derivation of this class of phenomena from a venereal source is not only involved in doubt, but that these secondary phenomena do not possess, like the primary symptoms, the capacity of transmitting the original infection. It is indeed true that these secondary phenomena do not clearly possess the characteristic signs which we have pointed out in a previous paragraph as *pathognomonic* of the venereal disease, we mean their *production by an* impure coït and their capacity to *reproduce* themselves in a *like form;* and even if we should succeed, in the further course of this work, in demonstrating their derivation from one or the other primary form by irrefutable arguments, we cannot accomplish this purpose until we shall have acquired a sufficient knowledge of the symptoms from which the *secondary* symptoms are derived, to become enabled in this way to form an *independent*, competent judgment concerning the relation and connection of the two classes of phenomena. Without troubling ourselves just now about the question whether *secondary syphilis* is a *venereal disease*, we will for the present confine ourselves to a consideration of the primary products of the *lues venerea primaria*, in order to ascertain the *undoubted* signs by which a venereal infection usually manifests itself. Inasmuch, however, as a number of authors, for the want of a fixed *diagnostic sign*, do not seem to know what symptoms ought to be considered as characteristic of a *primary* and what of a *secondary* disease; yea, inasmuch as not a few authors talk even of tertiary and quaternary forms, and some class the last-mentioned among the primary: we shall not be able to adopt any of the existing classifications of the different venereal products, and, guided by the light of our own judgment and experience, shall inquire for ourselves which of these products should be regarded as primary symptoms and which not.

Sec. 4.—Essentially Primary Forms.

Judging the so-called venereal products which are designated by different authors as *primary symptoms*, by our criterion of the undoubted derivation of these symptoms from an impure sexual source, we shall find that one of the most positive of these products is the so-called *gonorrhœa* concerning whose direct origin in an impure coït there can be but one opinion, although there are physicians who are unwilling to class even this affection among the venereal diseases. But since this opposition, as we have seen in § 1 and § 2, rests exclusively upon a confusion of the ideas which some physicians attach to the terms *gonorrhœa* and *venereal*, and inasmuch as we have explained to satiety our own meaning of the term *venereal*, every body will most likely admit with us that *gonorrhœa*, even if not a *chancrous syphilitic*, is at least a *venereal* disease. On the other hand, that *chancre* is in every case an undoubtedly venereal product, is admitted at the present time by all physicians, even those who do not admit the specific virus of chancre, and hence do not believe in the contagiousness of chancre in the strict meaning of the term; as regards the *bubo*, authors differ very much in opinion, some (among whom Rückert in his "*Klinische Erfahrungen*," vol. II. page 187) regarding it as a symptom of *secondary syphilis*, others, like Broussais' *Physiological School*, denying it every venereal characteristic, and declaring it a purely *consensual* glandular swelling which terminates in suppuration like any other inflammatory abscess. Now as we stated before, inasmuch as we understand by *primary* symptoms of venereal disease all those symptoms which still embody *both* characteristics of the venereal product, namely its evident derivation from impure sexual intercourse and its contagiousness, not obscurely as in secondary syphilis, but with such unmistakable clearness that they cannot be doubted or ignored; we believe ourselves justified, and indeed compelled by logic and science to regard the *bubo* as a demonstrably primary symptom of the venereal disease, although it may not always occur protopathically, but in most cases as a sequel of *chancre*. The same remarks apply to the so-called *condylomata*, and to mucous tubercles, with which the former are so frequently confounded, and which often constitute the only sign by which a recent venereal infection is known, yet are nevertheless classed by a number of physicians among the symptoms of *secondary syphilis* from no better motive than that of simple routine; they had never reflected what constitutes *primary* and what *secondary* symptoms of syphilis, and what a vast and deep gap separates these two classes of symptoms even from a *pathological* point of view. After having sufficiently considered, in the two first divisions of this work, all the *primary* and *secondary* forms, we shall, in the third division, when reviewing the general course of syphilis (§ 190–198), revert to this point with great fulness and demonstrate by *pathological* arguments drawn from the *essentially distinct* nature of the proximate cause of *secondary syphilis*, why this form of the disease should be considered as something essentially distinct from the *primary* disease, and why it should be considered strictly scientific to class among the primary symptoms of syphilis many that have been hitherto considered as secondary. For the present we shall content ourselves with the external *diagnostic sign* which we have pointed out as showing in all cases the undoubted origin of a given *venereal form;* this sign leads us to class *buboes*, *condylomata* and *mucous tubercles*, as well as *gonorrhœa* and *chancre* among the *primary phenomena*, not only because they all originate protopathically in the same cause, but likewise because, even if they manifest themselves at ever so remote a period after a gonorrhœa or a chancre, they evince a like origin by the absolute capacity inherent *in their secretions* of transmitting the infection, and likewise by their specific products; properties that are not possessed in the same manner by any other so-called venereal affection.

Sec. 5.—Questionable Primary Phenomena.

There is another point that will have to be settled before we can enter upon a more circumstantial description of the different primary phenomena; it is this, whether the above-mentioned symptoms, such as gonorrhœa, chancre, bubo, mucous tubercles, and figwarts, are the *only* ones that can manifest themselves as immediate products of venereal infection, or whether there are other symptoms that will have likewise to be considered as primary symptoms of this disease. In this respect it is undoubtedly true that several writers on syphilis, among whom we may mention Dr. *Cazenave*, of Paris, who has contributed so much towards a correct pathology and treatment of the cutaneous syphilitic diseases, have advanced the opinion that the first manifestation of syphilitic infection may consist in the breaking out of a *general cutaneous eruption*, though all such eruptions are regarded by those who believe in a *secondary syphilis*, as characteristic of this form of the disease. In proof of this assertion Cazenave mentions a number of cases where the poison, after having penetrated a more or less perceptible wound, does not develop a chancre, bubo, or mucous tubercle, but a *pustulous* eruption that had hitherto been regarded as a symptom of *secondary infection;* so that we may very properly ask the question whether *syphiloid eruptions* ought not to be classed among the primary syphilitic symptoms. This would undoubtedly have to be done, if such a supposed primary syphiloid eruption were accompanied by symptoms that would render it impossible to connect it with any of the already known forms of syphilis, and if its syphilitic nature were moreover as self-evident as that of the acknowledged primary symptoms. For, if such a syphiloid has the unmistakable diagnostic signs of one of the primary forms, it is not a new, but one of the already known forms which is distinguished from chancre, sycosic condylomata, and figwarts, only by the fact that it does not, as is generally the case, break out only at the place of infection, but spreads at once over a large portion of the surface of the body. If, on the contrary, such a syphiloid is to be classed among the symptoms that do not betray their undoubted venereal origin by positive diagnostic signs, and whose venereal nature is doubted by many even for the simple reason that they never make their appearance after an impure coït, nor ever show the least sign of contagiousness; this syphiloid, in spite of its primary derivation, at some prior period, from an undoubted syphilitic source, cannot be received in the class of undoubted venereal phenomena, until it has shown a capacity of *reproducing its specific form by contagion*, or, at any rate, one of the known primary symptoms; as is the case with the bubo, for instance, which produces a chancre by infection with its own specific secretion. But even supposing that some observer had described cases where such a syphiloid, unaccompanied by any of the positive primary symptoms, had not only originated in an indubitably venereal source, but had likewise communicated the infection to persons in health, such isolated cases, the real nature of which may be doubted until they are verified by additional observations, would not justify us to class them, without further proof, among the category of phenomena such as *chancre*, *gonorrhœa*, *buboes*, *mucous tubercles*, or *sycosic condylomata*, whose venereal nature is so self-evident that we recognize and believe in it, even in the absence of any positive knowledge of their derivation from *impure sexual intercourse.* Since the nature of the so-called *syphiloids* that have been observed hitherto, is destitute of any such positive certainty, we shall have to regard, for the present at least, in spite of the contrary opinion of certain authors, the true *gonorrhœa*, *chancre*, *buboes*, *mucous tubercles*, and *sycosic condylomata* as the only really positive and fixed *primary symptoms* of lues venerea, and, so far, as the only known *certain fundamental forms* constituting this malady.

III. COMMON CHARACTERISTICS OF THE VENEREAL FUNDAMENTAL OR TYPICAL FORMS.

Sec. 6.—Common Pathological Characteristics.

We have seen what are the undoubted and undisputed phenomena and representatives of the lues venerea emanating from impure coït. Since they all originate in *one* source and hence must be produced by *one* cause, they must necessarily have certain signs in common, by which, in spite of all other differences, they are distinguished as members of one family from all other families of diseases. However, if we examine these common characteristics for the purpose of establishing a *general* pathology of the undoubted lues venerea, we meet at the first glance a number of *essential differences* that may serve to lead to distinctions among those characteristics, but, beside their *origin from a common source* and their *contagiousness*, do not reveal a *single sign* that is peculiar to all of them. Looking, for example, at the different forms under which they appear, we find that each characteristic is distinguished by fixed forms of its own, not possessed by any other characteristic, and that these forms run their whole course without ever infringing upon, or running into other forms. It is indeed true that *chancre* may, in a given time, assume the form of figwarts; but inasmuch as figwarts never terminate in chancre, it is not at all certain whether this apparent identity of figwarts and chancre is not confined to the external form merely, without justifying the conclusion that they are *essentially* alike. The *cauliflower-shaped* excrescences of certain *cancerous ulcerations* may show a great deal of external resemblance to venereal growths; yet no one has as yet presumed to consider figwarts and cancer as essentially the same. We would be far more justified in inferring a certain pathological identity between chancre and gonorrhœa, since both are equally capable of developing *inguinal swellings;* but independently of the fact that gonorrhœal and syphilitic buboes are pathologically distinct, if a purely *symptomatic* similarity were sufficient, we should have to class *herpes præputialis*, which may be one of the accidental results of an *ardent coït*, in the same pathological class with chancre and gonorrhœa, so much the more as this herpes, if it should be very much inflamed, may, like chancre and gonorrhœa, cause *inguinal swellings*, especially in scrofulous subjects, in whom these frequently terminate in suppuration. This want of a perfect pathological identity becomes still more striking if we consider the *course* of these different phenomena, some of them, like certain *forms of gonorrhœa*, running an *acutely* inflammatory course at the termination of which they become extinct of themselves; others, on the contrary, like chancre, observing in every case a *chronic* course; added to which we have the additional difficulty that each of these forms seems distinct from any other as regards their specific power of reproducing the contagium; at any rate, the cases where the infection caused by one form is said to have developed the specific products of another form, of phenomena, such as the virus of chancre causing gonorrhœa, are still doubtful, and in need of further confirmation. Be this however as it may, it seems to be admitted that, for the present at least, a *general pathology* of venereal diseases is an impossible thing, and that we have to content ourselves with describing each of its fundamental forms as independent of all others.

Sec. 7.—General Therapeutics of the Lues Venerea.

Our remarks concerning the absolute impossibility of building up from the symptoms of the different venereal fundamental forms, a series of characteristics common to all of them, and from which a general pathology of lues primaria could be deduced, applies with equal force to a system of *general therapeutics*. In this respect we have absolutely nothing that might be regarded as equally applicable to the different fundamental forms of lues venerea, each of these forms having its own rules and laws both as regards its greater or less susceptibility of a spontaneous cure, as well as with reference to the size of the dose and to the remedial agents that are specifically adapted to it; even to the extent that a method of treatment which might be proper for one of these forms, would become a positive falsehood if it were to be applied to venereal diseases generally. If gonorrhœa, for instance, has got well of itself, without the interference of art, we should be greatly mistaken if we were to lay it down as a general rule that lues venerea generally is susceptible of a spontaneous cure. It may indeed be proper to infer the spontaneous curability of gonorrhœa from a few isolated cases of spontaneous cure of this disease; but we would be greatly mistaken if we were to infer from such cases that, because the venereal disease has become spontaneously extinct, this may likewise be expected of *chancre* or *mucous tubercles;* for these forms, though they likewise constitute forms of lues venerea, may indeed change to other forms or other localities, but can never spontaneously terminate in a radical cure in the same way as some forms of *infectious gonorrhœa.* We should commit a grievous mistake if, because *cannabis* has proved such a signally effective remedy in gonorrhœa, we were to infer from this that cannabis is one of the most effcient *anti-venereal* remedies generally. It would leave us utterly in the lurch if we would employ this agent against chancre or mucous tubercles, although we cannot deny its anti-venereal properties, since infectious gonorrhœa is a venereal disease equally as chancre or sycosis. The same remark applies to *mercurial preparations*, which, though they constitute one of the most powerful specifics against the different forms of chancre, cannot on that account be regarded as a general anti-syphilitic panacea, since they are far from exhibiting their anti-syphilitic virtues in many cases of gonorrhœa, as well as in a variety of sycosic condylomata. Our remarks likewise apply to the size of the dose. The two general propositions, for instance, that venereal primary symptoms can be cured both by low, material doses of the mercurial preparations, and likewise by their highest potencies, are both of them correct and both of them false, according as either of them is adopted as a universal guide for the treatment of all venereal primary symptoms, or is limited only to single forms like chancre, gonorrhœa, sycosis, etc; for, even if chancre requires for its cure the grosser, more material doses of mercury, this is not by any means true as regards the other forms of lues venerea. In no respect, therefore, does it seem possible to lay down, in the domain of venereal diseases, a general therapeutic principle adaptable to all forms of venereal diseases; each form having its own rules, a *general system of therapeutics* of the venereal diseases is just as impossible as a *general pathology.*

Sec. 8.—Conclusions.

It is this absolute impossibility of achieving a general system of pathology and therapeutics of lues venerea, which has led several physicians, among whom *Carmichael*, of England, to assert that there is no *idiopathic* lues venerea, but only venereal *phenomena* that have been combined in one general idea by a process of abstraction, but have nothing in common but the anatomical *locality of their origin*, and may, each of them, owe their origin to an entirely different contagium, even as the people united under one imperial sceptre may belong to the most *different races*. A similar idea seems to have prevailed in Hahnemann's mind when he distinguished the *common gonorrhœa* from the *syphilitic chancre* as well as from *sycosis*. Without being intimidated by the tendency that seems to prevail among many of Hahnemann's adherents to criticise his teachings, we do not hesitate to declare even here that many of his *views* require further confirmation. At the same time we would not reject all his statements with the disregard with which the *Hygea*, as the sovereign mistress of our school, sought to put them down thirty years ago, not so much by the scientific superiority of its arguments as by a tone of defiant bravado. Inasmuch as in the course of this work we shall have frequent opportunities, when discussing the views of different old-school practitioners, of reverting to this delicate point, we leave this subject for the present, and content ourselves with stating that, if we have not succeeded in reducing the phenomena of the lues venerea primaria to an unitary generalization, our failure is not to be attributed to our predilection for Hahnemann, but to the absolute impossibility of perfecting such a generalization from a scientific point of view. Forms cannot be forced upon Nature, which laughs at the pompous arrogance of modern criticism. However, while in the subsequent chapters we shall treat, 1) of the different forms of *gonorrhœa*, 2) of *chancre*, 3) of *buboes*, 4) of *mucous tubercles*, 5) of *sycosic condylomata*, together with the symptomatology, pathology, and therapeutics peculiar to each class, as if these different forms constituted so many distinct diseases having no sort of internal connection with each other; we still reserve to ourselves the privilege of discussing the question of an unitary generalization more specially in a subsequent chapter, but shall allude to it, as often as may be proper, in treating of each particular form of the venereal diseases. We shall not be able to reach a decision on this subject until we shall have considered the general forms in the present division, and canvassed in the second division all the symptoms that have been comprehended under the general designation of secondary syphilis, after which, having acquired a full knowledge of all the elements that constitute the series *syphilis*, we shall be able to define the essential nature of this disease with an unbiassed mind and perfect competency of judgment. This point will be more fully considered in the third division. Until then we shall confine ourselves to a knowledge of the concrete products, and shall proceed as if there existed neither syphilis nor lues venerea, but nothing but *isolated venereal symptoms.*

SECOND CHAPTER.

THE DIFFERENT FORMS OF GONORRHŒA.

I. OF GONORRHŒA GENERALLY.

Sec. 9.—Idea of Gonorrhœa.

FROM what we have said it is evident that we do not understand by the term gonorrhœa, as so many continue to do, every imaginable mucous discharge from the urethra, but only an *infectious*, *inflammatory* blennorrhœa, and that we regard it as a great calamity in the domain of science that recent practitioners, even medical authors, should ignore the meaning of a term which had been consecrated by the common vernacular, and should designate as *gonorrhœa* every kind of discharge from the urethra, admitting not only venereal and syphilitic, but likewise arthritic, hæmorrhoidal, catarrhal, and Heaven knows what other kinds of gonorrhœa. We cannot wonder, in the presence of such a horrible confusion of terms, that some physicians should pretend having cured gonorrhœa with remedies that will never remove a genuine gonorrhœa, and that others should still advance the doctrine that a gonorrhœa may not only be caused by any *acrid*, though otherwise perfectly *innocuous* leucorrhœa, but even by the menstrual blood. True, *discharges* from the urethra may be occasioned by such causes, as well as by irritating bougies or other foreign bodies, such as gravel, stone in the bladder, urethral calculi, worms in the rectum, hæmorrhoids, medicinal substances, etc. What distinguishes this form of blennorrhœa from a genuine, infectious gonorrhœa is, 1) that the former is not *contagious;* 2) that it does not pass through a definite inflammatory stage, no matter how violent the inflammatory irritation may have been; and, 3) that after the removal of the irritating matter the blennorrhœa ceases of itself *in a few days*. Where these three diagnostic marks exist, there is, according to our definition of the term elsewhere as well as in the present work, no *gonorrhœa*, but simply an innocuous *discharge*. Where these signs do not exist; where the discharge runs through definite stages, from the incipient, scarcely perceptible oozing of a serous fluid to that of a greenish-yellow purulent matter, attended with constantly increasing symptoms of inflammation, after which the discharge decreases in quantity while it continues to increase in thickness; in all such cases we do not diagnose a simple discharge, but a genuine, *contagious gonorrhœa*, and it is our positive conviction that, in all such cases, the female who had infected the patient, was not merely afflicted with a corrosive leucorrhœa, or had a too acrid menstrual blood, but an *infectious gonorrhœa*, and even other troubles which she was anxious to conceal. Nothing produces nothing; where an infectious disease is contracted, it must have been derived from an infectious contagium. Hence we cannot call to mind a more foolish illusion than the belief which is not only entertained by many laymen, but even by physicians, that a gonorrhœa may be communicated during a heated sexual embrace even by a woman in perfect health; a discharge may indeed be occasioned, which, however, will cease again in a few days provided the woman was really sound, but in no case an *infectious gonorrhœa* like that which constitutes the burden of our remarks.

Sec. 10.—Simple and Syphilitic Gonorrhœa.

Another remarkable confusion of terms prevails in the use of the epithets *simple* and *syphilitic* gonorrhœa. Some, especially French authors, designate by the term *simple* gonorrhœa one that is not infectious, hence a simple blennorrhœa, or what we have described as a simple discharge; whereas they apply the term syphilitic to every form of gonorrhœa capable of transmitting itself to others by contagion, or having been contracted by impure coït, without considering whether the virus that had occasioned the disease was simple gonorrhœic or syphilitic virus. Further on (§ 15), we shall see whether there exist two different kinds of virus, the simple gonorrhœic and the chancre virus, by which gonorrhœa may be caused; for the present we will simply observe that, in accordance with the distinction which we have pointed out between the terms *venereal* and *syphilitic*, we shall in the present work understand by the term *syphilitic* gonorrhœa one that is caused by the chancre-poison; whereas we shall apply the term of simple *contagious* gonorrhœa to a urethral discharge that is occasioned by the simple gonorrhœal *virus;* distinguishing both kinds by the term *venereal* from any other form that is neither non-contagious nor had been communicated by contagion. In this way we expect to prevent any misunderstanding at the outset, and by means of these rigorous definitions of terms, elucidate more fully our understanding of the different forms of venereal gonorrhœa, which, though essentially distinct, are yet frequently confounded with each other in consequence of an habitual confusion of terms, showing at the same time that one class can no more be infallibly cured by Cannabis than the other by Mercurius, and that those who designate *any* discharge from the urethra as *gonorrhœa*, have a perfect right to declare that they have cured gonorrhœa with *Agnus*, *Mezereum*, *Natrum muriaticum*, *Ferrum*, even with *Nux vomica.* Such a discrimination is not only of particular importance in regard to the different forms of gonorrhœa of the female, but even as respects *balanorrhœa*, which, to this day, is regarded by some authors as a harmless secretion caused by a want of cleanliness and scarcely worth naming, whereas others, especially modern French physicians, regard it in all cases as a *syphilitic* disease. Be this as it may, let us for the present endeavor to obtain a correct knowledge of the exact symptoms, course, accessory phenomena and different forms of the *infectious gonorrhœa of the male*, and of the most appropriate remedies for this disease; having obtained this knowledge, we shall find it comparatively easy to rectify our opinions concerning *balanorrhœa*, and to perceive even a ray of light in the obscure domain of *gonorrhœa of the female.*

II. GONORRHŒA OF THE MALE.

Sec. 11.—Symptoms.

So far we have shown with sufficient clearness that we understand by the term *gonorrhœa* a urethral discharge that had been caused by the action of some specific *infectious virus;* not any discharge occasioned and continued by the action of some internal or external irritation of the urethra. A gonorrhœal infection that may not only result from impure coït, but likewise from the use of instruments to which the gonorrhœal virus had remained adhering, generally becomes apparent after the lapse of four to seven days, or even two or three weeks after the infection had taken place. At first it may betray its existence by a slight titillation in the urethra which is not disagreeable and excites erections and a desire for sexual intercourse. This titillation is soon after succeeded, and very frequently accompanied by a scarcely perceptible secretion from the urethra (gonorrhœa incipiens), which closes more or less the slightly reddened and, but in a few cases, somewhat swollen orifice of the urethra, and leaves very small, slight stains on the linen. Almost always, as I have noticed in many cases, this appearance is preceded the day previous by a feeling of malaise, which either remains unnoticed or is attributed by the patient to some other cause. This feeling of malaise is in a very few cases attended with slight febrile shiverings, but is almost always accompanied by a feeling of goneness or weakness in the præcordial region, and excites in the patient a desire to take something stimulating. Very frequently we notice already at this period of the precursory symptoms a scattering of the stream, which is probably owing to the partial agglutination of the urethra caused by the as yet imperceptible secretion in this organ. This scattering of the stream disappears, together with the other precursory symptoms, in order to reappear again with much more violence after the lapse of a few days. In a few days, probably two or three, the above-mentioned voluptuous titillation changes to a more or less troublesome sensation of smarting or tension, while the erections become even now somewhat painful. At the same time the orifice of the urethra appears more or less swollen, pouting, and a clear serous discharge sets in; the inflammation at the same time increases and is attended with a frequent urging to urinate; urination itself is likewise beginning to become painful. Generally these phenomena increase within a short time, but sometimes only *in the second week.* At this stage of the disease (*gonorrhœa inflammatoria*) the glans swells up and assumes a dark or yellowish-red color; the discharge keeps increasing in quantity, sometimes to an incredible degree, acquiring a yellow or greenish tint, and in appearance and consistence resembling a thin pus, and leaving yellowish stains on the linen, which always have a *gray, sharply-circumscribed border* (of which the stains occasioned by the *non-contagious* leucorrhœa of females are always destitute). The swelling from the meatus urinarius to the glans communicates itself to the prepuce and body of the penis (with more or less phimosis or paraphimosis); the urging to urinate increases, becomes very troublesome, and is attended with violent erections, which sometimes become so painful, especially at night, that they deprive the patient of all sleep. These *inflammatory* symptoms, if the disease is left to itself, generally increase to the 15th, 25th or 30th day, after which they gradually decrease, simultaneously with the discharge, which loses its greenish color, becomes yellow and afterwards whitish, more consistent and viscid, and finally disappears more or less rapidly, according as the constitution of the patient and the employment of proper hygienic and dietetic rules and more or less suitable remedial agents may influence the course of the disease. Left to itself, a gonorrhœa scarcely ever terminates before the 30th or 40th day, but, if mismanaged by improper treatment, or interfered with by a wrong diet, may continue for months, or even years, in the shape of *gleet.*

Sec. 12.—Accessory symptoms accompanying Gonorrhœa.

The course of venereal gonorrhœa which we have described, and by which it is distinguished from all other discharges from the urethra, *usually* takes place in all uncomplicated, *non-syphilitic* forms of the disease. Not in all cases, however, is this course equally simple and regular. Even in cases where the inflammation sets in with more than ordinary intensity, the pain becomes extremely troublesome and is frequently felt along the whole course of the urethra as far as the neck of the bladder; in such cases the discharge is streaked with blood; the swelling of the urethral lining membrane causes a true dysuria, and the urinary discharges, which only take place in drops, are sometimes either preceded or succeeded by the discharge of pure blood. At the same time the erections become more frequent and painful, and, in case the inflammation involves the corpora spongiosa, are not unfrequently accompanied by a painfully tensive curvature of the penis (chordée). In many cases the prepuce becomes swollen and inflamed to such an extent that it cannot be drawn behind the glans (*phimosis*); or else the swollen prepuce remains drawn back behind the glans and cannot be drawn forward, so that the glans becomes constricted and gangrene may set in (paraphimosis). The inguinal glands may likewise become swollen (*consensual buboes*), or small *knotty swellings* may arise on the *dorsum* or on the sides of the *penis* occasioned by a swelling of *Cowper's glands* or of the adipose tissue surrounding the bulbus of the urethra. If the inflammation is very violent, these swellings may terminate in suppuration, but generally they disappear of themselves in proportion as the gonorrhœal inflammation abates. There are cases where the inflammation is so intense that the discharge is almost entirely suppressed in consequence (*gonorrhœa sicca*); in such cases the pain is very acute, the inguinal glands and even the scrotum may become swollen, and ophthalmia, swelling of joints and a high degree of fever may set in. A so-called *dry* gonorrhœa may exist as an idiopathic, primary form, without any signs of violent inflammation, or without any inflammation whatever, provided such a designation may be applied to a form of gonorrhœa without any real discharge, or where only a few drops of a serous fluid are secreted. In this form the patient, a few days after the infection, experiences a more or less sharp pain at some deep-seated spot in the urethra, from which a very small quantity of infectious matter is secreted, which, though scarcely sufficient to form a drop at the orifice of the urethra, is nevertheless sufficient to transmit the infection during sexual intercourse. Here, too, the pain, dysuria and the troublesome erections may likewise acquire a great degree of violence, and the glans as well as the orifice of the urethra will be found swollen.

Sec. 13.—Metastases of the Gonorrhœal Disease.

Metastatic changes may occur not only while the secretion is still existing, but likewise, and indeed much more frequently, in consequence of a sudden suppression of the same. The most important metastases are: *orchitis, prostatitis, ophthalmic gonorrhœa* and *articular rheumatism.*

1. ORCHITIS, INFLAMMATION OF THE TESTICLES.

This form of metastasis occurs more frequently than any other, and more frequently invades the left than the right testicle, very seldom both at the same time; in the same patient it is frequently seen to travel from one testicle to the other. A metastasis of this kind may be occasioned by any cause that has power to effect a sudden suppression of the discharge before it has run through all its different stages, or to exert a violent irritation of the testicles. Among such causes we number the abuse of astringent injections, cold baths, exposure to wet and cold, excessive bodily exertions, sexual intercourse, dancing, long marches, long standing, any kind of pressure on the testicles and spermatic cord, and a number of other similar circumstances. Generally, however, a gonorrhœal inflammation of the testicles takes place when the inflammatory stage of gonorrhœa is on the decline rather than at its commencement. The first perceptible sign of gonorrhœal orchitis is a slight swelling of the epidydimis with a sensation of dull pressure, after which the inflammation speedily involves the whole testicle, which sometimes swells up to four, six or eight times its size, with agonizing pain. Even the spermatic cord is sometimes involved in the swelling, and the hardness and painful sensitiveness extend over the loins.

2. INFLAMMATION OF THE PROSTATE.

This inflammation may not only occur while the running is still going on, but likewise after it has ceased. Very frequently it occurs during the inflammatory period in consequence of the irritation extending to the neighboring parts; very frequently, however, a swelling of the prostate may occur after the running has ceased, even months and years after the first occurrence of the disease. In the former case, that is if the affection occurs as a consequence of violent inflammation, the patient experiences a weight and heat in front of the anus, attended with a violent urging to urinate, tenesmus of the bladder and intense pain in the region of the neck of the bladder, which increases when an effort is made to urinate or to evacuate the bowels; when introducing a finger in the rectum, the swollen prostate becomes distinctly perceptible, the urinary secretions become difficult, and fever supervenes soon after. If the inflammation should reach the highest degree of intensity, it becomes a difficult matter to prevent suppuration, which is always a very troublesome complication.

3. GONORRHŒAL OPHTHALMIA.

This affection, which is generally occasioned by a metastasis of the gonorrhœal inflammation to the conjunctiva of the eye and lids, occurs very rarely, and almost always in one eye. It runs a rapid course, may attain a fearful height even in twenty-four hours, is attended with agonizing pains in the eye and head, violent photophobia, fever, and discharge of a yellowish-green purulent gonorrhœal mucus oozing from every point of the conjunctiva. The inflammation may likewise be occasioned by the eye coming in contact with gonorrhœal mucus.

4. ARTICULAR RHEUMATISM.

This always results from the sudden suppression of gonorrhœa, and generally invades the knee, elbow and tarsal joints, which become swollen and inflamed. The affection is generally attended with frightful pains and a violent fever, and may, if left to itself, continue for fifteen or twenty days, unless the discharge from the urethra should be restored before that time.

5. AFFECTIONS OF THE MUCOUS MEMBRANES.

In the absence of adequate testimony, we are unable to affirm, with some authors, that a sudden suppression of gonorrhœa may be followed by metastasis to the mucous membrane of the ear, nose, pharynx, larynx, etc., even to the *serous* membranes of the brain, whereby violent cephalalgia, hemiplegia, and mental disturbances may be caused.

Sec. 14.—Sequelæ of Gonorrhœa, Lues Venerea.

Among these sequelæ we distinguish more particularly, a) *secondary gonorrhœa* or *gleet*, which is often very tedious, and, b) *strictures* of the urethra. Gleet is undoubtedly a phenomenon deserving of our serious attention; for, although it may be nothing more, in many cases, than a symptom of weakness of the lining membrane, yet it may likewise originate in the presence of some hidden syphilitic taint, and may cause the so-called *strictures* or callous contractions of the urethra. As regards the *lues gonorrhœica* of which Ritter has furnished us a description, it would seem that, if the existence of this lues were as positive as the *lues syphilitica* which owes its origin to chancre, we ought to see much more of this disease than we do, especially in the capitals of Europe, where so many hundreds of thousands of cases of gonorrhœa are mismanaged from year to year. What Ritter cites as phenomena of lues gonorrhœica, such as, violent itching in the hairy parts without any falling off of the hair; non-contagious warts on the labia and small tubercles on the scrotum; bluish-white spots and ulcerous erosions in the male urethra, at the vulva, and afterwards on the lower lip and cheeks; rhagades, inflammations of the skin, spots and herpes; affections of the periosteum covering the articular extremities of bones and in their neighborhood, attended with slight pains which recur only at long intervals, and a perceptible swelling of the bones without caries; affections of the lungs and eyes; all these phenomena may be observed in *syphilis* and the *mercurial disease*, as well as among persons who may indeed have had gonorrhœa once in their lifetime, but where the above-mentioned affections cannot be traced to gonorrhœal infection with as much positive certainty as the sequelæ of syphilis, all of which are distinguished by unmistakable, characteristic, pathognomonic signs, can be traced to their source. As for the other symptoms which Ritter regards as symptoms of the continued progress of the disease, such as, steatomata of a greater or less size on the neck and breast, as well as in and on the viscera of the thorax and abdomen, attended with physconia, deranged digestion, heart-affections, nocturnal headache, depression of spirits, feeling of exhaustion, a pale-yellowish complexion, slow fever, increasing tension of the abdomen, progressive debility and sometimes sudden death; all these symptoms may indeed occur among persons who have been afflicted with gonorrhœa, but likewise among those who never had this disease; whereas, on the other hand, thousands of individuals had gonorrhœa not only once, but ten times, and were treated with injections, yet never manifested any of the above-mentioned symptoms. All this is different as regards the well-established symptoms of secondary syphilis. The only phenomena of secondary or chronic gonorrhœa which, beside the above-mentioned metastases, are so far established as undeniably positive sequelæ of the original infection, are, *strictures* of the urethra, chronic *swelling of the prostate*, and other local affections, such as *gleet*, which last-mentioned trouble may likewise arise from excessive weakness of the mucous membrane of the urethra.

Sec. 15.—Relation of the Gonorrhœal to the Syphilitic Virus.

Although, even at this day, a number of physicians regard, with Girtanner, Hunter, Harrison, and most French authors on syphilis, both miasmata as identical, yet a more matured judgment and correct observation must lead us to deny the correctness of their opinions. For, although it cannot be denied that the gonorrhœal virus, when inoculated upon a sound mucous surface, may produce chancre, mucous tubercles and other syphilitic phenomena; yea, though it is perfectly positive that the gonorrhœal virus has produced all the symptoms of secondary syphilis which are generally attributed to the operations of the chancre-virus; it is, on the other hand, equally certain that there are cases of *contagious* gonorrhœa where none of these symptoms occur; from which we conclude that there exists a special gonorrhœic virus which has nothing in common with the virus of syphilis; but that, on the other hand, the syphilitic virus may cause gonorrhœal discharges which, in such cases, take the place of chancre, provided that the two poisons have not coalesced, which may and does occur here and there. In addition to all this, we have to state that the cases where, as I myself have had occasion to observe, a so-called contagious gonorrhœa is afterwards succeeded by all the symptoms of constitutional syphilis, occur much more frequently among women than among men, probably for the reason that, if the internal parts of the female were more frequently examined, we should find that what was supposed to be gonorrhœa, was nothing else than a profuse secretion from syphilitic erosions caused by the chancre-poison, with a liberal admixture of leucorrhœal matter. It is very likely that similar erosions may occur in the urethra of the male, where they likewise occasion a gonorrhœal discharge which is mistaken for a *common* gonorrhœa; this may even be considered as certain, if, simultaneously with the gonorrhœa, we perceive such erosions on the glans in company with balanorrhœa (see below), or if, at a later period (see Sec. 73), we not only notice *figwarts* but real *chancre.*

Sec. 16.—Diagnosis.

We consider it, therefore, as an established fact that there are two kinds of *contagious* or venereal gonorrhœa, both of which result from impure coït and differ greatly in their results, one of which, constituting a more or less local affection and confined to the sexual organs, runs the above-described course without leaving any other than local symptoms after the cessation of the discharge; whereas the other form, which might be designated as chancrous, or, in a more restricted sense, as syphilitic gonorrhœa, may be accompanied by, or cause the appearance of, all the phenomena which a chancre may be capable of occasioning. We have shown above in what way these two kinds of gonorrhœa are distinguished from other innocuous non-contagious urethral discharges; but it is much more difficult to show by what signs a simple venereal local gonorrhœa is distinguished from the *syphilitic* form. In the absence of such signs as chancre or syphilitic erosions, Ricord knows of no better diagnostic proof than *inoculation* in order to find out whether it will produce chancre or not. This is undoubtedly correct; for all the other signs are altogether uncertain, and may equally occur in both forms of gonorrhœa. It being, however, impossible, in most cases, to employ Ricord's method of ascertaining the syphilitic character of gonorrhœa, we shall be compelled, in many cases, to remain in doubt regarding the true nature of the discharge. From my own observations I have deduced the following points, which, if they do not afford diagnostic certainty in all cases of female gonorrhœa, yet will justify the suspicion that we have not to deal with a simple venereal gonorrhœa, but with a discharge that had been caused by the poison of chancre.

1. The *more purely* the true, specific gonorrhœal symptoms, with or without the local consensual affections that are peculiar to them, manifest themselves, and the more uncomplicated their course through their different stages, from the first moment of their increasing inflammation to the gradual decrease and final

termination of the discharge, the less need we suspect the presence of a secret chancrous virus.

2. The less distinctly marked the course, and more especially the inflammatory period of gonorrhœa; in other words the *more torpid* a gonorrhœa, and the longer a copious discharge continues, even after the disappearance of all inflammatory symptoms, the more we have a right to suspect that the existing discharge is owing to the presence of chancre-virus.

3. This probability becomes positive certainty, if, during the course of the disease not only chancre, but suspicious erosions and even figwarts break out upon the mucous lining.

4. The most suspicious in this respect are the so-called torpid gonorrhœas, consisting of a very slight painless discharge, with scarcely any inflammation either preceding or still accompanying the discharge; for, as we shall see afterwards, inasmuch as the syphilitic erosions caused by the chancre-poison are almost always painless, the presence of such erosions in the urethra, may very readily lead to such a gonorrhœal discharge.

Sec. 17.—The Contagiousness of Gonorrhœa.

As a matter of course, we do not speak here of discharges that owe their origin to the chancre-poison, but of a local gonorrhœa caused by a *specific virus*. It is an established fact that this form of gonorrhœa is likewise contagious, and capable of exciting a similar pathological product in a person in perfect health. The question here is not whether venereal discharges are contagious, but in what degree the contagiousness of the non-venereal, inflammatory non-syphilitic gonorrhœa exists, and to what stage it continues. Regarding this point, I can refer to six cases in my own practice, where wives were infected by their husbands at a stage of the disease when there was scarcely any perceptible discharge, and only a little redness of the orifice of the urethra, and a secretion leaving only a few scarcely observable stains on the linen and slightly closing the urethra by agglutination, on account of which the patients came to consult me, admitting that they had had sexual intercourse with their wives all the time in spite of these appearances; of course, the consequences of such conduct did not fail to show themselves in 6, 10 or 14 days. It is difficult to say, however, how long after the disappearance of the inflammatory period gleet may still continue to remain infectious; all I know in this respect, is, that I have been consulted by men who had been for years afflicted with more or less considerable mucous secretions from the urethra consequent upon gonorrhœa contracted at that remote period, who finally got married without communicating to their wives any trace of disease. On the other hand, cases have come to my knowledge where women who had been perfectly sound previous to getting married, and whose husbands had been afflicted with gonorrhœa, which, about the period when the marriage took place, still left a secretion of a few drops of serous liquid behind, experienced various irritations of the orifice and neck of the womb, which, in consequence of the continuance of contagious irritation through the sexual act, became very obstinate. In cases where the secretion that had been regarded as a simple inflammatory gonorrhœa, is really a syphilitic discharge arising from the presence of chancre, it is evident that this question must be involved in great doubt, and it may be regarded as certain that, as long as there is the least remnant of a discharge, the danger of contagion is not entirely passed; hence it is advisable to impress all such patients with the conviction that the infection may be communicated even by the least quantity of secretion remaining after gonorrhœa; and that young men who are afflicted in this manner, had better not get married until all traces of the disease, and the remaining secretion, are effectually removed.

Sec. 18.—Prognosis.

From what we have said, it must be evident that the prognosis must not only depend upon the individual constitution of the patient (which, however, is of very little moment in the purely inflammatory form of gonorrhœa), but likewise upon the *nature of the discharge.* The purely inflammatory non-syphilitic gonorrhœa, if left to itself, and if the patient observes a careful diet, generally gets well in six or seven weeks, without leaving any other difficulty than a disposition to *stricture* and swelling of the prostate. But if the strictest dietetic rules are not observed; if the patient indulges in beer, coffee, but more especially in spirituous beverages; if he fatigues himself by excessive bodily exertions, long standing, forced marches, etc.; if he exposes himself to catarrhal influences, or indulges in sexual intercourse before the discharge is entirely removed; it may not only pass into the form of a most obstinate gleet, but may occasion many additional sufferings. Irritating injections or other influences by which the discharge may become suddenly suppressed, not only occasion the metastases described in § 13, but, even if these metastases do not result, the discharge, which they only suppress palliatively, may return again, in which case its radical cure becomes more and more difficult, and the most obstinate gleet is the consequence. Another circumstance, which is rarely taken notice of, but is of the utmost importance and exerts a powerful influence upon the prognosis, is this, whether the gonorrhœa was the result of a *single* accidental contact with the gonorrhœal virus, or whether the patient had repeatedly had connection with the infected female before he became aware of the contagion. Baffled in all my efforts to cure an apparently simple gonorrhœa with remedies that had always exerted a specific curative influence, I have been finally led to conclude, after the most careful observations, that the obstinacy with which the disease, even when of an apparently simple character, resists the effect of the usual remedial agents, is owing to the fact that intercourse with the infected female had been repeatedly indulged in; in other cases, where the disease had been transmitted by one single act of coïtion, I have effected a cure of the most violent inflammatory gonorrhœa in from fifteen to at most twenty-one days. My experience has led me to establish a rather unfavorable prognosis in all cases where the act of coïtion had been exercised with the diseased female in repeated succession. As regards the prognosis in the case of *syphilitic* gonorrhœa (or such as had been caused by the chancre-poison) it is quite the same as in any other case of syphilitic products; a definite prognosis as regards the duration or the possible consequences resulting from such forms of gonorrhœa cannot well be established, though even such forms, if not *mismanaged* by improper treatment, can be radically cured after a longer or shorter lapse of time, without leaving any untoward consequences behind. The greatest difficulties in the treatment of gonorrhœa will be met with in cases of *gleet* resulting from so-called desiccating injections; such injections, even if not succeeded by metastases, *never* cure, but only *mask* the disease for a time, which is evident from the fact that the discharge, if the injections are discontinued for a few days, re-appears, generally at once, until finally the injections likewise cease to be of any effect.

Sec. 19.—Treatment of Gonorrhœa.

Every homœopathic physician who has acquired some experience in the treatment of venereal diseases, must have become aware of the difficulty of selecting the *specifically characteristic* remedy adapted to every case of gonorrhœa. This difficulty will be found much less, if, in selecting a remedy for any particular case, we keep in view the remarks we have offered in previous paragraphs, relating to *diagnosis*, and the essential points to be considered in establishing our *prognosis*. Starting from this position, I commence the treatment of gonorrhœa in every case by interdicting the use of spirituous beverages, coffee, beer, excessive bodily exertions, long standing, and more particularly all sexual intercourse until the discharge is entirely stopped; I warrant a speedy and rapid cure only on condition that all these rules are strictly complied with. As regards the medical treatment, if the case is non-syphilitic, not occasioned by the chancre-virus,—

1. I give the patient, if he presents himself for treatment before there is any actual running, and he only complains of titillation at the orifice of the urethra, with slight redness and a scarcely perceptible secretion, barely sufficient to close the orifice of the urethra by agglutination (*gonorrhœa incipiens*), *Sepia* 30, two pellets morning and evening dry on the tongue, by which treatment I frequently effect a cure without any inflammation supervening, or, at most, without any other increase of symptoms than perhaps a more profuse secretion.

2. If, at the time when the patient presents himself for treatment, the secretion is already quite copious, or if the inflammatory period is already more or less advanced, or if *sepia* has had no effect within six or seven days in diminishing the incipient symptoms, I at once give in all cases *Cannabis* 3, two pellets morning and night, without *paying any attention to consensual symptoms* (such as pains in the testicles, phimosis or paraphimosis, swelling of the inguinal glands, difficulty of urinating, painful erections, etc.); by persevering in the use of this agent, two, or, in very few cases, three weeks, at most, suffice to radically cure every case of gonorrhœa, together with all the consensual symptoms, provided the patient does not commit any of the above-mentioned errors in diet, and the disease is not complicated with

syphilitic taint, and does not primarily owe its origin to chancre-virus.

3. If the patient presents himself after the inflammatory symptoms have entirely disappeared, and is still affected with a continual, painless, more or less profuse discharge, I commence the treatment with *Cannabis* in every case where this remedy has not yet been used, and from which I have derived excellent results in this form of gleet. In cases where *Cannabis* had almost effected a cure, but where the disease had again become aggravated in consequence of errors in diet, I again restore the normal condition of things by means of a few doses of *Cannabis.* If *Cannabis* should prove of no avail, I give in either of these two cases half a grain of the second trituration of *Mercurius vivus*, repeating this dose every three or four days, a few doses being in most cases sufficient to remove every trace of the discharge.

4. It is only cases where *a few* scarcely perceptible *drops* are still secreted that are quite unmanageable, and seem to resist all treatment. In such cases *Sepia*, *Sulphur*, *Pulsatilla*, and, if the secretion is of a milky whiteness, *Capsicum* and *Ferrum*, and in some cases *Tussilago* and *Natrum muriaticum* have rendered me excellent service. Regarding such remedies as Agnus, Agaricus, Copaivæ balsamum, Cantharis, Cubebæ, Petroselinum, Fluoris acidum, Polygonum, Mezereum, etc., I have no experience to offer; but, if I may judge from what I have seen of *Cannabis* in the treatment of gonorrhœa, it is my opinion that those who use all sorts of remedies for one or the other accessory symptom, waste their time and cure gonorrhœa much more slowly on that account. It is only when intense inflammations threaten dangerous results, such as gangrene, where *Arsenic* would have to be used, that intercurrent remedies become necessary.

5. As a matter of course, where gonorrhœa is evidently complicated with syphilitic symptoms (such as erosions, chancre, figwarts, etc.,) the remedies which have to be advised for chancre, figwarts, etc., will have to be resorted to.

[*Sepia* and *Cannabis*, as recommended by Jahr, are relied upon by many of our most prominent homœopathic physicians in the treatment of gonorrhœa; but there are vast numbers of cases where other means have to be resorted to, as we shall see by-and-bye. Even in cases where cannabis is the remedy, it may have to be given in massive doses. In a case where chordée was a very prominent and very painful symptom, we effected a perfect cure by means of large doses of the tincture of *Cannabis*, beginning with five drops of the tincture the first day, and gradually increasing the quantity to thirty drops in the course of a day; a cure was effected in a fortnight; our patient was a member of the Legislature, and had to transact a large amount of business every day. —Hempel.]

Sec. 20. Treatment of the Metastases and Sequelæ of Gonorrhœa.

1. INFLAMMATION OF THE SCROTUM AND TESTICLES, ORCHITIS.

This inflammation generally yields to *Pulsatilla* (a solution in water, a teaspoonful every three hours); and if *Pulsatilla* should not prove sufficient, *Mercurius vivus* 12, given in the same manner, will do the rest. In former years I used to obtain good results from *Aurum*, but latterly I have got along with *Pulsatilla* and *Mercurius*. For the *induration of the testicles*, which sometimes remains for years after mismanaged gonorrhœa, the most efficient remedies in my hands have been *Aurum* and *Clematis*, though they may leave one in the lurch in some cases.

[In phlegmonous inflammation of the testicles, *aconite* is an agent of paramount importance. We have cured such cases with *Aconite* 30. Cases may arise where *Belladonna* may be necessary. We have employed successfully the lower attenuations and even the tincture internally, at the same time applying compresses soaked with a strong solution of the fluid extract in water, externally. If the inflammation is extensive, involving the spermatic cord, and is moreover attended with cerebral symptoms, torpor, slight delirium, etc., Belladonna will be found indispensable.—Hempel.]

2. METASTASIS OF GONORRHŒA TO THE EYES.

Here we give at once *Aconite* every three hours, after which, if the inflammation is less, but the discharge is not restored, we resort to *Pulsatilla* or *Mercurius sublimatus*. After the danger is

5

removed, and *Mercurius* should not have wiped out the disease, we finish up the treatment with *Acidum nitricum*. *Belladonna* and *Tussilago* have likewise done me good service in all such cases.

[In the case of a blacksmith, whose right eye had become inflamed by being brought in contact with the gonorrhœal virus, one pellet of *Acidum nitricum* 200 in half a tumbler of water, effected a perfect cure. The inflammation set in suddenly during the night. The day previous both eyes were perfectly sound. The affected organ seemed like a disorganized mass of a dirty-looking yellow-greenish pus. The pain was agonizing.—Hempel.]

3. INFLAMMATION OF THE PROSTATE, PROSTATITIS.

The first remedy to be employed against this always extremely painful affection is *Pulsatilla*, and if this should either totally or partially fail, we may resort to *Thuja*. *Merc. viv.* and *Nitri acid* have likewise rendered essential service, and, in two cases, I have obtained good results from *Tussilago*, recommended by Rosenberg. [The Hydriodate of Potash should not be forgotten in this affection.—Hempel.]

4. ARTICULAR RHEUMATISM.

In one of the most desperate cases of this kind, where the patient was a female, and the sudden suppression of the discharge by astringent injections not only induced inflammation of one knee, as is most frequently the case, but inflammation of the knee, elbow, tarsal, and wrist-joints, *Pulsatilla*, preceded by a few doses of *Aconite*, had a marvellous effect, and restored the discharge, which was afterwards cured, together with the remaining symptoms of articular inflammation, by means of *Mercurius vivus*. In a few other badly managed, less acute cases, I have seen good effects from *Thuja*, and sometimes from *Sarsaparilla*, but *never* from *Clematis*, which has been recommended for this affection.

5. GLEET.

If painless, and not very copious, gleet is generally nothing more than a symptom of weakness of the mucous lining, which had been occasioned by this disease; in such a case *Ferrum*, *Phosphori acidum*, and *Sulphur*, have proven more efficient in my hands than any other remedial agent.

6. STRICTURES.

Whatever remedies I may have used against these callous contractions of the urethra, as consequences of the gonorrhœal disease, I have never yet succeeded in superseding, by internal treatment, the use of bougies, by the systematic introduction of which into the urethra, this organ is gradually dilated to its natural dimensions. In a single case, where I had administered *Aurum*, for a considerable period of time against mercurial symptoms, and where a bougie had to be introduced at least once a week, the stricture, with which this patient was afflicted, improved at the same time so far that, for the last three years, the patient has been able to urinate without any pain or difficulty, only the stream is a little thinner than usual.

NOTES BY DR. HEMPEL.

[Jahr's remarks on the treatment of gonorrhœa are undoubtedly judicious, and the remedies he proposes for the treatment of this disease may be sufficient in a large number of cases. Nevertheless, a few additional remarks may not be out of place.

If the testicles, one or both, should be much swollen and inflamed, it will be found necessary to wear a suspensory bandage for the purpose of alleviating the pain caused by the dragging weight. At the same time the patient should remain in a state of perfect rest until the inflammation is removed.

If a sudden suppression of the discharge, consequent upon exposure to wet, a draught of air, etc., or occasioned by violently astringent injections, should result in violent inflammation of the urethra and neck of the bladder, or the bladder itself—accompanied by excruciating burning pain and an agonizing dysuria or ischuria, violent chills and fever, discharge of blood from the urethra—it will be found nesessary to give *Aconite*, of which, in all such cases, I mix a few drops of the tincture in half a tumbler of water, giving a dessert-spoonful of this solution every five or ten minutes until the pain is relieved. Some practitioners, among others Yeldham, in his "Homœopathy in Venereal Diseases," propose to alternate Aconite with Cantharides. I prefer giving each remedy by itself: *Aconite* as long as it is specifically indicated, and, if necessary, follow it up with *Cantharides*, if this agent seems to be specifically indicated by such symptoms as violent priapism, agonizing chordee, delirium, etc.

I have not the heart to give Copaiva and Cubebs the go-by, as Jahr and other Homœopathic physicians are in the habit of doing. Any one who will consult the second edition of my Materia Medica, will find that both Copaiva and Cubebs produce a discharge from the urethra, which, in addition to the other symptoms accompanying the discharge, would seem to justify the inference that these agents must be possessed of powerful curative virtues in gonorrhœa. But they must not be given in small doses. Copaiva is evidently adapted to the primary or acute, and Cubebs rather to a chronic, form of the disease, or to gleetish discharges with simple burning and a slightly increased desire to void the bladder. If used in the acute stage, *Copaiva* need not be given in larger doses than ten or twelve drops three or four times a day; when the inflammatory symptoms have subsided and a whitish discharge remains, with more or less burning, urging to urinate, etc., I give larger doses, adapting their size to the tone of the patient's stomach. This method frequently leads to a cure, and as frequently, perhaps, leaves us in the lurch. In such cases other remedies have to be chosen. If Ricord's opinion that Copaiva does not act dynamically, but by virtue of a mechanical contact with the urethral lining membrane, is correct—and he seems to have substantiated it by a number of observations—it is evident that Copaiva, if given at all, should be given in large doses. A very convenient mode of administering the balsam is the frequent introduction into the urethra of a bougie smeared with Copaiva.

* * * * * * *

In the Report of the Medical Statistics of the United States Army, Assistant-Surgeon Hammond, in his report on the diseases of Socorro, New Mexico, mentions a new remedy for gonorrhœa, the Exhedra occidentalis, called by the natives *popilote.* The taste is terebinthinate and astringent, yet agreeable. It is a stimulant diuretic, and does not constipate the bowels. It is prepared for use by macerating two ounces of the branches, cut into small pieces, in a pint of hot water, in a close vessel, for three hours, and then straining. A pint of the infusion may be drunk during the day. It acts with surprising promptness, and is an efficient and valuable medicine. The shrub is an evergreen, and grows in great profusion throughout the country.

In the first volume of the North-American Journal of Homœopathy we find the Nitrate of potash recommended by Dr. J. S. Henry, of Montgomery, Ala., for gonorrhœa. He prescribes one grain three times a day, with a little sugar of milk; sometimes he gives ten grains three times a day. Recent cases yield in a week; old cases in two or three weeks.

Professor Hale, in his work entiled "New Remedies," has added the following to the list of those that homœopathic physicians have been in the habit of employing in this disease:

Alnus rubra, or tag alder, recommended by Lee.

Asclepias incarnata, or swamp milkweed. Dr. Hauser recommends it strongly for gonorrhœa and syphilis. He gives a table-spoonful of the tincture three times a day, before breakfast, dinner, and supper. [See Tilden's Journal of Materia Medica, vol. i. page 41.]

Asclepias syriaca, silkweed. It has long been in use among the Negroes of the South for gleet, gonorrhœa, scrofula, etc. The most usual mode of administration is in powder or infusion, the latter made with water and whiskey. Old cases of gleet, of many years' standing, have been reported cured, after other medicines had failed, by taking a wine-glassful of an infusion of the fresh root, three times a day, before meals.

Chimaphila, pipsissewa, and Caulophyllum, blue cohosh; our experience in the use of these agents is limited.

Erigeron canadense, Canada flea-bane. Recommended by Coe. "It allays the scalding of the urine, and assists materially in cutting short the disease."

Eryngium aquaticum, button snakeroot. "Two ounces of the pulverized root, in doses of two or three grains, have effected cures in obstinate cases of gonorrhœa and gleet."

Gelseminum sempervirens, yellow jessamine. A case of cure is reported at page 448 of Hale's "New Remedies."

Hydrastis canadensis, golden seal. Dr. Brown cured a case of gonorrhœa with five-drop doses of a saturated tincture three times a day. It is also used as an injection.

Phosphorus. Dr. Meyer of Leipzic reports a case of secondary gonorrhœa, complicated with hypertrophy of the prostate gland, which was cured by the persistent use of this agent in the space of seventy-one days. Both the discharge and the hypertrophy yielded perfectly to the treatment instituted.

Aloes. Dr. Gamberine, of Bologna, treats gonorrhœa very successfully with injections of diluted tincture of aloes. His formula is as follows:

Aloës, 4 drachms;
Water, 4 ounces.

He injects the urethra three times a day.

In the twenty-third volume of the British Journal two new remedies are recommended for gonorrhœa by Dr. Thomas B. Henderson; one of them is obtained from the wood of the tree, *Sirium myrtifolium.* Dr. O'Shaughnessy writes: "Sandal wood, in powder, is given by the native physicians in ardent remitting fevers. With milk it is also prescribed in gonorrhœa." The other remedy is the Gurjun or Gurgina balsam, or wood oil. It is the product of the *Dipterocarpus turbinatus*, an immense tree growing in different parts of India. Thomas recommends both medicines very highly. [See British Journal.]

* * * * * * *

Regarding injections, it may be said that opinions among homœopathic practitioners are divided. Some reject the use of injections entirely, others resort to them even to the extent of adopting the French "abortive plan." I have known this plan to succeed to the perfect satisfaction of both the physician and the patient. Sometimes the gonorrhœal inflammation is cured upon the principle of Trousseau's method of substitution: the nitrate of silver inflammation being substituted in place of the gonorrhœal inflammation. The former, running a definite course, carries off the disease, leaving at most a weakness of the urethral lining membrane, which is afterwards removed by the use of tonic astringents, such as *tannin*, a solution of quinine, the sulphate of zinc, the sub-acetate of lead, hydrastis canadensis, etc. An excellent agent to inject is the *sulphate of hydrastin*, which may, at the same time, be administered internally. In all cases where a gleetish discharge remains, more especially in debilitated and cachectic individuals, mild astringent injections, like those mentioned, may be of great use. Even cold water injections may prove expedient and beneficial. The injection-syringe should be provided with a long nozzle that should be well inserted in the urethra. The liquid injected has to be retained in the urethra for several minutes. For this purpose the penis has to be held in a horizontal position, and, at the same time, compressed between the thumb and index finger of the left hand, while the syringe is drawn out with the right. Injections, if they prove suitable and beneficial, may be repeated three or four times in the twenty-four hours.

The muriate of iron is likewise useful in this stage, both in the form of an injection and by the mouth. Internally I give ten to twelve drops in water three times a day, and when used as an injection, mix fifteen to twenty drops to an ounce of water.

In the ninth volume of the North American Journal of Homœopathy, the late Dr. J. C. Peterson, of St. John's, N. B., publishes an interesting article on gonorrhœa, where he recommends the following injections of the chloride of zinc during the initial stage of the disease: Three drops of the liquor chlorid-zinc. to eight ounces of water. Before the patient uses the injection he is directed to void his urine, after which half a drachm of the solution is thrown up the urethra, and retained until it produces a smarting sensation; the liquid is then allowed to escape, and is followed in a few minutes with an injection of cold water. In the third stage, when all inflammatory action has ceased, he uses injections of the nitrate of silver, chloride of zinc, or the acid nitrate of mercury. In the fourth stage, or that of gleet, he uses injections of rose water and port wine, and of the iodide of iron; four ounces of the wine to two ounces of water; and two grains of the iodide of iron to six ounces of distilled water.

Peterson's injection of chloride of zinc was first mentioned by Gaudriot. His formula is:

Liquid chloride of zinc, 24 to 36 drops.
Distilled water, 4 ounces.

Two injections a day, for two or three days, will generally suffice for a radical cure of gonorrhœa; the first injections are almost always followed by more or less swelling of the glans penis, but this does not contraindicate their continued use.

For gonorrhœa in females suppositories may be used composed of

Liquid chloride of zinc,	5 drops,
Sulphate of morph.,	½ grain,
Mix with 3 drachms of paste made of mucilage of gum-tragacanth,	6 parts,
Starch powder,	9 parts,
Powdered sugar,	6 parts.

Make into vaginal suppositories, one suppository every day, or every third day. Four or six in all will effect a cure; the first suppository generally causes a swelling, with more or less heat of the vulva, which soon subsides.

Thomas Evans, of London, uses very frequent and very weak injections of the sulphate of zinc, one grain to the ounce, to be still further reduced if pain is felt. They are simple but efficacious. He repeats them every half hour during the day. Slight cases are cured in twenty-four hours, severe cases in three or four days.

Velpeau prefers nitrate of silver to sulphate of zinc, one grain to the ounce; in old-standing cases two grains may be used.

Carmichael prefers a quarter of a grain to one ounce of water; he seldom increases to one grain. He recommends three or four injections a day.

Alum injections are used by Dr. H. Collis exclusively in all stages of gonorrhœa. In the most acute form the patient is directed to pour a small jug of cold water on the organ; and immediately inject a syringeful of alum solution, one-half of a grain to an ounce of water. The first day the injection is to be repeated every half hour; at night as often as the patient wakes. In old cases the injection may be increased to one drachm of alum in eight ounces of water, three or four times a day. [See British Journal, vol. xxiv. page 183.]

Injections of *Merc. corr.* and *Arg. nitr.* are used by some French physicians in quantities equivalent to our first or second centesimal attenuation. Many cases are reported by them as having been cured by these injections without the aid of any other remedial agents.

* * * * * * *

Gonorrhœal ophthalmia, when resulting from metastasis, may have to be treated like any other severe inflammation of the eyes, with Aconite, Belladonna, Bryonia, Pulsatilla, etc., the specific treatment for gonorrhœa being continued all the while, if the gonorrhœal discharge is not suppressed. For an interesting cure of such a case I refer the reader to page 275 and further, in the tenth volume of the British Journal of Homœopathy.

An interesting cure of gonorrhœal rheumatism is reported at page 23 of the fifteenth volume of the British Journal. It occurred in consequence of a gonorrhœal discharge having been suppressed in three weeks by means of copaiva [? Ed.]. Soon afterwards he experienced a tearing pain in the left knee, with swelling and stiffness of the joint. The patient took the Schlangenbad, one of the Teplitz baths. The rheumatism left him entirely after the discharge had reappeared ; it gradually ceased entirely.

* * * a * * *

Beside the sequelæ of gonorrhœa, mentioned by Jahr, we have "irritable bladder," a most annoying symptom. In a case of irritable bladder, of several years standing, which had remained after a gonorrhœa treated allopathically with caustic injections, and where the patient was troubled with painful urging to urinate, the urine dribbling off in drops; and where quantities of mucus were discharged with the urine, and the patient complained of debility, loss of appetite, etc., we effected perfect relief by the persistent use of Copaiva and the tincture of Cinchona. Owing to circumstances, the patient mixed both ingredients in one bottle, in the proportion of one ounce of Copaiva to two ounces of Cinchona, of which preparation he took a teaspoonful three times a day. After using it for a week he considered himself cured.]

III. VENEREAL BALANORRHŒA.

Sec. 21.—Symptomatology,

As we have a venereal, *contagious* blennorrhœa, superinduced by venereal infection, and another form of blennorrhœa which is non-contagious, and may have been induced by irritating stimuli, so we have a so-called balanorrhœa or external gonorrhœa. The non-contagious form, which frequently befals individuals who do not keep themselves clean, or whose prepuce is very long and narrow and covers the whole glans, is a simple affection, that may occur in young as well as old people, and may even be occasioned by the friction in sexual intercourse. As in gonorrhœa the matter is discharged from the urethra, so in balanorrhœa it is secreted between the prepuce and glans, sometimes attended with swelling of the prepuce, increased redness of the glans, and partial excoriations, which, however, are merely superficial, and, in a few days, heal of themselves. *Venereal* balanorrhœa acts in a similar manner, with this difference, that it never gets well of itself, and that the erosions, which, in simple non-contagious balanorrhœa, scarcely look like redness such as may be produced by simple irritating stimuli, in the syphilitic form, which always results from an infection by the chancre-virus, are more or less ulcerated and characterized by the diagnostic signs of other syphilitic products. What distinguishes the contagious from the non-contagious balanorrhœa, are the complications that either exist or may occur in the course of the disease, such as chancre, buboes, figwarts, mucous tubercles, etc. Regarding its origin, it may exist as a secondary disease, consequent upon constitutional syphilis, or as a primary disease induced by an immediate, direct or primary infection by the chancre-virus. In this case it commences exactly like simple balanorrhœa, the patient experiencing at first, under the prepuce, a simple titillation, burning and unusual itching; the under surface of the prepuce and glans looks red and swollen; an increased secretion arises between the prepuce and glans, at first of a sero-mucous character, and afterwards, as the inflammation increases, assuming an increased degree of thickness, and finally changing to gonorrhœal matter. If the inflammation is violent, it may induce a true inflammation of the vein along the dorsum of the penis, and even a severely-constricting phimosis, in which case the pus, instead of running off, remains behind the glans, and the whole of the integuments of the penis become involved in the inflammation. In such a case, the above-mentioned erosions, pustules or chancre arise at a later period, whereas, in the *secondary* form of syphilitic balanorrhœa, these phenomena generally precede that affection for a certain period of time.

Sec. 22.—Diagnosis.

In the presence of other symptoms of syphilitic infection it is not difficult to distinguish a syphilitic from a simple non-contagious balanorrhœa; but such a distinction is almost impossible, if the balanorrhœa sets in as a primary, acute disease, and the erosions are only slight and superficial. In such cases *inoculation* affords the only true *diagnostic sign;* nevertheless, the following points may facilitate the diagnosis:

1. A non-contagious balanorrhœa, whether caused by a want of cleanliness or heated coït, gets well of itself in a few, or at

most, in from eight to ten days, simply by frequent washing of the parts; this result is never obtained in the syphilitic form.

2. The erosions which may take place in simple balanorrhœa, are neither as broad, nor as numerous or red as in the syphilitic form; at the same time the surrounding mucous membrane is never as much inflamed, nor does the inflammation extend over as large a surface; nor is the discharge as copious.

3. The preputial herpes, which, located on the inner surface of the prepuce, may likewise occasion a sort of balanorrhœa, and may cause erosions by the bursting of its vesicles, never exhibits such a red inflammatory border round the ulcerated spots as the syphilitic erosions, and is moreover accompanied by itching both before and after the appearance of the vesicles, which itching is wanting in the syphilitic products.

Sec. 23.—Treatment.

In every form of balanorrhœa, no matter what its pathological nature may be, it is advisable to keep the parts as clean as possible, by washing them quite frequently with tepid water, or by injecting this fluid between the prepuce and glans. It may likewise be an excellent proceeding to insert linen rags moistened with water between the prepuce and glans. In non-contagious balanorrhœa this method will prove sufficient in most cases to remove the trouble in four, five, or, at latest, eight days. If there should be violent inflammation, a few doses of *Sepia* or *Mercurius vivus* will speedily remove it. Care must be had not to apply externally to such erosions remedial agents that have a specific relation to syphilis, lest the removal of such erosions by external means should lead to the breaking out of syphilitic phenomena in other places. The solutions of lunar caustic which are applied by allopaths between the glans and prepuce, are sometimes the most dangerous things to be used. If the phimosis or paraphimosis should become so violent as to result in *gangrene*, *Arsenic* will have to be used.

If the *syphilitic* character of balanorrhœa is evidenced by the presence of suspicious erosions, figwarts or chancre, we have to resort to the treatment that will be described hereafter.

[The non-contagious form of balanorrhœa does not always yield to mere washing. In highly scrofulous individuals the disease may not only become troublesome, but even disgusting, in consequence of the enormous secretion of purulent matter, which threatens to result in a partial disorganization of the parts. In such cases, we have succeeded in arresting the disease promptly by the external application of a solution of the *Muriate of Ammonia*, at the same time administering the medicine internally in the form of a weak solution.—Hempel.]

IV. GONORRHŒA IN THE FEMALE.

Sec. 24.—Symptomatology.

Nothing probably is more difficult than to furnish a full and correct symptomatic description of female gonorrhœa and its various forms. For the sake of correctness, not only the different varieties of non-contagious leucorrhœa, but likewise both kinds of gonorrhœa, the simple contagious or venereal and the syphilitic gonorrhœa which owes its origin to the chancre-virus, should be grouped in accordance with their distinctive phenomena; which is the reason that some authors have classed all these different forms more or less under one head. In addition to this, there is no portion of the mucous membrane, from the pudendum to the uterus, that may not become the seat of infectious gonorrhœa just as well as it may be the seat of the most innocuous leucorrhœa. Though some authors contend that the gonorrhœal infection starts from the orifice of the female urethra, whereas others are of opinion that its primary seat is the vagina, it seems, on the contrary, to be an established fact that the infection may arise from various points indiscriminately; so that the *seat* of the inflammation, if the affection should emanate from other parts than the urethra, can shed but a feeble ray of light upon the nature of the affection. What we know to a certainty is, that in every case of contagious venereal, though even not syphilitic gonorrhœa, a few days after the suspected coït a feeling of heat, smarting and tension, together with a sensation of increased dryness, is experienced in the more immediately affected parts. If the vulva is affected alone, or in company with other parts, they are swollen either partially or totally, so that, especially if the vagina is involved in the inflammation, the introduction of the finger becomes either difficult or painful, or even intolerable, and the patient is sometimes unable either to walk or to seat herself. These symptoms are attended with a great deal of itching, and occasionally with such a powerful irritation in the sexual organs that the patient experiences a strong desire for sexual gratification. The parts covered with mucous membrane, are dark-red, dry and tense; the redness being sometimes visible only here and there, with or without slight excoriations, or granulations which arise from the swelling of the mucous glands. During micturition, the last drops are attended with the most intense burning pain, though the urethra may not be involved; if this, however, should be the case, its orifice is red and swollen, and, when pressing upon it, a drop of purulent matter escapes from it; urination, in such a case, is painful from beginning to end. Very frequently the appearance of the local phenomena is preceded by other sympathetic symptoms, such as colic, constipation or diarrhœa, etc., which may continue even after the discharge has commenced. In many cases the color and consistence of the menstrual blood are altered. The discharge, as soon as it makes its appearance, has the color and consistence of purulent mucus, leaving sharply-circumscribed stains of a yellow, green or brown color upon the linen, by which it is generally distinguished from the ordinary leucorrhœa with which the patient may have been affected heretofore; toward the termination of the disease this discharge assumes a milky-white appearance.

Sec. 25.—Particular Forms.

As has already been stated, gonorrhœa in females may be seated in the vulva, vagina, and at the neck of the uterus as well as in the urethra. If the *vulva* is the seat of the disease, the inflammation may be confined to single parts such as the papillæ, labia, clitoris and its prepuce, etc.; in most cases the whole of the vulva is involved. In such a case we notice very often an erythematous redness without any perceptible alteration of the secretion; such an alteration always takes place if the inflammation becomes more deep-seated, in which case it may assume a phlegmonous character. In some cases this affection, which is very much like the balanorrhœa of the male, seems more particularly confined to the mucous and sebaceous follicles. In such a case the itching is generally very violent; œdema or an inflammatory swelling of the affected parts, and even abscesses frequently supervene; in some cases the phlegmonous swelling may become so extensive that it may close up the entrance of the vagina and may render the emission of urine difficult and painful. The inflammation may even extend to the external pudendum and the surrounding integuments, in which case they become œdematous, the epidermis softens, and the parts assume the appearance of a suppurating blister. In all these forms of gonorrhœa of the pudendum the secretions always have a fetid odor.

In most cases gonorrhœa remains confined to the pudendum; but frequently it gradually progresses through the vagina as far as the uterus, more particularly if it lasts a long time; after having disappeared in every other part, it may localize itself in the uterus, and, without causing any other ailments, may occasion those *uterine catarrhs* which are often of such an equivocal nature, and which, without betraying their true character by any external signs, are nevertheless capable of transmitting the venereal infection by coït.

In the female gonorrhœa, the inflammation may extend to the ovaries, as in the male to the testicles; who knows whether a number of ovarian affections in old prostitutes do not owe their existence to such a cause?

Another complication, which can only take place in females, is the spreading of the inflammation to the anus and the lower border of the rectum; these organs being so situated that, when the female is lying on her back, the discharge from the vagina must necessarily gravitate towards them, and must corrode them to a greater or less extent. Such an invasion of the back parts by the gonorrhœal disease frequently develops a true *anal* gonorrhœa (as I know from personal observation), with extensive soreness of the surrounding parts, profuse secretion, frequent tenesmus, and very frequently such violent pains during an evacuation that they cause the patient to scream and tremble.

We hardly need allude to the fact that the metastases of which mention was made when treating of the gonorrhœa of males, such as *ophthalmia, articular rheumatism*, may likewise occur among females. Among the latter, however, they seem to be less frequent than among the former.

Sec. 26.—Diagnosis.

If it is difficult, in the case of males, to have a correct opinion of the nature of the discharge, this difficulty sometimes becomes insurmountable in the case of females, who are troubled with so many different kinds of discharges, the most varied of which are grouped together under the general denomination of *leucorrhœa.* During the inflammatory period, when the affected parts can still be subjected to close observation, the physician may be enabled, either by the period when the inflammation supposed to have resulted from an infectious coït, took place, or by other circumstances that are communicated to him by the patient, who must necessarily be interested in being cured as speedily and radically as possible, to decide with more or less probability or even certainty whether the existing discharge is, or is not, of a contagious nature. But what is to be done if the inflammatory period is passed (though it may be advisable in all cases not to relinquish our suspicion that the discharge is contagious), and the affection has reached the stage which, in the male, corresponds to the period of *painless gleet*, and where, even if the affected parts show ever so little redness, a contagious discharge still continues to be secreted, though neither the microscope nor chemical reagents are capable of determining its contagious nature or the difference between it and the most harmless leucorrhœa? It is true that in some cases, especially when the inflammatory period is still running its course, a gonorrhœal discharge in the female does not leave uniform and diffuse stains on the linen, as is the case with innocuous leucorrhœa; but that these stains, when caused by a gonorrhœal discharge, exhibit a dark *nucleus* in the centre, and have a grayish, sharply-circumscribed border. Or, in other cases, where females are not only afflicted with ordinary leucorrhœa but at the same time with contagious gonorrhœa, we may discover, in addition to a slight, scarcely perceptible redness of the affected parts, a few yellowish particles in the white mucous secretion, the presence of which, as long as it continues, furnishes evidence of the infectious character of the discharge. Nevertheless, although all these phenomena are observed in cases of undoubted gonorrhœa, they, as well as the inflammation of the affected parts, may result from the action of entirely different, extremely harmless causes, and hence can at most only justify suspicion, but not, by any means, infallible conclusions. And lastly, supposing the contagious nature of the discharge is fully established, how are we to determine whether the discharge is *simply venereal* or owes its origin to the virus of chancre? In this latter case, if we do not confine our examination to the pudendum, but likewise investigate the condition of the vagina as far as the uterus, we may perhaps discover suspicious products resulting from the action of the chancre-virus; these products may, however, be wanting, since they sometimes occur at a later period. Adding to this that the true *syphilitic* gonorrhœa, we mean the gonorrhœa caused by the chancre-poison, not by its own specific virus, is very frequently quite painless and only attended with very little inflammation, we cannot fail to comprehend how the most dangerous forms of gonorrhœa, even those causing chancre in the male, and, in the female developing every symptom of syphilitic disease among their ulterior consequences, have been utterly misapprehended, and have been regarded as *insignificant leucorrhœa.* From my own practice I have now more than ten cases of constitutional syphilis before me, where the patients were not aware of ever having had a chancre, but attributed their trouble to an *entirely painless leucorrhœa*, which the physician whom they consulted, had declared harmless, and had treated with injections composed of an infusion of walnut-leaves. In the presence of so much uncertainty, inoculation furnishes in such cases the only certain *diagnostic sign*, although it sheds no light on the question whether a discharge that is incapable of producing a chancre, is caused by the specific gonorrhœal virus, and therefore is, or is not contagious; for it is a well-known fact that the specific gonorrhœal virus is incapable of causing syphilitic products, although it has power to transmit its own infection by contact with the sexual organs.

Sec. 27.—Prognosis.

When the allopaths, among whom we mention more particularly *Ricord* of Paris, maintain that gonorrhœa in the female is most easily cured if it only affects the vulva; less easily if it is located in the urethra; still less easily if the vagina is invaded by the disease, and least easily if the cavity of the uterus is involved in it: this radical error is in the first place owing to the fact that French pathologists comprehend by the term gonorrhœa, without regard to *specific* causes, all such inflammations of the sexual organs as are attended with secretions from the affected parts, distinguishing the inflammation according as this or that part is affected, by such special names as *vulvitis*, *vaginitis* and *urethritis*; in the second place the error arises from their faulty system of treatment, which leads them to suppress the symptoms (the inflammation and the discharge) by external applications. Any one who knows what is meant by a radical homœopathic cure, not a mere removal of the symptoms but of the specific cause of the disease itself, must know that the locality of the disease neither facilitates nor impedes its cure, and that, howsoever difficult it may be to heal many other uterine catarrhs and vaginal blennorrhœas occasioned by *non*-contagious causes, affections of the female organs depending upon the gonorrhœal or upon the chancre-virus, are, all of them, easily cured with their *specific* remedies, as soon as the poison which sustains their existence is annihilated in the organism. Where a cure is delayed, as may be the case with *syphilitic* uterine or vaginal catarrhs, the cause is not to be sought in the anatomical relations of the affected parts, but in the peculiar nature of the malady. In this respect we offer the following distinctions: Simple *acute gonorrhœa*, whatever the affected parts, is most easily cured; next, we cure most easily gleetish discharges remaining after the acute form of gonorrhœa has passed away; by far the greatest difficulty is experienced in the treatment of truly *syphilitic* discharges and products, or such as are traceable to the action of the chancre-virus, especially if they are of a secondary nature, provided always that there is such a thing as *secondary* gonorrhœa. This point, however, will be discussed in the third division of this work.

Sec. 28.—Treatment.

What has been said (Sec. 19,) of the kind of diet that should be pursued in the treatment of gonorrhœa, is equally applicable, and just as rigorously, to the treatment of gonorrhœa in the female. Taking this point for granted, we depend upon *Cannabis* as our chief remedy in the treatment of *simple acute gonorrhœa*; this remedy will effect a cure in most cases, in the space of two or three weeks, provided its use is persevered in and the patient abstains from all improper dietetic indulgences.

As regards female *gleet*, with or without non-syphilitic erosions, we have in *Sepia* a remedy whose curative virtues in this affection are unsurpassed, no matter whether the discharge is localized in the pudendum, the vagina, or the uterus. *Mercurius*, *Nitri acidum* and *Thuja* may likewise have good effect, even if there is no suspicion of chancre-poisoning. In simple excoriations, however, Mercurius and Nitri acidum sometimes aggravate the disease instead of benefiting it, in which case we have to resort again to *Sepia.*

If such a gonorrhœa owes its origin to chancre-virus, the treatment of syphilis that will be indicated in the next chapter comes into play. In such cases, beside *Mercurius*, *Nitri ac.* and *Thuja*, we may have to use, and frequently do use with good effect, *Lycopodium* and *Phosphori acidum*, likewise *Zincum.*

If, towards the end of a cure, the disease seems to remain stationary, as is frequently the case both with males as well as females, and the discharge seems to resist all further treatment without diminishing either in quantity or consistence, this want of success should not always be laid to the charge of the remedies used, but will have most frequently to be accounted for by the sexual or dietetic excesses committed by the patients who fancy themselves cured before a cure is really completed. In such cases all that the physician, who has it not in his power to lock his patients up, can do, is to try to influence them by the weight of argument; in spite of all he may say or do, he will never learn all the imprudences that they may commit behind his back. Be this as it may, it is indispensably necessary that the patient should be impressed with the importance of avoiding all dietetic irregularities until the cure is complete; lest he should be afflicted with remnants of his disease for months to come. From a single cup of coffee or from a single coït, I have seen the discharge return worse than ever, even after it was all but stopped.

V. VARIOUS REMEDIES FOR GONORRHŒA, PROPOSED BY OTHER PHYSICIANS.

Sec. 29.—General Remarks on the Different Stages.

Not every thing that is recorded in our books on the homœopathic treatment of gonorrhœa, is the result of clinical experience; a good deal of it is based upon *theoretical hypotheses.* Let us try to separate as much as possible the chaff from the wheat.

1. *First stage.*—At this period, Wahle has used with distinguished success, *Bignonia rad. min.*, provided the discharge had not yet made its appearance, and the patient only complained of titillation, burning and itching during micturition. He effected a cure with the 20th to the 30th potency in from three to seven days. Drs. Mueller and Noack (in the All. hom. Zeit., vol. 15), and Stapf (in Arch., vol. 18, no. 3), confirm the curative power of this agent. Regarding the curative virtues of *Cannabis* in this stage, most practitioners seem to agree. As for Hartmann's praise of the curative virtues of *Copaiva* in this stage, I have never seen them verified in my practice, no matter in what dose this agent was used.

2. *Inflammatory stage.*—Most practitioners recommend *Cannabis* as the best remedy in this stage. Beside Cannabis, other practitioners have used with more or less good effect: *Copaiva*, *Cantharides*, *Mercurius*, *Petroselinum* and *Polygonum* (see § 32). *a*). For painfulness of the neck and region of the bladder: *Cantharis*, Capsicum, Petroleum, *Pulsatilla; b*). for *dysuria: Cannabis*, *Cantharis*, Mercurius, *Petroselinum; c*). for suppression of the discharge: Cantharis; for painless discharge: Cubebs, Capsicum, Ferrum; for bloody discharge: Cannabis, Cantharis, Tussilago; for thin discharge: Cannabis; for thick discharge: Capsicum, Mercurius; greenish discharge: Cannabis, Mercurius, Cubebs, Petroselinum; white: Capsicum, Ferrum.—For phimosis: Cannabis, Mercurius; for violent, painful erections: Cannabis, Cantharis, Mercurius.

3. *Syphilitic* gonorrhœa, with or without figwarts.—In a case of balanorrhœa: Merc. corr.—for figwarts: Nitri. ac., Thuja.

4. *Metastasis.*—For *orchitis:* Agnus, Aurum, Clematis, *Mercurius*, *Pulsatilla*, (Tussilago); and for *induration* of the testicles and the inguinal glands: Clematis. For *affections of the prostate:*

Pulsatilla, Selenium, Nitri ac., Sulphur, Thuja.—For gonorrhœal ophthalmia: Aconitum, Pulsatilla, Nitri ac., Merc. subl.—For rheumatism: Merc., Sarsaparilla.

5. *Gleet.*—Agnus castus, Cannabis, Capsicum, Cubebæ, Ferrum, Fluoris ac., Merc., Mezereum, Natrum mur., Nitr. ac., Petroleum, Sepia, Sulphur.

This is a general list of the remedies that have been used by homœopathic physicians in the different stages of gonorrhœa and its sequelæ. In the following paragraphs we will furnish more special information concerning their therapeutic value and use.

Sec. 30.—Remarks concerning the Remedies that have been employed by Homœopathic Physicians up to the present time.

1. *Agave Americana.*—Rosenberg has cured with the extract of this plant one of the worst cases of gonorrhœa, accompanied by violent erections, chordée, strangury, and drawing in the testicles.

2. *Agnus castus.*—Recommended by Attomyr, theoretically or speculatively only for gleet and induration of the testes.

3. *Bignonia.*—Used, with great success, by Wahle, Haubold, Müller, Noack and Stapf, for gonorrhœa in the initial and inflammatory stage, and likewise for gleet.

4. *Cannabis.*—This agent has been employed in the initial and inflammatory stage of gonorrhœa more frequently than any other. Kreussler justly observes that two doses of it administered morning and night, frequently cure gonorrhœa in eight days. It may be said that it will cure any case of gonorrhœa, though not always so rapidly; we should not, however, as Hartmann advises in his Therapeutics, change to Cantharis or some other remedy if the cure is not completed in eight days; nor should we allow ourselves to be deceived by the presence of such accessory phenomena as *difficulty of urinating*, *phimosis*, *inguinal swellings*, *hæmaturia*, *inflammation of the glans*, *painful erections*, etc., and to be induced to employ some intercurrent remedy for the removal of these symptoms. All these accessory phenomena yield to the continued use of Cannabis, even more readily than to any other agent. It is only when the discharge has become suppressed, either by accident or by artificial means, that Cannabis seems to be powerless; against *gleet* it is very often more efficacious than any other remedy. The alternate use of Cannabis and Sulphur,

recommended by Bernstein, leads to no good results, and retards the cure rather than hastens it.

5. *Cantharis.* Hofrichter does not think much of this remedy. Attomyr's and Hartmann's remarks on the appropriateness of this agent in gonorrhœa, are based upon theoretical grounds rather than upon experience. It is only when the accidental or violent suppression of the discharge causes trouble about the bladder, difficulty of urinating or even hæmaturia, that this agent may become of real value; I pity those who can be induced by the symptomatic erections or urinary difficulties which are present in every case of gonorrhœa to substitute Cantharides, which are so uncertain in their action, for Cannabis which is reliable and certain.

6. *Capsicum annuum.*—What Attomyr writes concerning this agent, is likewise hypothetical rather than founded upon fact. C. Hering's remarks, however, concerning the curative virtues of Capsicum in *gleet*, if the discharge looks like fat milk, and the patient complains of a burning during urination, and of a stinging and cutting pain between the acts of urination, have been verified by me on numerous occasions.

7. *Clematis.*—What Stapf relates of the efficacy of this remedy in inflammation and induration of the testicles (Arch. 7, no. 3), is confirmed by Attomyr (Arch. 19), and likewise by Rosenberg (All. hom. Zeit., vol. 35), who not only cured with this remedy inflammation of the testicles and a *pain* in these organs (without swelling) but likewise old indurations of the inguinal glands.

8. *Copaiva.*—Beside an incipient gonorrhœa for which Hartman found this remedy useful in one case, we have no clinical experience to refer to; when Attomyr states that this agent has never been of much use to him in his practice, most practitioners of our School will most likely be found willing to confess to a like experience.

9. *Cubebæ.*—According to Hirsch, Rosenberg and Wurda they are of little or no account in the inflammatory stage of gonorrhœa; in *gleet*, however, they have derived essential benefit from this agent. This has likewise been my own experience.

10. *Ferrum.*—Attomyr's remarks concerning Ferrum (Arch. 18) are simply hypothetical. Hering's statement, however, that Ferrum is useful in gleet, when the discharge is whitish, like milk, is based upon fact. Rosenberg confirms this statement by a case (All. h. Zeit. 35).

Sec. 31.—Continuation of the same subject.

11. *Fluoris acidum.*—Rosenberg states (All. h. Zeit., 35) that this remedy effected a speedy cure in a case of gonorrhœa that had been treated with Tussilago, and where the following symptoms remained: burning urine, painfulness of the bladder, discharge of a yellow drop from the urethra every morning, and an oily exhalation from the genital organs, having a pungent smell.

12. *Kali jodatum.*—Rosenberg's case, which he describes as a complication of syphilis and lues venerea, resulting from neglected gonorrhœa, and which he cured with this agent, is not very clear; it seems altogether to have been a discharge traceable to the action of the chancre-virus (see § 14).

13. *Kreasotum.*—Rosenberg cites another case where this agent, after previous treatment with emulsions of flax-seed, almonds, and hemp, cured the remaining *gleet*, together with a debilitating fever, exhausting sweats, increasing emaciation, and excessive secretion of a colorless, very fetid urine. These symptoms may, however, have resulted from the excessive action of hemp; I have noticed them even after the somewhat liberal use of Cannabis.

14. *Mercurius.*—Hartmann's (Therapeutics), and Attomyr's (Arch. 18) remarks about this remedy are purely hypothetical. According to the experience of most practitioners, with which my own experience agrees in all respects, the true sphere of action of Mercurius is a form of *gleet* over which Cannabis has no influence whatsoever; it is more particularly indicated, if, as Hering observes, the discharge continues of a greenish-yellow color. If administered at the commencement of gonorrhœa, or even during the inflammatory period, its sole effect, especially if the doses are continued too long or too frequently, seems to be to render the cure more protracted and more difficult. It is only in cases where chancre and gonorrhœa are combined that *Mercurius* should be given from the very commencement, when it is often alone sufficient to effect a cure. Rosenberg's case of balanorrhœa (related in the All. h. Zeit.), which he cured with *Corrosive Sublimate*, was most likely of a syphilitic nature. In cases of *metastasis* of the gonorrhœal discharge to the *testes*, the *prostate* and *eyes*, *Mercurius* (or Corr. Subl.) is, next to Pulsatilla, an indispensable remedy.

15. *Mezereum.*—Rummel (All. h. Zeit., vol. 3) says that this remedy has been of much use to him in some cases of gleet; and Attomyr (Arch. 18) alleges that he has found it useful in *hæmaturia.* What he says of the specific virtue of Mezereum in female gonorrhœa, needs further confirmation.

16. *Natrum muriaticum.*—Stapf recommends this remedy as useful in *gleet;* Lingen and Hering have found it useful in simple, non-venereal blennorrhœa, owing its origin to acrid menstrual blood (see §§ 9 and 10).

17. *Nitri acidum.*—We have to repeat that Attomyr's remarks on this agent are purely speculative. Hahnemann's recommendation of this remedy for sycosic gonorrhœa is essentially founded upon experience; so are Goullon's, Stapf's, and Greter's remarks about its curative power in painless, simply *contagious* gleet.

18. *Nux vomica.*—Although Rosenberg relates a case (All. h. Zeit., 35) where this remedy has cured a kind of gleet; and although others recommend it for similar kinds of blennorrhœa resulting from piles, yet it is more than probable that this agent has nothing whatsoever to do with the *true contagious gonorrhœa*, and holds curative relations only to harmless or non-contagious discharges from the urethra.

Sec. 32.—Continuation.

19. *Petroleum.*—Although Schrœn (All. h. Zeit., 6), as well as Trinks (Griessel. Skizzen, p. 52), praise this agent, if administered in drop-doses of the original substance, not in an attenuated form, as one of the best remedies for gonorrhœa; my *own* experience leads me to doubt its efficacy in gonorrhœa, except, perhaps, in gleet, which, after all, it does not cure more speedily than any other drug. Attomyr's remarks (Arch. 18) about the curative relation of this drug to gonorrhœa are purely theoretical, and require further confirmation by practice.

20. *Petroselinum.*—Those who have used this substance in gonorrhœa, will agree with Vehsemeyer, and others, that its boasted curative virtue in gonorrhœa is, to say the least, very problematical, and that it would be very wrong, while speaking of this agent, to lose sight of *Cannabis;* at any rate, during the inflammatory period. In cases of *gleet*, where *Cannabis* seemed insufficient, I too have found it useful; more particularly when the patient, as Hahnemann likewise observed, was troubled with

frequent urging to urinate. Nevertheless, it would be ill-advised to employ this agent before we have become perfectly convinced, by a fortnight's use of *Cannabis*, that this medicine will neither remove the discharge nor the urinary difficulties. To alternate Cannabis with Petroselinum, might be like jumping from the frying-pan into the fire. This would be mismanagement, as I can testify from personal experience, which might result in delaying the cure of gonorrhœa, which another week's use of Cannabis would have completed, beyond even the period of six weeks.

21. *Polygonum maritimum.*—Rosenberg (All. h. Zeit., 35) cured a case of gonorrhœa in a man who was habitually afflicted with urinary difficulties, renal calculi, and the most horrid pains when urinating, with a few drops of the saturated tincture.

22. *Phosphori acidum.*—Rosenberg furnishes (All. h. Zeit., 36) several more or less hazardous theoretical speculations, concerning this agent. He recommends it for the *gleet* of debilitated individuals whose system has lost its tone and reactive energy, and who are afflicted with impotence and affection of the testicles. From personal observation I can admit that this remedy is somewhat useful in gleet of an exceedingly chronic nature, but I do not consider it as one of the most important remedies for gleet, and never employ it as long as I can fall back upon some other remedy that is more intimately related to gleet. Bernstein, in his "Mosaik," mentions a case where, after the cure of gonorrhœa, a few whitish drops were secreted every morning from the urethra of a man who had become weakened by self-abuse. The discharge was attended with the loss of quantities of prostatic fluid. This disease yielded perfectly to Phosph. ac., which was undoubtedly a specific curative agent in this case.

Sec. 33.—Continuation.

23. *Pulsatilla.*—This medicine has not been much in favor with homœopathic practitioners as a remedy for gonorrhœa. We must wonder that Attomyr should think much of the curative virtues of this medicine in gonorrhœa, since he himself reports a case where it only helped to quiet the general vascular excitement, to restore the appetite, and to remove the evening-chills and the increased thirst, but where the discharge remained entirely unaffected by the drug. For a discharge of this kind, Pulsa-

tilla will never be of any use; it is so much more powerful as a remedial agent in all cases of *suppressed* gonorrhœa, especially when resulting in *orchitis*, *gonorrhœal ophthalmia* and *swelling of the prostate*. This fact has been confirmed by the experience of other physicians, as well as by my own.

24. *Sarsaparilla.*—Rosenberg relates a case (All. h. Zeit., 35), where *articular rheumatism* consequent upon suppression of gonorrhœa was rapidly cured by this remedy. Similar results have been obtained in my own practice.

25. *Selenium.*—Attomyr's suggestions (Arch. 18), concerning the curative virtues of this agent in affections of the prostate, are problematical, and require further confirmation.

26. *Sepia.*—One of the most important remedies for *gleet*, especially in the case of females, and likewise for incipient gonorrhœa, although Seidel is as yet the only one who has published a case of cure with this remedy (see Annal. I.); Lobethal has published an observation concerning this drug (All. h. Zeit., 13).

27. *Sulphur.*—From my own practice I am able to confirm Attomyr's, Bernstein's and Lobethal's remarks concerning the curative virtues of this agent in *chronic gonorrhœa*. Nevertheless, I would add that I prefer *Sepia* to Sulphur in this affection, and that the *painless*, exceedingly chronic forms of gleet seem to constitute this agent's chief sphere of action. Attomyr's observation that *Sulphur*, if given too soon, increases the burning in the urethra and other symptoms of inflammation, is undoubtedly correct. Personal experience, likewise, leads me to confirm the curative virtues of *Sulphur* in *chronic articular rheumatism*, *chronic gonorrhœal ophthalmia* and *inveterate affections of the prostate*, where these affections have resulted by metastasis from the suppression of gonorrhœa. In accompanying hæmorrhoidal affections, Sulphur is likewise eminently useful.

28. *Thuja.*—The observations of our practitioners concerning the curative virtues of Thuja in *gleet*, especially when accompanied by *affections of the prostate* (Attomyr), by figwarts (Habermann), a thin, greenish discharge, etc., and its particular adaptation to such diseases in the case of *female* patients, find abundant confirmation in my own practice. Nevertheless, except in sycosic gonorrhœa, and in gonorrhœa attended with diseases of the prostate, *Sepia* seems to me to deserve a preference over Sulphur.

29. *Tussilago petasites.* Although recommended by Schwei-

kert sen., Wahle and Küchenmeister, as an excellent remedy for gonorrhœa both in the acute and chronic form: yet, so far, it has only been used by Rosenberg in several cases; by means of a watery infusion this practitioner has cured not only chronic, but likewise acute gonorrhœa; likewise ophthalmic affections and indurations of the testes when resulting from suppression of the discharge.

30. *Aurum.*—Although this remedy has really no connection with gonorrhœa, properly speaking, yet it deserves mention. More than once I have removed with this agent a *swelling of the testes* attended with slight inflammation, when resulting from a suppression of the discharge, which was re-established at the same time; in another case, the use of *Aurum* was incidentally attended with considerable diminution of an old stricture.

THIRD CHAPTER.

THE VARIOUS FORMS OF CHANCRE.

I. OF CHANCRE GENERALLY.

Sec. 34.—General Properties.

NOTWITHSTANDING that the *Hunterian chancre* is no longer, as formerly, at Hunter's and even afterwards at Hahnemann's time, considered as the only primary syphilitic ulcer; and although several chancres are known at the present time which differ more or less by their anatomical relations: yet all these different forms have so many pathological properties in common that it seems logical to regard them as different varieties of one and the same species, and to apply the term *chancre* to all of them, that is, if we understand by this term the characteristic ulcer by which *syphilis*, which, in the more restricted sense of the term, is so entirely distinct from the gonorrhœal disease, generally first manifests its existence. This ulcer, which may likewise show itself as *consecutive* chancre in the course of the syphilitic disease, breaks out in its *primary* form, that is, as the primary manifestation of the syphilitic infection, in six or seven days, sometimes sooner, and sometimes in two or three weeks, or even at a later period, at the very spot that first came in contact with the poison; whereas *consecutive* chancres appear more or less remotely from the original place of infection, sometimes only several months after the disappearance of the first, primary ulcer. In their primary form these ulcers most generally break out on the glans or prepuce, or on the labia minora or majora, the clitoris, or at the entrance of the vagina, or even, according to some authors, on the neck of the uterus. By accidental contact, primary chancres may likewise break out on other parts, such as the lips, nose, etc.; though most of the chancres which break out in the mouth, throat, eyes, on the scrotum, umbilicus, etc., are frequently of a secondary nature. Chancre, in its primary form, generally begins in the shape of small, red, more or less inflamed spots, which cause little or no itching. Soon after, we see whitish, transparent vesicles start from the middle of these spots, which burst and discharge a reddish, acrid, serous fluid, after which, in most cases, the ulcer caves in in the middle, like a funnel-shaped depression, and is surrounded by a red, hard, callous border, with a whitish-gray and lardaceous base; whereas, in other cases, the base is raised, and, instead of forming a depressed, forms an elevated ulcer, which shows in all cases a well-defined tendency to spread, if not in depth, at least in circumference, in which latter case it may cause extensive disorganizations.

Sec. 35.—Various forms of Chancre.

Regarding the anatomical relations of chancre, we discover a great diversity, not only as regards their development, but likewise with reference to the forms which chancres may adopt in their course. So far from always first breaking out as vesicles or pustules, chancres, if the poison comes in contact with a wound or a spot deprived of its epidermis, may at once assume the form of ulcers; whereas, if the poison touches a lymphatic vessel or a ganglion, they may assume the shape of pustules. Sometimes they commence like slight, superficial excoriations, which soon penetrate to greater depth and assume all the characteristic properties of chancres. In other cases, again, the virus is so violent and active that the ulcer spreads immediately and penetrates to a great depth before the pain caused by this destructive process, leads to a suspicion of its existence. We have already stated that some chancres are depressed and deeply-penetrating, whereas others, on the contrary, are more elevated. Beside these, there are other varieties which render it difficult to bring all their pathognomonic characteristics under one generalization. Even the properties which so far have been considered as common to all chancres, such as the lardaceous, whitish-gray surface; the more or less raised, red, almost perpendicularly circumscribed borders, and their hard base, etc., admit of exceptions. Chancres, for instance, that are located on the glans, do not show a fatty, ash-colored, but a claret-colored base; the surrounding parts are neither hard nor swollen, and their borders are soft and flat rather than raised and sharply circumscribed. Other chancres are indolent, not much inflamed and almost painless, whereas others again are intensely inflamed and cause intolerable pain, which increases from nine o'clock in the evening until two in the morning, and deprives the patient of all sleep. Finally, there are chancres which, after having attained a certain size, cease to spread either in circumference or depth, whereas others penetrate to, and destroy the subjacent tissues, and others again spread more in circumference, like serpiginous ulcers, and while cicatrizing at one end, continue to spread at the other. These differences have led modern writers on syphilis to adopt several varieties of syphilitic ulcers, such as 1, the *regular*, *simple Hunterian chancre;* 2, the *soft* or *raised* chancre; 3, the *phagedenic* or *serpiginous* chancre, and 4, the *syphilitic erosions.* Whatever may be alleged, however, in favor of such a classification, it has, after all, only a *diagnostic* value, since, as I know from my own experience, any of these different forms may cause a chancre of the other class, and may entail the same *constitutional* symptoms as any of the other forms. All these different forms should not be regarded as symptoms of essentially distinct venereal diseases, but only as members of one and the same family, distinguished from each other by external diagnostic signs. Since it is of importance, however, in order to acquire a correct knowledge of the various syphilitic products, that all their forms should be known, we shall, in the subsequent chapters, consider more particularly not only the different pathological forms under which syphilitic products manifest themselves, but likewise the differences resulting from their different anatomical localities.

II. DIFFERENCES IN THE FORM OF CHANCRES.

Sec. 36.—Regular, Simple and Hunterian Chancre.

[*Ulcus regulare, simplex et induratum.*]

This chancre, which forms the real type of the primary syphilitic ulcers, and which is generally located on the frenulum, corona glandis, or even on the glans itself, consists, if manifesting itself upon the skin or upon a mucous membrane, in a simple, not very extensive ulcer, that usually penetrates every layer of the integuments, until it reaches the subjacent cellular tissue that serves it as a base. Its shape is generally round, except in cases where the ulcer rests upon two tissues of a different kind, for instance, partly on the glans, and partly on the prepuce; although even in these cases its round shape is distinctly recognizable, as much so as where this rounded form seems more or less obscured by the position of the affected parts, such as the anal fissure, the folds of the prepuce, etc. The base of the ulcer is usually lardaceous, whitish-gray, rough and uneven; its abruptly-rising borders, which are somewhat shaggy on their inner surface, are in most cases gaping and everted, which communicates to the ulcer a funnel-shaped appearance; the parts around the ulcer are either red or dark-brown, according as the attending inflammation is more or less intense. The ulcer secretes a thin ichor, which is sometimes mixed with blood, has an alkaline reaction, and sometimes contains small animalcules. If it is secreted in large quantity, for instance, on the glans, the prepuce, the pudendum, the anus, it is very apt to assume a fetid odor; upon mucous membranes that are not accessible to the action of atmospheric air, it preserves its liquid form; upon the external skin it dries up, forming crusts which are sometimes sunk deeply into the integuments.

This appearance has led some authors to adopt another peculiar form of chancre, under the name of *soft* chancre. The ulcer may persevere in this shape for several days without showing a *hard base.* But if the inflammation continues and increases, the ulcer never fails to become dense and *hard*, so that this induration, which is always sharply circumscribed, can be felt under the ulcer as if it had the shape of half a pea (Hunterian chancre). If resting upon loose cellular tissue, the induration has always a circular form; but if seated upon denser tissue, where it is more or less compressed, the induration may assume an elongated, or otherwise more or less altered form; in every case, however, it offers to the exploring finger a peculiarly elastic resistance by which it can readily be distinguished from any other kind of swellings.

Those who have distinguished this chancre into two kinds, namely, a soft and an indurated chancre, assert that the induration is not only perceived at the first breaking out of the ulcer, but even before this takes place. This assertion evidently rests upon erroneous observation. Every *indurated*, genuine *Hunterian* chancre, is at first soft; the induration generally only showing itself five or six days afterwards, although it may likewise appear in the first twenty-four hours. What distinguishes both these ulcers *in common* from all other ulcers, is, in the first place, their funnel-shaped, depressed form, with abruptly-rising, everted edges; and, in the second place, the fact that, after a short period, the above-mentioned characteristic *induration* never fails to show itself.

Sec. 37.—The Raised Chancre.

This chancre may be located upon the integuments of the penis, or upon the inner and outer side of the prepuce, even on the scrotum. When first breaking out, it looks like a small whitish ulcer of the size of a small split pea to that of a dime. In eight or ten days, or even sooner, the edges of this ulcer, together with its base, become raised, forming an elevated, projecting, whitish-gray ulcer, of a spongy appearance. These ulcers generally are of an oval shape; they secrete a purulent serum, are not very, or even not at all painful; neither the edges nor the base are *indurated*. If fully present, they do not change, neither penetrating to the subjacent tissues nor extending perceptibly in circumference. When healing, they lose their whitish-gray color, first in the *centre*, and afterwards from the centre towards the circumference; at the same time they gradually become flatter, so that, after their cicatrization, a small white elevation remains, which finally disappears without leaving the slightest trace of a scar. In this last respect they likewise differ essentially from the *regular*, simple, and indurated chancre. In the case of this chancre, the first sign that the healing process has commenced, is the diminution of the red areola surrounding the ulcer; the edges flatten and gradually exhibit a paler appearance, while cicatrization extends in concentric circles from the circumference to the centre, the base becomes cleaner and is covered with healthy granulations, but generally leaves a cicatrix of greater or less depth. In addition to this, the regular, simple, and Hunterian chancre usually forms a single isolated ulcer, whereas the elevated chancre very frequently consists of several ulcers. In one case I have seen the folds near the border of the inner surface of the prepuce covered by these ulcers like a wreath, so that the prepuce itself seemed divided into several patches. In all the cases that have come under my observation, I have never seen them single, but always two or three together, and always in the case of individuals who had been infected with chancres at some former period and still exhibited their badly healed and distinctly perceptible cicatrices; so that I am to this day in doubt whether this form of chancre is not a product of recent infection, but modified by a pre-existing constitutional syphilitic taint. In other respects this form of chancre which breaks out at the outset such as it shows itself at a later period, should not be confounded with the vegetations which, after the ulcerous stage has run its course, likewise manifest themselves with the Hunterian chancre when the vegetative stage sets in. In their case the base may likewise become raised and form a more or less prominent ulcer; but the base of such an ulcer has no longer the lardaceous and ash-colored appearance which characterizes the elevated chancre of recent origin; but is rather copper-colored throughout its whole extent.

Sec. 38.—Phagedænic Chancre.

This form, like the preceding one, has no induration; if the edges or the base should appear swollen, such swelling is nothing else than a malignant œdema. The ulcers penetrate less to the subjacent tissues than they spread in circumference; they may preserve their round shape, but in most cases they spread about irregularly, assuming a *serpiginous* character. Their base is generally uneven, covered with a sort of whitish-gray false membrane, or secreting a pulpy matter which, diffusing itself over the surface, shows here and there new granulations that, however, become decomposed again very speedily. The edges of these ulcers are generally very thin, irregularly indented, and, in places where they are gaping and detached, very frequently perforated by the ulcer. When first breaking out, the ulcer begins with a scarcely perceptible swelling and slight excoriation of the surface. This excoriation soon becomes putrid, shows a yellowish base and secretes a watery, brownish ichor. Any tissue upon which this ulcer rises, may be destroyed by it; although the cellular tissue is more rapidly destroyed by it than the skin of the prepuce and the body of the penis. For this reason, when concealed under the integuments of the penis, the ulcer may spread onward towards the corpora spongiosa which it detaches from their covering, after which it continues to spread even as far as the pubes, so that it becomes impossible to completely lay bare the base of the ulcer. In such a case the visible portion of the ulcer is sometimes quite clean and even cicatrized, while the hidden portion is yellow and putrid, and secretes a copious quantity of a thin, brown ichor. This hidden portion is surrounded by the usual swelling, which can be felt externally like a hard ring surrounding the penis, and which, in proportion as the disease progresses, approximates more and more to the root of the penis. As long as this thick enlargement can be felt, so long does the hidden ulcer continue to progress; in proportion as the ulcer heals and cicatrizes from its base, the enlargement disappears with corresponding rapidity and certainty. Usually the progress of the ulcer is marked by putrid disorganization; accidental circumstances frequently convert it quite suddenly into a *gangrenous sore* (*ulcus syphiliticum gangrenosum*), causing the destruction and detachment of large patches of the prepuce, glans, or the corpora spongiosa. Very frequently a portion of the urethra becomes involved in the destruction. These phagedænic ulcers always secrete a copious ichor, which, however, does not seem to affect the parts with which it comes in contact, since the glans and prepuce are constantly seen inundated by this secretion without showing any signs of ulceration; or since the ulcer may be exclusively localized on the body of the penis, without the prepuce, which is in perpetual contact with the secreted ichor, being affected by it. The pain is seldom acute, and the inflammation not very violent. Nevertheless there are cases, especially if gangrene supervenes, where the inflammation may become intense, and the pain intolerable. On the other hand, the constitutional symptoms are often very prominent, the pulse accelerated, the skin hot, the appetite diminished, and the sleep uneasy and disturbed.

Sec. 39.—Syphilitic Erosions.

These erosions, which, in most cases, are of a secondary order, occur in their primary form, in the case of males, most frequently as an accompaniment of syphilitic balanorrhœa, and, in the case of females, supervene as an accompaniment of gonorrhœa of the vulva. They are distinguished from benign erosions by their greater depth, by their sharply circumscribed border, their rounded or oval form, and a border which is either whitish with a red centre, or red with a whitish centre. If continuing for a longer period, such erosions, if primary, very readily change to simple or even *Hunterian* chancres, from which they are usually distinguished by being less penetrating. They never occur singly, but always several together, and may not only produce an infectious chancre by coït, but, if suppressed by external means, may develop symptoms of constitutional syphilis. As a general rule, these erosions do not secrete a great deal, though, in the case of males, they are frequently attended with balanorrhœa, and, in the case of females, with a suspicious blennorrhœa. In one case, that of a girl, I have seen them mixed with mucous tubercles, and in the case of another girl, where they had almost become quite dry, they were accompanied by funnel-shaped, depressed, chancrous ulcers, the deepest of which, of about two lines in diameter, was seated on the clitoris, but did not secrete scarcely anything, and did not seem to leave the least stain on the linen. There were, at the same time, perceived, wart-shaped blotches on the hands, and light, transparent spots resembling syphilitic *roseola*, of a yellowish-brown color on the neck and around the axillæ. A young man who had had connection with her, had been infected by her (or perhaps by some other female ?) with balanorrhœa and figwarts; six months previously, the girl had had a hard, elastic swelling on the right labium, which was attended with violent itching and had yielded to a small dose of *Mercurius*. Of leucorrhœa she had never seen a trace either before or after. The phenomena in the vulva were rapidly cured with *Merc. præc.*, and the wart-shaped blotches in the palms of the hands with *Nitri ac.*

III. DIFFERENCES OF CHANCRES WITH REFERENCE TO THEIR LOCALITY.

Sec. 40.—General Remark.

We have already remarked in a previous paragraph that primary chancres generally break out at the spot where the poison has come in contact with the parts; in the case of males more particularly on the glans and prepuce, or on the scrotum and dorsum of the penis; and in the case of females on the pudendum;

we have likewise stated that chancres appearing on other parts are generally of a secondary nature. *Primary* chancres may, however, likewise break out elsewhere in consequence of accidental contact; for instance, on the mouth after being kissed by persons who have venereal ulcers in the mouth or throat; on the breasts of nurses who suckle infants which, born of syphilitic parents, are affected with ulcers in the mouth; at the anus of people who indulge in unnatural criminal intercourse, and so forth. These chancres do not essentially differ from those that are seated on the sexual parts, but precisely on account of their unusual locality, may easily be misapprehended and confounded with innocuous ulcers, on which account it may be advisable to devote a little additional space to their consideration.

Sec. 41.—Chancres at the Anus.

These chancres, if occurring as *primary* ulcers, always result from direct infection caused either by criminal intercourse, or by transmission of the virus from the sexual organs to the anus, which may easily occur in the case of females while in a recumbent position, when the matter flowing out of the pudendum touches the neighboring parts and this contact continues for a certain time. The longitudinal folds of the skin and mucous membrane of the anus generally impart to these chancres an oblong shape, sometimes even the form of *rhagades*, with which they must not, however, be confounded. In most cases all doubt regarding their true character will be readily removed by their simple appearance, by their edges and base, in which respect they are altogether like other chancres, likewise by their size, which far exceeds that of simple rhagades, by the lesser pain during stool, and by a careful investigation of all prior circumstances. They are seldom indurated, still less frequently phagedænic, but generally belong to the category of the so-called *simple*, soft chancre, and seldom leave distinctly-perceptible cicatrices, but may be complicated with *buboes*. Such chancres may not only occur at the anus, but likewise in the rectum, in which case they are generally located not far from the sphincter ani. They have generally a rounded, irregular shape, with edges that are more or less indented. As a general rule they are superficial; frequently, however, they involve the whole thickness of the mucous membrane and the subjacent cellular tissue. The accompanying pain is not very considerable, and the expulsion of fæces is not interfered with.

Sec. 42.—Chancres in the Mouth and on the Lips.

These chancres, when resulting from a primary infection, are always produced by direct contact with the infectious matter. Such a contact may occur while kissing with a chancrous tongue or lips, or by the insertion of a finger to which some of the chancre-virus is adhering, or by touching the parts which are affected with chancre, with the mouth. If located on the tongue, or at the tip of the tongue, they are generally round and indurated, with an ash-colored, lardaceous base; if seated along the edges of the tongue, they appear more elongated. They generally cause an extremely violent pain, and not unfrequently they impede mastication and speech, or cause a more or less considerable swelling of the tongue. On the *lips*, they always occupy the free border, more frequently that of the lower than the border of the upper lip; sometimes they are seen on the inside of the lips, but never in the corners of the mouth, where only secondary chancres can break out. They are either round or oblong, generally belong to the class of the simple, soft chancres, and only become indurated or phagedænic if they are treated with irritating agents. They cannot very well be confounded with ordinary *rhagades*, for these are always long and narrow, in the direction of the folds of the lips; nor with *cancer of the lips*, the edges of which are everted, with stinging pains. It is with *mercurial ulcers* that they might be confounded most readily; these, however, are scarcely ever, if ever, located on the free border of the lips, and have moreover a whitish base, which is on a level with the vermilion border, in addition to which we have swelling of the gums, and the peculiar mercurial fetor.

Sec 43.—Chancres on the Eyes, Ears, Nose and Skin.

Nothing can be said regarding the form of chancres in the eye; for if the chancre-virus penetrates the eye, the destruction which immediately results from its presence is so violent that a practitioner has no time to attend to any thing but to the preservation of the organ. Chancres occurring on the lids, being much less destructive, ought, therefore, to be considered as secondary.

Primary chancres have even been seen on the ears, or in the inner ear, where they may be caused by inserting a finger to which some of the virus is adhering. Upon the whole, such chancres are very scarce; where they do occur, they are very easily misapprehended, and, at most, can only be confounded with secondary syphilitic ulcers.

The same remarks apply to *primary* chancres at the entrance of the nostrils, which differ but slightly from the not unfrequently occurring secondary chancres, except that they are much more virulent.

Primary chancres upon the external skin are likewise characterized by all the signs generally characterizing other chancres, from which they differ almost exclusively by the manner in which they had originated. If these chancres are caused by the virus penetrating a *denuded surface*, or open wound, they generally adopt at once the form of an ulcer; if *inoculated*, they look like the *pustules* in variola, with a depression in the centre, and are caused by a protracted contact of the skin with a part affected with chancre; for instance, of the thighs with the diseased penis during sleep, the pustules generally soon breaking and showing a fully-formed chancre. In most cases they belong to the class of *regular*, simple, or *Hunterian* chancres, but may likewise assume the form of *phagedænic* chancres.

Sec. 44.—Chancres on the Female Organs.

As primary ulcers, they are most frequently seen at the lower commissure of the labia majora or in the fossa navicularis; but about as frequently on the clitoris or on the inner wall of the labia majora or minora; somewhat less frequently in the neighborhood or even at the orifice of the urethra, or at the entrance of the vagina; and least frequently, perhaps, on the outer side of the labia majora or minora, high up in the vagina, or at the os tincæ. Nevertheless, according to some authors who have paid particular attention to diagnosis by inoculation, chancres appear much less frequently at the os tincæ than is generally supposed; and even here they are frequently misapprehended by those who make frequent examinations with the speculum, except where the Hunterian chancre-form is exhibited. All these chancres may occur in both sexes as regular, simple or indurated, or as elevated and phagedænic chancres, and may cause more or less extensive disorganizations. Not unfrequently the labia majora and minora are perforated and corroded by them, but the lower commissure and the fossa navicularis are likewise lacerated by them; they penetrate even through the perineum as far as the anus, where they cause ulcers, inflammations, and purulent discharges. Frequently they are accompanied by œdematous swellings, considerable inflammations, extremely violent pains, and more or less copious discharges from the vulva, urethra, and vagina, which do not by any means always justify the belief in a simultaneously existing gonorrhœal infection. Chancres located at the os tincæ are sometimes quite painless, but may speedily superinduce the nervous disorders which so frequently accompany other affections of this organ. Chancres situated at the entrance of the vagina, in the neighborhood of the small papillæ, may readily be confounded by inattentive observers with lacerations that may have taken place during sexual intercourse, for this additional reason, that, in all such cases, it is not very easy to discriminate between the two series of phenomena. Nevertheless, errors of diagnosis may be avoided in most cases by co-existing inguinal swellings, which, it is true, are not always very considerable in the case of females; and, in addition, by a careful investigation of all the circumstances that had preceded the outbreak of the disease.

Among women, especially while nursing children at the breast, primary chancres are frequently discovered at the *nipples*, where they are caused by the contact with the infant's diseased lips. They are generally seated close around the nipples, or on the areola, and may be confounded by an inattentive observer with the ulcerated fissures and rhagades that so often break out on these parts.

IV. DEVELOPMENT, COURSE, AND TERMINATIONS OF CHANCRES.

Sec. 45.—Development of Chancres.

We have already stated in a previous chapter, that chancre generally breaks out in six days to a fortnight after infection. Most physicians had agreed on this point until the *inoculators* made their appearance, maintaining that a so-called *period of in-*

cubation, which had heretofore been universally admitted, did not exist, and that the development of the product of infection commenced at the moment of contact, and continued uninterruptedly until the breaking out of the first vesicle. In their opinion, the difference in time intervening between infection and the first appearance of the vesicle, in one case or another, depends entirely upon different degrees of susceptibility inherent in differences of organization; and likewise upon the important circumstance that most patients do not heed the first changes at the place of infection, nor do they notice the infection until the chancre has already caused extensive destructions, and hence are led to imagine that the period intervening between infection and manifestation seems longer than it really is. It is indeed true that it is very difficult, in practice, to determine the number of days that elapse between the moment of infection and the first breaking out of the disease. I have heard patients affirm that they had been with a woman three days ago, and had been infected by her with a big chancre; an examination, however, showed that this woman was perfectly sound, and that the chancre must therefore have been caused at a much earlier period. As a general rule, therefore, the cases where a chancre is said to have broken out immediately after the infection had taken place, do not prove any thing. They could only be looked upon as reliable testimony in case the patient had not seen a woman for months after the last coït. As regards the experiments of the inoculators, with which they seek to combat the incubation-theory, we have to remind these gentlemen of the fact that all that their experiments prove is, that when the virus is introduced into a wound, or placed upon a denuded surface, the local inflammation generally begins in 24 hours, and certainly before the third day, as may be seen in the case of all poisoned wounds resulting from a bite, or in consequence of surgical operations; or in all cases of infectious coït when the virus comes in contact with a denuded surface, without epithelium, either on the prepuce or glans. I have often observed that in such cases, on the second or third day a suspicious irritation is seen on the affected part, which very soon changes to a regular chancre. Where this is not the case, the virus is received by the lymphatics and mixed up with the general circulation, after which the local symptom only shows itself in consequence of a general reaction of the organism that seeks to cast out the poison at the original place of infection. In sensitive individuals, this process is often preceded for one or two days by a general malaise and slight febrile motions, which sometimes remain unheeded, or are attributed to other accidental circumstances.

Sec. 46.—Possible duration of the period of Incubation.

Except the cases where the poison is brought in contact with a wound or a denuded surface, it may be said that chancre, generally, breaks out six or seven days after infection, most frequently a fortnight after, sometimes even at a much later period; I know of cases where it did not break out until one or two months after infection had taken place. A ship captain, who could not have been exposed on the voyage from Buenos Ayres, which had lasted two months, consulted me on the third day after his arrival in Paris, on account of a chancre that had broken out six weeks after his departure from Buenos Ayres. A young Englishman, who had hurt his foot during the passage to France, had been compelled, through allopathic mismanagement, to keep his bed for six weeks. A week after I had taken charge of him, and when he had not yet been able to leave his room, one of the worst phagedænic chancres I had ever seen broke out on him. One of the most remarkable cases, where I had a chance to observe the whole course of the disease from the first moment of the infection to the breaking out of the ulcer, is the following. One of my patients, an abstemious young man of excellent conduct, being in company with a few friends and several girls of an equivocal character, had been induced to have connection with a strange female, who, as he learned the following day, had already infected several men. Having been concerned about his health for some time past, he came to me the next day, begging me to examine the young woman with whom he had had connection, and whom he promised to send to me the next day. Contrary to my expectation, the woman came, confessing that she had done wrong in a moment of intoxication, and asking me whether I could cure her. An examination revealed a large Hunterian chancre on the inside of one of the labia majora, a bubo in the right and left groin, and on each thigh a moist excoriation of the size of a dollar, so that I cannot conceive it possible, even now, that this woman should have been willing, even in a moment of intoxication, to give herself up to a man for purposes of debauch. In six weeks she was all but cured, before even a trace of disease could be discovered in the young man, who presented himself every four days for examination, with the most conscientious fidelity. His general health remained unimpaired, except a certain dulness of spirits which I attributed to the anxiety which tormented him; not till the end of the seventh week he began to complain, on his regular visiting day, of a general feeling of languor in all his limbs, a peculiar feeling of weakness and emptiness in the stomach, and some chilliness. Next day already he came again, showing me on the prepuce, not far from the frænulum, a small, roundish, red-brown spot that had come out over night, and which, without the previous frequently-described vesicle, and after destroying the epithelium, had become converted into a *simple* chancre without any induration. I cured him in ten days.

Sec. 47.—The Initial forms of Chancre.

The above-described case shows that the original chancre-vesicle neither is, nor need be, in every case, the primary beginning of chancre. I have seen this vesicle once in my practice; in this case the appearance of the vesicle was soon after followed by elevated chancres on the margin of the prepuce. The patient was a Spaniard, who, although he had a Hunterian chancre that was not yet entirely cured, had not been able to restrain himself from sexual intercourse, had connection with a diseased female, came to me, ten days after this event, with two new white vesicles on the margin of the prepuce, seated upon a red base. While talking about this thing, and I was on the point of examining them with a glass, he scratched one of them open, so that I was able to discover beneath it a small, lardaceous, somewhat depressed base of equal size, which, however, together with the vesicle that had not been scratched open, changed within forty-eight hours to a distinctly-recognizable elevated chancre. If, according to Ricord's observation, inoculation first develops a slight swelling upon which a little papula shows itself, which is succeeded by a vesicle, and that this vesicle in four or five days increases to a pustule, which, after breaking, gives rise to a fully developed chancre: this course of development may take place upon the epidermis, but is not to be accepted as a criterion for the development of chancre upon the epithelium. In the case which I have related above, the vesicles were not seated on the inner, but on the *outer* surface of the prepuce, near the margin, where the epidermis is still intact; and it is very likely that, where a chancre breaks out on the epidermis, for instance, on the body of the penis, or on the outer surface of the prepuce, its development takes the above-described course, from the vesicle to the pustule. On the other hand, it is equally probable that, when a chancre develops itself on the mucous membranes, vesicles never arise; and that the ulcer, according to Castelnau's very correct and incontrovertible observations, emerges in most cases from red or brown spots by the gradual destruction of the epithelium. Ricord's description of the formation of chancre from a small abscess, I have seen verified in one case, where the chancre was located upon the dorsum of the penis, at a spot where the skin had become chafed by mere accident; five days after I noticed the little abscess, the chancre broke out.

Sec. 48.—Course and Terminations of Chancres.

If recent authorities assert that it is wrong to regard chancre as an ulcer that never heals *spontaneously*, this probably arises from the circumstance that physicians are not agreed on what they understand by a cure. If we mean by a cure a mere cicatrization of the ulcer, those who maintain that a chancre can heal spontaneously, may perhaps be correct. It is indeed true that some chancres may cicatrize without the interference of art; but no one who has seen these cicatrices, as they remain, for instance, after cauterization, will be tempted to consider them as evidence of a cure. How great soever the loss of substance; if the chancre is *really cured*, there must not remain the least induration, nor any discoloration of the cicatrix; the skin must have a natural, healthy color; where the cicatrix remains hard, copper or violet-colored, a cure is out of the question. If the chancre is left to itself and is not phagedænic, a period arrives sooner or later when the ulcerative process ceases, when the ulcer loses its syphilitic characteristics, its lardaceous base, everted edges and cup-shaped form, and either changes to a brown or violet-colored *induration* or is transformed into *condylomatous growths*. In such a case we may, if we choose, regard the ulcer as healed, or, in other words, the ulcerative process is stopped; but, that this does not mean a cure, is evident from the fact that almost at the very moment when the induration or the condylomatous growths set in; that is to say, at the very moment when the chancre loses its syphilitic characteristics, its lardaceous base and everted edges, and there remains nothing of the chancre than a copper-colored or violet-red surface: the first symptoms of constitutional syphilis, such as roseola, syphilitic itch or ulcerations in other parts, especially in the throat, make their appearance. In a true cure of chancre the ulcer first becomes cleansed at its base, secretes a laudable pus, and forms new, healthy granulations, by which means the hardness and the swollen edges gradually decrease, and the ulcerated surface covers itself with a sound skin from the circumference to the centre in gradually decreasing concentric circles, thus forming at last a somewhat depressed, but otherwise perfectly smooth cicatrix of the same color as the sound skin. Phagedænic as well as Hunterian chancres may terminate in *gangrene*, which, however, is very seldom the case. On the other hand, recent chancres frequently become transformed into obstinate, malignant *indurations.* Such a case has occurred in my own practice, where, after treating an incipient chancre with *Arnica*, a violet-colored, stone-hard swelling became perceptible on the prepuce, without any trace of an ulcer, but associated with various symptoms of constitutional syphilis.

V. DIAGNOSIS OF CHANCRES.

Sec. 49.—General Remarks.

Although any one who has seen the different forms of chancre once, can scarcely ever fail to recognize them again: on the other hand, nothing is more difficult than to point out the general characteristic signs that will render the dignosis of chancre certain beyond all doubt. This difficulty arises from the fact that not one of these signs, such as the funnel-shaped appearance, the coppery color, the everted edges, the lardaceous base, the indurated border, etc., is uniformly present in every case; and that one or the other of these signs, according as the form of the chancre varies, is, and indeed must be wanting without the ulcer ceasing to be a chancre. If we ask ourselves what diagnostic sign which no one can gainsay, distinguishes the primary chancre, whatever its form, from a *non*-syphilitic ulcer, we have but one answer: its inherent faculty *to cause constitutional syphilis.* As regards its contagious character, chancre shares it not only with the small-pox pustule, but likewise with all diphtheritic and other ulcers; and in its serpiginous or deeply-penetrating character, or in its property never to heal spontaneously and radically without the interference of art, it resembles cancerous ulcers so closely that it might readily be confounded with them. For this reason inoculation does not decide any thing; it only proves that the ulcer from which the matter is taken, is of a contagious nature; whether the ulcer is *syphilitic*, can be doubted until symptoms of constitutional syphilis develop themselves. We might go further, and ask: If those who regard *inoculation* as the sole diagnostic sign, decline to impart the name of chancre to any ulcer, the matter from which does not produce a like ulcer; by what *diagnostic* sign do they know, after inoculation more than before, that the new ulcer, resulting from the inoculation, as well as the old, is necessarily a *syphilitic* chancre and not some other *contagious* ulcer? In order to remove this uncertainty there must be other *diagnostic signs* which, if not isolatedly, but taken together, must render the diagnosis certain even without inoculation. The case is similar to that of the itch, where modern pathologists will not recognize any other diagnostic or truly pathognomonic sign than the acarus. Here, too, we have a right to ask: if the acarus is indeed the *only* sign the presence of which justifies us to impart the name of *itch* to an eruption where the acarus is found: how do these modern pathologists know that the eruption where the acarus is found is really the very same eruption as that which has hitherto been designated as the itch? Although it may be difficult to establish a fixed diagnosis of chancre for such as are anxious to carry on an argument on the subject, nevertheless there are, fortunately for the practical physician who means to help his patient and free him from a loathsome disease, other diagnostic signs which, if they do not convey absolute certainty, yet render the recognition of chancre exceedingly probable, and point out a certain road to a cure.

Sec. 50.—Diagnostic Signs.

To the statement which we have made in the preceding paragraph that the simultaneous presence of several diagnostic signs is required in order to establish a reliable diagnosis of chancre, we desire to subjoin the remark that a careful examination of the following points will render this diagnosis all but certain:

1. The general aspect of the ulcers, and their comparison with the different forms which chancres may assume (§ § 36–39).

2. The seat of these ulcers, and their comparison with other more or less similar phenomena that may manifest themselves on the same parts.

3. The anamnesis, or a consideration of the circumstances that may have preceded the breaking out of the ulcers.

Chancres occurring on the sexual organs, cannot well be confounded with other similar appearances, since the only two kinds of eruption with which chancres might possibly be confounded in some one of their different stages, *herpes pudendorum* and the *aphthæ pudendorum*, only occur in little girls. As regards herpes, it may cause more or less extensive erosions and ulcerated surfaces both on the prepuce and on the labia; but in the case of herpes, these ulcerated surfaces are always very superficial, and never penetrate to the subjacent tissues; moreover, its base has a smooth surface and its edges are not the least indurated; the ulceration is, moreover, from the first, more extended than in the case of chancre. In addition to this, chancre always arises from a single isolated vesicle; even where several vesicles exist, they are nevertheless detached, whereas herpes, at its first origin, forms a surface of several densely-crowded vesicles. In females it is much easier to confound the ulcerated surface of *herpes intra-vulvaris* with chancre; more particularly since, as I have seen in my own practice, herpes, when very much inflamed, may occasion a slight swelling of the inguinal glands. But even in this case an erroneous diagnosis is impossible, provided we remember that the ulcerations of the herpes intra-vulvaris are always irregular, imperfectly circumscribed, and more extensive than chancre, which, even when *phagedænic*, always rests, if not upon an indurated, at least upon a swollen base as upon a bed, and has hard edges. These diagnostic signs enable us to distinguish herpes from *syphilitic erosions*, which are likewise sharply circumscribed, surrounded by red and hard borders, and never heal, like herpes, in ten days or a fortnight, by resorting to no other means than washing. As regards the aphthæ pudendorum, which, in the case of feeble and cachectic children, may likewise break out on the inner surface of the vulva; their dirty appearance when in a state of ulceration, may indeed lead us, at first sight, to confound them with small chancres, and if reasonable grounds for suspicion exist, may induce us to believe that the ulcerations were the result of violent abuse by some diseased person; but a closer inspection soon shows that these apparently depressed, whitish-gray ulcers are exceedingly superficial, and that the depression is occasioned by an exceedingly soft border, which is raised up like a wall, consisting, as it were, of a fold of mucous membrane, and exhibiting but slight redness, or none at all.

Sec. 51.—Mercurial Ulcers.

In the case of chancres that break out on other parts than the sexual organs, it seems scarcely possible to confound them—unless we except those the diagnostic characteristics of which we have recited in previous paragraphs (§§ 40 to 43)—with any other form of ulcer, with the exception of *mercurial ulcers.* We deem it so much the more incumbent upon us to offer a few remarks on this subject, since it is from this source that the most pernicious consequences frequently arise in a twofold manner. For, while on the one hand there are practitioners who falsely look upon every chancre that proves somewhat obstinate and cannot be influenced by Mercury, as a mercurial ulcer, and owing to this mistake, allow the chancre to cause the most horrid destruction; on the other hand there are practitioners, not only among the allopaths, but likewise among the homœopaths, who smile contemptuously at the aggravations supposed to result from large doses of Mercury, and, whatever course the ulcer may take, deem it necessary to pile on the Mercury in increased quantities, fancying that the organism had not been sufficiently saturated with this metal; and yet, the phenomena which they desire to combat, are most generally nothing else than the effects of large doses of Mercury. Mercurial ulcers being, therefore, an established fact, we will offer the following advice, by means of which they may be correctly known and distinguished from chancre. As a general rule, the mercurial ulcer is never as painless as chancre; on the contrary, it is very sensitive and painful to the touch, but is never accompanied by the nightly stinging and boring pains that sometimes attend the Hunterian chancre when very much inflamed. The ulcer spreads very rapidly, almost like a phagedænic chancre, but never like a serpiginous sore; its base is of a milky-white, gray or livid, very frequently with bluish-white edges, sometimes superficial like simple excoriations, secreting a purulent serum, or else covered with a cheesy layer; sometimes the ulcer dips to the subjacent textures, with a dirty-looking, even lardaceous base, but always of an *irregular*, *indistinctly-circumscribed shape*, with unequal circumference, and always healing from one side of its border, whereas a chancre first becomes cleansed on its base and afterwards cicatrizes from its circumference in concentric circles. These ulcers most frequently break out in the mouth, or on the inside of the lips, on the edges of the tongue, or on the sexual organs and in their neighborhood. Very frequently they break out in existing wounds, in cicatrices or on ulcerated surfaces, which, in such a case, spread rapidly and become painful, phagedænic, ichorous, and bleeding. Sometimes this kind of ulcer shows itself on hairy parts (especially on the hairy scalp) under the form of a superficial ulcer, with a rough, uneven surface and lardaceous, fungous growths, without any malignant character, and dissolving into a purulent liquid, after which the ulcer disappears without leaving a scar, but reappears again sooner or later on other parts.

VI. PROGNOSIS AND TREATMENT OF CHANCRES.

Sec. 52.—Prognosis.

In giving the prognosis of a chancre, we always have to take into consideration the following two points:

1. The greater or less degree of curability of a given chancre; and

2. The greater or less danger that this chancre may terminate in constitutional syphilis.

As regards the first of these two points, it is an undoubted fact that a simple chancre is most curable; so is the Hunterian chancre, provided the treatment is properly conducted; for if mismanaged or neglected even ever so little, it is apt to terminate in chronic indurations or condylomatous growths, the appearance of which is inevitably followed by general syphilis. The *simple* chancre, if neglected, is very apt, on the other hand, to pass in two or three weeks into the Hunterian chancre, with all the danger accompanying this form of the syphilitic disease. If properly treated at the outset, both can be cured in ten to fifteen days; but if the treatment only commences fifteen days after their first appearance, it will take from twenty to thirty and even more days, to cure them. The ulcus elevatum likewise heals very rapidly, if properly treated; but, if badly treated, may readily assume the character of a *phagedænic* chancre. This is undoubtedly the worst form of the primary syphilitic ulcer, not only on account of the difficulties encountered in its treatment; on account of its ready termination in gangrene, and of the terrible destruction it may cause in the tissues; but likewise on account of the violence of the secondary phenomena by which it may be succeeded. If this chancre cicatrizes spontaneously, it always leaves behind it hard, uneven, rough cicatrices of a blue and brown-red color. The assertion that syphilitic *erosions* are easily healed, and that they often disappear of themselves, is incorrect; it is almost certain that those who offer these statements, have confounded the erosions with the harmless herpes intra-vulvaris, whose resemblance to erosions is exceedingly deceitful. According to my experience there are no more tedious, and hence no more deceitful or more dangerous phenomena, than those very erosions; for if they continue for any length of time, they may superinduce secondary syphilis, even while they are still out upon the skin. The danger of a primary chancre terminating in constitutional syphilis, not only depends upon the treatment, but likewise upon the *age* of the chancre. Chancres that are only treated externally, readily induce constitutional syphilis; neglected chancres produce this result in six or eight weeks. Ricord's statement that an incipient induration is a sure sign that constitutional syphilis has already set in, may apply to all chancres that commence as *simple* or *elevated* chancres and afterwards become indurated; in the *Hunterian* chancre, however, where the induration exists at the outset, the danger only begins after the ulcer passes from the *ulcerated* stage into that of *condylomatous growths*, which, at the earliest period, takes place in from four to five, and, at the latest period, in from six to eight weeks. Regarding the promises which a physician can safely make to his patient when first taking charge of his case, *it is of the utmost importance that the physician should first inquire of his patient how long the chancre has been in existence; if the chancre has been out four weeks, it would be rash to promise that secondary symptoms may not supervene in spite of the best treatment; if the ulcer has already lost the characteristic appearance of the primary chancre, or has been treated by external means exclusively, no promise of any kind can be made.*

Sec. 53.—General remarks on the treatment of Chancres.

If Ricord and his disciples maintain that every chancre that has not yet become indurated, hence in the first four or five days, can be safely treated by cauterization, my own experience justifies me in contradicting this statement most positively. It is indeed true that in these cases of suppression of primary chancre, symptoms of secondary syphilis do not occur as readily as when the chancres have already existed for some time. But these gentlemen never see the consequences of their doings which frequently break out three, six, and even eighteen months after the first destruction of the chancre. From my own practice I might fill volumes with what I have seen of the consequences of such criminal proceedings. Every chancre, no matter what its primary form, is a sort of *noli me tangere*, whose appearance upon the external skin, even where an appropriate internal treatment is pursued simultaneously, is never disturbed in its course by external means without such criminal encroachments being succeeded by terrible consequences. In every case, and at all times, it should only be treated with internal means, until such treatment has resulted in the destruction of the contagium, after which it disappears, as it were, of itself, without leaving a single suspicious-looking cicatrix. The only thing that can be applied externally, is pure water, for the purpose of keeping the parts clean. Cleanliness must not be neglected by any means; the patient may wash the affected parts as often as he pleases, and may even apply lint moistened with fresh water. In all other respects the treatment must be conducted by internal means; only it is to be regretted that we are not acquainted with any remedy which, like Apis and Phosphorus in diphtheritic, non-syphilitic ulcers of the throat, will extirpate a *primary* chancre even when administered in the smallest dose. For, although *Mercurius*, which is as yet our chief remedy in syphilis, is capable of rendering eminent service in secondary syphilis, even when given in the 30th potency; yet, on the other hand, it is an established fact that, in the acute form of this disease, we have to administer repeated doses of the first centesimal trituration, at least half a grain morning and evening, if we desire to make sure of a radical and speedy extirpation of the syphilitic virus. This necessity is to be regretted, in so far at any rate, since this agent, which, if used in such cases in accordance with specific indications, does not cause any perceptible inconvenience, yet, on the other hand, if not specifically indicated, may cause considerable aggravations which it may afterwards be found exceedingly difficult to remove. For this reason we advise the physician, in case Mercurius should seem to aggravate the symptoms during the first eight days of the treatment, to stop the exhibition of this agent, and to look for a more specific remedy among those that will be described in subsequent paragraphs.

Sec. 54.—Treatment of the regular (Simple and Hunterian) Chancre.

In this form of chancre the leading remedy is, and always will be, *Mercurius*. According to my experience, it is the *Mercurius solubilis Hahnemanni*, half a grain of the centesimal trituration of which, given morning and evening, will in all cases prove sufficient to effect a cure. If the cure proceeds as it should do, signs of an incipient cure will be speedily perceived, sometimes already in twenty-four hours, but scarcely ever at a later period than four days; the base of the ulcer will become cleaner; at first it may bleed a little, but healthy granulations will at the same time begin to start up; the edges of the ulcer will flatten down, and the hard foundation upon which the ulcer seems to rest, will become more and more diminished in circumference. If the ulcer takes this course, all we have to do is to continue the Mercurius, and the ulcer, provided the treatment commences one or, at the latest, eight days after its first appearance, will heal perfectly in fifteen to twenty days without the use of Nitri acidum or any other agent than Mercurius; the general health will remain unimpaired. Among my own customers, who generally apply for treatment one or two days after the products of infection manifest themselves, I have cured both the simple and the Hunterian chancre, even when the induration of the base was already fully present, in the space of ten days; incipient signs of a cure often showed themselves in twenty-four hours.

It is not in all cases, however, that patients present themselves for treatment at the earliest period; two or three weeks sometimes elapse before they apply to a physician. In such cases, if the patient has already received large doses of Mercury from the hands of an allopathic physician, and the chancre has already passed from the first or ulcerous stage into the second stage, or that of condylomatous growths, I give Nitri acidum, one drop of the first attenuation morning and night, and, by this means, accomplish my end in most cases. But if, at the time when I take charge of the patient the ulcer has still preserved its primary aspect, I give *Mercurius solubilis* even if the patient should already have been drugged with it under allopathic treatment; and, if no improvement takes place in seven or eight days, I resort to the *red precipitate*, (*Mercurius præcipitatus ruber*,) which I employ in the same dose as Merc. sol., and, by this means, accomplish a cure in most cases without resorting to any other remedy. For neglected chancre I employ *Cinnabaris*, which, in such cases, I prefer to all other mercurial preparations.

Even in cases where the chancre, either simple or Hunterian, has already lost its primary, lardaceous aspect, and exhibits a copper-colored surface with tendency to adventitious growths, I pursue the same treatment with *Merc. sol.*, *Merc. præc. rub.*, and *Cinnabaris*, provided the patient has not yet taken any mercury; in almost every case this course of treatment leads to the most satisfactory results without any other agent, like Nitri. ac., for instance, being required.

In general, I cannot sufficiently caution the physician against the premature employment of Nitric Acid in primary chancre. If administered before the ulcer is perfectly cleansed by *Mercurius*, and for the purpose of effecting cicatrization more speedily, I have frequently seen the use of this acid followed by symptoms of secondary syphilis, and a general *constitutional* taint, on which account I only have resort to the acid in chancres that are not complicated with *inflamed buboes*, in the following cases: 1) if the patient who is affected with chancrous condylomatous growths, has already taken much mercury; 2) if, under my treatment, the ulcer assumes the form of condylomatous growths; and 3) if chancrous condylomatous growths, in cases that had not been treated with Mercury allopathically, do not improve under my own treatment with *Merc. sol.*, but, on the contrary, get worse; in all such cases, I have had every reason to be satisfied with the good effects of the acid.

Sec. 55.—Treatment of the other forms of Chancre.

In all these forms *Mercurius* remains the leading remedy, with this difference, that it may be necessary to employ other mercurial preparations.

1). For *elevated chancre* (ulcus elevatum)—which is not, as some suppose, an accidental elevation of the simple chancre, but constitutes a more or less special variety of chancre, and may not only pass into the *Hunterian*, but, according to circumstances, into the *phagedænic* chancre—the principal remedy is not *Cinnabaris* (as has been improperly, or hypothetically inferred, from this ulcer being confounded with the *regular* chancre, which likewise assumes an elevated form in the second stage), but *Mercurius solubilis*, an agent that will undoubtedly prove most specifically curative, as long as the chancre still preserves its ash-colored, lardy appearance, and will even surpass in curative power any other agent, in cases where the ulcus elevatum has already passed into the Hunterian form of chancre. It is only where, by neglecting the first or lardaceous period, new condylomatous growths develop themselves, that *Cinnabaris*, which, however, is in all cases inferior to Nitri ac., may be indicated. If, however, the elevated ulcer should terminate in *phagedænic* chancre, we have at once to resort to *Corrosive Sublimate*, and pursue the treatment that will be found described in the following paragraph.

2). *Phagedænic chancre.*—Nothing can be more ill-advised than to lose one's presence of mind in this form of chancre, although it is undoubtedly a most dangerous and destructive ulcer; and to follow Hartman's advice, who counsels in his system of Therapeutics that the patient be treated with *Mercurius* until his system is thoroughly drenched with it. Even allopathic practitioners advise the cautious use of Mercury in this disease, for the reason that it will often aggravate the symptoms. I am able, from my own observation, to confirm the fact that even half-grain doses of Mercury of the first centesimal trituration may aggravate the case. The main object is to employ a mercurial preparation that will of itself arrest the ulcerative stage as rapidly as possible. This preparation is *Mercurius corrosivus.* Even in cases where any other preparation of this metal would seem to produce a most rapid and danger-threatening progress of the ulcer, *Corr. subl.* has never left me in the lurch, although I never give it in larger doses than one-half of a grain of the first centesimal trituration, morning and evening. This agent very speedily arrests the ulcerative progress, but should not be repeated too often after symptoms of improvement have begun to set in, lest cicatrization should take place too rapidly and only superficially. For this reason it may be advisable to follow it up with some other mercurial preparation, such as *Merc. præc. ruber.*

3). For the syphilitic *erosions* described in § 39, *Præc. rub.* has always rendered me most excellent service; they often resist most obstinately any remedy that may be employed against them; on the other hand, in spite of this obstinacy, their continuance is less dangerous than that of any other form of syphilitic ulceration. I should regard them, without hesitation, as secondary products, if I had not likewise seen them break out simultaneously with *primary chancre.*

Sec. 56.—Treatment of complications and sequelæ of Chancre.

The complications that may occur during the presence of chancre, are either *purely local*, such as *gangrene* of the affected parts, phimosis and paraphimosis, or other accidental occurrences, such as inflammation and suppuration of buboes, gonorrhœal discharges from the urethra, and mucous condylomata. In most of these cases, I do not suffer myself to be influenced by these accessory phenomena in my general management of chancres; only if *gangrene* sets in, I give *Arsenic;* and if this agent has removed the gangrene, which it always does, I return to the mercurial preparation that is specifically adapted to the case; the phimosis and paraphimosis, which are dependent upon the chancre, improving in the same degree as the chancre itself, all we have to do is to use the remedy that will prove most specifically curative in the case. If the chancre is complicated with gonorrhœa, I leave this last-mentioned symptom unnoticed as if it were not present, only attending to the chancre; in by far the largest number of cases *Mercurius* will be sufficient to cure them both. The same result is obtained, if numerous tubercles or buboes are present with the chancre; it is only when the buboes become intensely inflamed and threaten to break (as to inconsiderable consensual swellings of the inguinal glands, I do not heed them), I substitute *red precipitate* in the place of *Merc. sol.*, or I give *Cinnabaris*, which is sometimes preferable to the precipitate; and I only resort to *Nitri ac.*, or to some remedy indicated for buboes in § 66, if the chancre has been sufficiently cleansed, or the condition of the buboes should render it necessary that a *direct* treatment be instituted against them. If fig-warts are present, I leave them for further treatment until the chancre is entirely healed.

Regarding the *sequelæ* of chancre (which occur very frequently under the allopathic treatment; and under homœopathic treatment only if it is improperly conducted), we must be permitted to offer a few remarks. These sequelæ are, 1. *indurations* of the prepuce or of the spot where the chancre had been located; 2. *new ulcers* which are sometimes very superficial, sometimes, however, of considerable depth; or *re-opening* of *old cicatrices.* The indurations are generally the result of the extirpation of chancres by external means, and are of a *syphilitic* nature; I generally treat them with *red precipitate*, or, if the patient had already taken more or less Mercury, use the *Cinnabaris;* in all cases, however, they require a long period for their radical cure, and, in order to prevent an excess of mercurial action, I give a dose of *Mercurius* only every other day.—For *subsequent ulcers* or *re-opening cicatrices* which may likewise occur under violent homœopathic treatment, I generally, especially if no syphilitic discoloration of the skin is any longer present, give with the best effect *Nitri ac.*, or *Sulphur*, sometimes *Lachesis* or *Phosphorus;* but if symptoms are still present, such as permanent indurations, discolored cicatrices, etc., that might lead us to suspect remaining traces of syphilis, I commence the treatment with some mercurial preparation that had not yet been given to the patient, (most generally *Cinnabaris* or *Mercurius vivus*,) and only resort to *Nitri ac.* or *Sulphur*, if the former should remain without effect or even induce aggravations.

If *aphthæ*, which must not be confounded with chancres, should break out on the mucous membrane of the lips or on the edges of the tongue, in consequence of too liberal a use of Mercury, or even while this agent is still being given, we have to treat them with the remedies mentioned at the end of this work for *mercurial syphilis.*

Sec. 57.—Remarks on the different modes of treating Chancre recommended by others.

It must be evident, from a simple review of the lists of cases and remedies mentioned in Rückert's "Klinischen Erfahrungen," that in both schools, the allopathic as well as the homœopathic, there is so much theory and hypothesis mixed up with the genuine results of practical experience, that a beginner who reads all these things might easily be misled into a labyrinth of errors, without some reliable guide. For this reason we will add a few remarks to our previous paragraphs concerning the practical treatment of chancre.

1. Hahnemann. Hahnemann's remarks on the efficacy of the smallest doses of Mercury in chancre, are undoubtedly correct if applied to *secondary* syphilis, or to discolored cicatrices remaining after badly managed or suppressed primary chancres, or to other chronic sequelæ. Most probably these secondary phenomena occurred in his practice more frequently than primary chancre. In the former, small doses of Mercurius do more good than large ones; but in acute *primary* chancres, comparatively large doses will have to be employed, for the present, at any rate.

2. Attomyr. (Varieties of Chancre, pages 23–27). This author's remarks on his three varieties of chancre, the first of which comprehends the Hunterian chancre, and the second the ulcus elevatum, are in so far correct as the chief remedy for the first class is indeed *Merc. sol.;* but we must modify the author's proposition

to employ *Nitri ac.* for chancres of the second class, by stating that, for recent *primary*, elevated ulcers, several of which may break out at the same time, the chief remedy is likewise *Merc. sol.;* taking it of course for granted that his second variety, so far from being a chancre, is not rather a *mucous condyloma*—(see Sec. 72). Only in cases where the improper treatment of a chancre with excessive doses of Mercury, results in the breaking out of elevated ulcers, *Nitri ac.* is in its place; whereas, if *Merc. sol.* is not sufficient in a case of recent ulcus elevatum, *Cinnabaris* is preferable to Nitri ac. The same remark applies to the author's so-called third form, the more perfectly developed *ulcus elevatum*, where neither Thuja nor Nitri ac., nor Staphysagria have yielded me the same good effects that I have derived from *Merc. sol.*, or, in appropriate cases, from the *red precipitate.* As regards the author's fifth variety, which breaks out with violent itching on the external surface of the prepuce and covers itself with a scurf that only becomes detached after the complete healing of the ulcer, and for which *Sulphur* is said to be the principal remedy: I have met with such *scurfy* chancres in my own practice, on the prepuce, the dorsum of the penis and the scrotum, but have never known Sulphur to do any good in such cases, but have always found *Merc. sol.*, *Merc. præc. ruber*, and in some, perhaps secondary cases, *Aurum*, efficacious. Moreover, since it is an established fact that true syphilitic ulcers do not itch, I am almost inclined to believe that Attomyr's fifth variety is nothing else than an external preputial herpes, so much the more as this eruption, if very much inflamed and far-spreading, may cause swelling of the inguinal glands, and yields to the internal use of *Hep. sulph.* Finally, in Hunterian chancre, *Thuja* and Causticum should never be used, as Attomyr advises, as intercurrent remedies; we should only lose time if we were to allow ourselves, by such a proceeding, to interrupt the highly important employment of *Mercurius.* Regarding this author's fourth variety, for which he recommends Corallium, we have to remark that it most probably coincides with the *syphilitic erosions* that have been described, Sec. 39. But inasmuch as he admits that Corallium is not always capable of preventing the passage of this variety into Hunterian chancre, we infer from such an admission that it would be much better to commence the treatment at once, instead of with Corallium, with *Merc. sol.*, *Merc. præc. rub.* or *Cinnabaris.*

3. Buchner (Hygea, vol. 13), utters *golden* advice which should be thundered into the ears of every physician, when he says that, although *Mercurius will cure a chancre in the reproductive stage, yet we should administer the smallest justifiable doses of this agent, and thus guard against a too rapid cicatrization of the ulcer, lest the disease should be merely suppressed, and continue to spread in the organism, as is often the case after the persistent employment of Merc. corrosivus.* (See also Sec. 59, Vehsemeyer.)

Sec. 58.—Continuation of the former subject.

4. Hartmann. (Theory and treatment of chronic diseases.) As a general rule, the remedies for the different forms of chancre are very correctly and appropriately indicated in this work; we would simply add that, if *Merc. sol.* does not act promptly in a case of Hunterian chancre, the *red precipitate* or *Cinnabaris* will almost always prove sufficient, so that we need not resort to the equivocal and unreliable *Iodide of Mercury*, which, besides, is much more adapted to chronic secondary ulcers. Regarding Thuja, which Hartmann recommends for the ulcus elevatum, we can only repeat what we have already said on this subject, when commenting on Attomyr's recommendation of this agent for the Hunterian chancre. In fully-formed chancre, the employment of this agent would involve an irreparable loss of time; how far Nitri ac. may here subserve our purpose, has already been shown in § 55. Hartmann's remarks on the persistent employment of *Merc. corr.* in *phagedænic chancres*, and upon the danger consequent upon the irrational alternation or change of remedies in this disease, deserves the greatest attention, since all these remarks are founded on experience; but if the same author teaches, in a subsequent paragraph, that, in phagedænic chancre, this agent should not be exhibited in an attenuated form, but in substance, until the organism is thoroughly saturated with it, we have to oppose this advice most positively. As we have said before, in this form of chancre, nothing is more dangerous than an excess of mercurial action, which sometimes superinduces the most horrid aggravations and destructions; and since *Merc. corr.*, if administered in half-grain doses of the first centesimal trituration, morning and evening, proves sufficiently powerful to control this disease, and too weak to develop material aggravations, it seems proper to administer it also in this form of chancre in the above-mentioned dose.

5. Clotar Müller. (All. hom. Zeit., vols. 34 & 57.) What this excellent practitioner observes regarding the curative powers of *Merc. præc.* and *Cinnabaris*, which he considers as far superior to those of Merc. sol., is likewise founded in experience. For myself, I prefer those remedies to *Merc. nitros*, which is so highly praised by Dr. Trinks, but, on account of its intense action, is attended with more or less danger; more particularly since I personally have never yet met with any cases, even of inveterate primary chancres where the *red precipitate* or *Cinnabaris* has not accomplished every thing that could be desired. Nevertheless, I never use these remedies in recent primary chancres, where I have found *Merc. sol.* sufficient in every case; but for all mismanaged and neglected chancres, I consider them as the best preparations that can be used. More especially they become indispensable (more particularly *Cinnabaris*) when recent chancres, whose appearance still counter-indicates the employment of Nitri ac., at the outset are accompanied by buboes. In this case, Cinnabaris frequently becomes an indispensable remedy, which often cures chancre and buboes at the same time. In old chancres, complicated with buboes, I likewise prefer using *Cinnabaris* before I resort to Nitri acidum. In *recent* chancres on the glans and prepuce, Clotar Müller always employs the *red precipitate;* and *Cinnabaris* in the cure of *old* chancres on the same parts, especially if they dip down to the deeper textures, are indurated, suppurate a good deal, and the individual has already been infected a number of times; for chancres on the scrotum and dorsum of the penis he employs *Aurum mur.* (which I likewise recommend), and for chancres in the throat, *Corr. subl.* He neglects to mention whether it is for primary or secondary chancres.

6. Rosenberg (All. hom. Zeit., vol. 35) asserts that, in cases complicated with scurvy, he has been unable to effect any thing with Mercurius; that, after the use of this agent, the ulcers became worse, assuming an appearance of increased malignity and disorganization. I have met with such ulcers, where the diagnosis was made difficult and uncertain by a complication of syphilis, mercurial poisoning and scorbutic taint. But if Rosenberg proposes for this condition *Mur. ac.*, *China*, *Camphora*, *Carbo*, *Ferrum*, *Kal. nitr.*, *Kreasotum*, *Manganum*, *Sabina*, *Secale*, and *Sarsaparilla*, without particularizing the indications, the beginning practitioner

who can be induced to try all these remedies, one after the other, on good luck, deserves to be pitied; according to my own experience, he had better try *Nitri ac.*, if Merc. should aggravate the symptoms; after which he may use *Sulphur;* he will be much more satisfied with the result.

Sec. 59.—Continuation of the same subject.

7. VEHSEMEYER. The best thing that has ever been published in the literature of our school, is to be found in "Vehsemeyer's Jahrbüchern," vol. 3, page 134 and following, by the editor of this publication; we fully accept what he says in this article: "Chancre exhibits in its course two stages, an *ulcerative* and a *reproductive* stage. The character of the first stage is *loss of substance*, that of the second *adventitious growth.* The syphilitic ulcer, if taken charge of by a physician at the very outset, leaves this stage under the persistent use of *Mercurius sol.* in ten or twelve days, at the latest in a fortnight. (V. gives every day two or three doses, of one to five grains each, of the second or third decimal trituration). On the sixth or eighth day, an improvement becomes evident; the ulcer is arrested in its course, ceases to spread, and begins to cleanse itself from the circumference to the centre. If this change does not take place within the time indicated, another remedy will have to be chosen." In such a case, if the ulcer spreads rapidly, V. gives *Corr. subl.*, and if the ulcer is indolent, *Merc. phosph.*, but warns the physician against the too long continued use of the sublimate, lest it should produce a deceitful cure. He says: "Instead of becoming cleansed from the circumference, the cleansing process of the ulcer proceeds from the centre; the edges become raised, grow like condylomata, and in a few days, under the continued use of the sublimate, the chancre cicatrizes. . . . . If this result should take place in spite of the most cautious treatment, the method recommended for the second stage should at once be pursued, and should be *persistently* continued until the cicatrix assumes a natural appearance." For the second stage, V. recommends *Nitri ac.*, two or three drops of the second watery dilution morning and evening, but advises (and this cannot be repeated too often) never to use it *too soon*, but to first await the full setting in of the *reproductive process;* on the other hand, where *adventitious growths* have begun to make their appearance, the employment of *Nitri ac.* should not be delayed for a moment.

Except the doses of Mercurius, which are unnecessarily large (for half-grain doses of the first centesimal trituration, given morning and night, are entirely sufficient), Vehsemeyer's advice may be safely followed by any practitioner. If the author afterwards states in a note that, although chancre is often treated with *Mercurius* alone, cicatrization does not take place as rapidly as when Nitri ac. is used, he certainly can only mean cases where the *condylomatous growths* had already shown themselves, or where the chancre had not been healed in the first stage. For if the chancre is healed in the ulcerative stage, the process of cicatrization and the arrest of loss of substance progresses in the same ratio, so that, at the moment when the *process of reproduction* is completed, the cicatrix is likewise perfect; whence it follows that, where Mercurius has healed a chancre in the ulcerative stage without the supervention of adventitious growths, no Nitri ac. will be found necessary to complete the work of cicatrization.

8. Rummel. See his very remarkable case, in the chapter on "*Sycosic condylomata*," § 78.

9. Other authors. We might have quoted a number of other authors, such as Aegidi, Bernstein, Buchner, Fielitz, Goullon, Hartlaub, Knorre, Kurtz, Kreussler, Rummel, Schelling, Schade, Sommer, Thorer, Trinks, Wahle, Wolf, etc.; but inasmuch as we deal in the present chapter with the *primary* chancre, and shall, when treating of the other forms of chancre in subsequent chapters, do full justice to the observations of other practitioners, we have deemed our present quotations sufficient, if for no other reason than that they give the most important data. At the same time we refer the reader to the last chapter of this work, "*General pharmaco-dynamic observations*," (§ 227–236,) where he will find the views of other authors, who have only furnished isolated remarks concerning one or the other of the remedies that have been recommended so far.

10. Hale. *Apocynum androsemifolium* or dog's-bane. The Choctaw Indians regard this drug as a specific for secondary syphilis; they chew the root.

Asclepias tuberosa, pleurisy-root. Professor Hale has employed this remedy with uniform success in constitutional syphilis.

Iris versicolor, blue-flag. Recommended very highly for mercurial syphilis. Dose: one or two fluid drachms of the tincture, six or eight times daily.

Lobelia inflata, Indian tobacco; this remedy is used by the Indians for syphilis.

Phytolacca decandra, poke. Recommended by the Eclectics for bone-pains and mercurial syphilis. It is likewise said to have been used with good effect in primary chancre.

Stillingia sylvatica, queen's-root; is extensively used by Eclectics in primary and secondary syphilis; they regard it almost as a specific in this disease.

FOURTH CHAPTER.

SOME OTHER PRIMARY FORMS OF SYPHILIS.

I. BUBOES.

Sec. 60.—General Definition.

In former times, by the term *bubo*, physicians always understood a swelling of the inguinal glands; afterwards the term was likewise applied to glandular swellings in the arm-pits, on the neck, etc.; more recently, beside the bubo of the plague, this term has been limited to a *syphilitic swelling of the inguinal glands*, in regard to which we distinguish (a) *sympathetic* and *essential*, and (b) *primary*, *secondary*, and *constitutional buboes*. Sympathetic buboes are in fact nothing else than simple, more or less painful, inguinal swellings, which may arise not only from chancre, but likewise from every somewhat intensely inflamed herpes, or other ulcers, and likewise from gonorrhœa, and are caused not so much by the transmission of the poison as by an extension of the inflammatory irritation to the neighboring lymphatic vessels. These sympathetic swellings, which are scarcely ever entirely wanting if the chancre is more or less inflamed, do not properly come under our consideration at this place, since they disappear of themselves after the chancre is healed. The case is different as regards inguinal swellings that are occasioned by the *direct action of the poison*, and which alone are meant by the term *syphilitic buboes*. A bubo is a more or less inflamed, and painful, and sometimes very extensive tumor, comprising several glands in one swelling, and showing an extraordinary tendency to suppurate. When first originating, the bubo announces itself by an unpleasant feeling and a slightly painful tension in the groin, resembling the sensation which is sometimes experienced after long walking, or after excessive bodily exertions. An examination with the hand shows that one or more glands are swollen, sensitive to pressure, and even painful. Soon after, the neighboring glands and the cellular tissue become irritated, in consequence of which a hard swelling of considerable size develops itself, whose surface appears red, and which interferes a good deal with walking. Suppuration is preceded by a violent throbbing pain, and the bubo discharges, sooner or later, according as the inflammation was more or less intense. If the swelling of the inguinal glands is not *essential*, but *sympathetic*, it is mostly painless and not sensitive to pressure, at least not much so; the glands involved in the swelling remain detached for a long time, and the skin retains its natural color. This condition may continue for weeks and months, according as the ulcer from which the irritation proceeds continues; a sort of induration may even develop itself as an accompaniment of such sympathetic swellings; and if a general infection of the organism should take place, these sympathetic swellings may even terminate in suppuration, without, however, secreting a contagious virus, as is the case with the genuine bubo when it discharges and suppurates. Usually the bubo shows itself while the chancre is still existing, particularly if the ulcer is treated with external irritants; if chancres are made to cicatrize by cauterization, the bubo sometimes shows itself all at once after the cicatrix is fully formed; in some cases it shows itself at once, directly, without any previous chancre, as the first sign of primary syphilis.

Sec. 61.—Primary, Consecutive, and Constitutional Buboes.

Recently a good deal has been argued, pro and con, whether there are *primary* buboes, or such as occur without any previous chancre; or truly *constitutional buboes*, or such as arise in the course of constitutional syphilis as one of the symptoms of this disease; or whether every bubo is not either a secondary or consecutive phenomenon, that is, a phenomenon which always occurs *after* the breaking out of the chancre, although as one of its immediate consequences. As regards constitutional buboes, I must confess that I have never seen them occur as symptoms of secondary syphilis, and that, according to what I have read on this subject in different authors, they understand, all of them, by constitutional buboes those that do not develop themselves while the chancre is still running its course, but after its cicatrization, provided the aforesaid authors did not mean by buboes an induration of purely sympathetic inguinal glandular swellings, that had remained behind after the primary chancre had healed. But, if we inquire into the manner in which the primary chancre had disappeared, we shall find that it was through some external agency, such as cauterization, after which the bubo remained, not as a symptom of constitutional infection, but as a *vicarious product*, standing in the place of the primary chancre; that is to say, a swelling where the secreted pus retains all the characteristics of the *non-modified* and still *contagious* secretion. If, after the fashion of some French pathologists, we extend the term bubo to every painless inguinal swelling, even to a mere kernel, we can indeed find buboes in the secondary form or second stage of syphilis, which, after all, are nothing else than slight indurations remaining after former sympathetic swellings. If, in accordance with the present more rigid interpretation of the term, we understand by bubo a large, inflammatory, inguinal tumor, produced by the direct action of the poison, it is perfectly proper to consider such a bubo as one of the characteristic products of the *primary* period of syphilis, and therefore endowed with a faculty of transmitting the infection. Whether a bubo may occur all at once, as the primary *protopathic* sign of syphilis, without any previous chancre or syphilitic gonorrhœa, is quite another question that is always settled in the affirmative by those who have met with such an occurrence, but is denied by those who have not yet witnessed it; and will hereafter be denied as long as its possibility is not theoretically established. All we can say on this point is, that those who deny protopathic buboes, affirm in support of their opinion, that, where such buboes seem to exist, there must have been some previous chancre which the patient did not heed, and which had been made to cicatrize through some accidental influence, or by the action of some ointment, before the patient had been aware of the true nature of the ulcer. This is indeed possible. I have seen such buboes arise after the breaking out of ulcers on the glans, which the patient regarded as simple excoriations contracted during coït, and which were removed at the outset by the use of lead-water. Cases of this kind may occur; yet they do not afford an argument against the opinion entertained by many physicians, that buboes may likewise arise *protopathically* without any other symptom of syphilis having been present previously.

Sec. 62.—Various Kinds of Buboes.

Modern writers on syphilis have attempted to describe several varieties of the syphilitic bubo. Although they are in reality nothing else than the same bubo in different stages of development, yet they deserve a more attentive consideration, in so far as they enable us to recognize the true character of these swellings, and to distinguish them from tumors of a different class. Agreeably to their classification, we have two large classes of buboes: 1) *Phlegmonous* or *inflammatory;* and, 2) *Indolent* or *non-inflammatory buboes.* In accordance with their periods of development, these two classes are again distinguished: *a*) in *fluctuating; b*) *suppurating;* and, *c*) *chancrous buboes.* A cursory review of this classification shows that these supposed varieties are not distinct buboes, of essentially different natures, but that these differences are purely accidental, depending merely upon the different stages of development through which such a syphilitic product has to run. As regards *indolent* buboes, they coincide with the sympathetic inguinal glandular swellings that have been described § 60, and likewise may become indurated, so far as not to deserve more special attention until they assume the form of real buboes, in other words, become inflamed, in which case they come under the head of *inflammatory* or *phlegmonous* buboes, and belong to the first class. For this reason, our business here is with the *genuine, essential* buboes, of which we have the following varieties, or rather stages, as described by modern authors:

1) *The non-fluctuating inflammatory buboes.*—The swollen gland is not movable, as is the case when the swelling is purely sympathetic; the cellular tissue, likewise, becomes swollen, forming a more or less dense layer around the gland, where the inflammation progresses much more rapidly than in the tissue of the gland, and which offers a peculiar elastic resistance to the feel. The swelling assumes a dark or violet-colored redness, that sometimes is confined to the middle region of the swelling, but very

frequently spreads as far as the circumference. The pain may be violent, with a moderate degree of inflammation; or it may be slight, while the inflammation is intense.

2) *The fluctuating inflammatory swelling.*—According as the pus collects in the cellular tissue, or in the gland, or in both at the same time, the examining finger discovers either a soft, doughy swelling, or distinct fluctuation. As this change sets in, the inflammation and pain become less; as long as the suppurating process remains confined to a few spots, and the skin retains its violet redness, a cure by resorption still remains within the bounds of possibility.

The suppurating glandular swelling.—If the bubo is of a syphilitic nature, the margins of the opening, after the bursting of the abscess, will appear unequal, gray, more or less indurated, indented, abrupt, and everted, gaping; the bottom of the ulcer rests upon the tissue of the gland, shows the same phenomena, and the surrounding cellular tissue is more or less indurated. Altogether, the surface of such an ulcer may exhibit all the phenomena observed in the case of simple, indurated, elevated, or phagedænic chancres; the same remark applies to the course, cicatrization, and healing of these ulcers, whose cicatrices are generally most prominent and depressed when seated in the bend of the groin. If the whole body of the gland has been involved in the inflammation, it may have been entirely destroyed by suppuration; in such a case, the cicatrix may rest upon the subjacent cellular tissue.

Sec. 63.—Diagnosis.

Although our previous remarks point out the diagnostic signs of a syphilitic bubo, with so much evident correctness that it seems impossible to commit an error of diagnosis in cases where a chancre has preceded the appearance of a swelling; yet we must not overlook the fact that buboes may, although in rare cases, occur *protopathically*. If they do, it is of the utmost importance to be able to diagnose their true nature before suppuration and fluctuation set in. Syphilitic buboes follow the same general course, like any other inflammatory swelling, even to the period of suppuration, so that this fact alone would be sufficient to cast a doubt on their true character, wherever no positive signs of a previous syphilitic infection are present. If these signs are wanting; if the patient does not show any other symptoms of primary syphilis; if no ulcer can be discovered, and the patient is perhaps unwilling to admit that he has had intercourse with a suspected female, the diagnosis is sometimes very difficult. In such cases, we risk to confound buboes with scrofulous swellings, or even, if the inflammation is still inconsiderable, with aneurisms of the femoral artery, or even with inguinal hernia, or vice versa. The last-mentioned mistake occurred quite recently to a Professor of Surgery in the Medical Faculty of Paris, who, mistaking an inguinal hernia for a bubo, cut into the swelling, when he found, to his amazement, that, instead of laying open a bubo, he had ripped open a portion of bowel. This shows that, whereas on the one hand preceding and accompanying circumstances may shed light on the diagnosis, in case a genuine bubo is before us, we may on the other hand be led into grave errors, if circumstances favor the suspicion that the existing tumor is a syphilitic product. Nevertheless, a close examination ought to prevent mistakes like that which happened to the French professor; for a hernial swelling is always indolent, the color of the skin remains unaltered, the integuments over the swelling are immovable; in a recumbent posture, the bowel either reënters the abdominal cavity spontaneously, or is easily replaced by the taxis; all of which does not occur in the case of a bubo. Nor is it generally difficult to distinguish a bubo from aneurism of the femoral artery, although the throbbing pains which are experienced in a bubo, during the period of suppuration, may lead to false conclusions in cases where all symptoms of syphilis are wanting, and where the patient obstinately asserts that he never had any connection with a diseased female. Yet, even in such a case, we may obtain some certainty from the circumstances that, during its earlier period at least, an aneurismal swelling can be compressed with the finger, the removal of which is succeeded by a return of the pulsations; that an aneurismal tumor enlarges, and that its pulsations become more distinct, if the artery is compressed above the tumor; whereas the swelling caves in, and the pulsations cease, if compression is effected between the aneurism and the heart. What is most difficult, is, to distinguish a bubo from a scrofulous swelling; if we may give credence to Ricord's statement, inoculation affords in all such cases, in the absence of any other directing circumstances, the only sure diagnostic evidence of the true character of the tumor. Nevertheless, we will endeavor to show in the next paragraph that there are other means to establish, even in such dubious cases, a tolerably reliable diagnosis.

Sec. 64.—Differences between Scrofulous and Syphilitic Buboes.

One bubo might possibly be confounded with another, if the syphilitic bubo is without a sign of inflammation, and there are no circumstances present that might justify the suspicion of any syphilitic taint; in such a case a scrofulous bubo might easily be mistaken for a non-inflammatory syphilitic bubo, and vice versa; although, even in such a case, the appearance and course of the bubo, and other symptoms, may render the diagnosis comparatively easy to an attentive observer. For, in a case of scrofulous as well as of syphilitic bubo, we have to depend in our diagnosis upon a careful examination of the general phenomena characterizing the condition of the patient; the leading circumstances of the patient's childhood and youth, etc.; the presence of other glandular swellings that may denote the existence of a general scrofulous diathesis; and, on the other hand, upon an examination of the bubo itself, which, if scrofulous, progresses much less rapidly than the syphilitic bubo; scarcely ever invades the surrounding cellular tissue, preserves for a long time its mobility, and, instead of the elastic hardness of the syphilitic bubo, is soft to the feel, remains unchanged for a long period, and only involves the integuments little by little, which, in such a case, change to a violet-red color, without any perceptible signs of inflammation, and become thinner, until the tumor bursts and discharges a granulated, serous pus, thus becoming converted into a scrofulous ulcer. Such an ulcer, in regard to its slow course and obstinate character, has all the signs of a scrofulous sore; the surrounding skin is seldom red, generally livid; the subjacent cellular tissue is neither hard nor swollen, as in the syphilitic bubo. It is true that a scrofulous ulcer likewise often sends out fungous growths, and is of a whitish-gray color, on which account they may readily be assimilated to syphilitic ulcers. But, in the case of these last-named ulcers, the grayish-yellow, lardy appearance always depends upon the formation of a false membrane lining their surface, and which can easily be removed by rubbing; whereas, in the case of scrofulous ulcers, the grayish-yellow color adheres to the cellular tissue itself without showing a trace of false membrane. In the case of syphilitic buboes the destructive ulceration progresses very rapidly until it is arrested; whereas scrofulous ulceration remains at the same point, with the same characteristic signs, so that its course is not marked by two essentially distinct periods, like that of the syphilitic ulcerative process, namely, a substance-destroying and a substance-repairing period, or the period of adventitious growths. Moreover, in a scrofulous bubo, the ulcer is always seated on the surface of a more or less extensive tumor, formed by swollen and very hard ganglia; whereas the ulcer of the syphilitic bubo always rests upon the cellular tissue, and, of itself, neither induces hypertrophy nor induration of the inguinal ganglia. There are cases where the scrofulous and syphilitic miasms are united in one bubo. In such a case we first notice a simple inguinal swelling, without any enlargement of the glands; this thickening or enlargement occurs at a later period, increases more or less rapidly, and imparts to the tumor an irregular shape, while the sore remains fistulous and ulcerated, the vivid redness of the skin, with the earlier symptoms of inflammation, disappears, and only the livid color of the evidently scrofulous bubo remains behind.

Sec. 65.—Prognosis and Terminations.

With a correct, homœopathic treatment the prognosis is never unfavorable, although, if the swelling has already progressed to a certain size before the physician is applied to, cases may occur under homœopathic treatment where neither the bursting of the tumor, nor the supervention of gangrene, which, however, is not of itself the most dangerous symptom, can be prevented. It is the buboes consequent upon superficial or simple chancres that most readily terminate in suppuration, whereas the most deep-seated buboes, or those that succeed the Hunterian chancre, incline to *induration*. Suppuration rarely takes place without the cellular tissue, which surrounds the glands, becoming previously involved in the destructive process; and, vice versa, the near approach of suppuration must be apprehended, if the skin on the glandular tumor, that had been free and movable heretofore, and the subjacent tissue, become firmly adhering. Where the prognosis is most dubious, is in the case of buboes consequent upon phagedænic chancre; for the consecutive ulcers are very apt to assume the same character. If this should happen, the ulcer invades with more or less rapidity a considerable portion of the surrounding tissues. This fungous ulcer, which is lined with a copious exudation of a grayish, papescent matter, may preserve its peculiar appearance and its infectious power for years, provided its syphilitic nature, after a shorter or longer period of time, does not undergo an essential alteration, as may readily occur with scrofulous individuals; in consequence of which the destructive ulceration ceases to spread, becomes circumscribed, and even shows some inclination to cicatrize. In the case of scrofulous individuals this cicatrization, provided there is no mismanagement, may continue more or less rapidly, until the wound is closed; if the treatment, however, is improperly conducted, or if the scrofulous diathesis is more or less manifest, the syphilitic virus may become active again before the process of cicatrization is completed; the wound breaks open again, enlarges, spreads over the surrounding tissues, and frequently covers a considerable surface of the abdomen and thighs. This ulcer is, moreover, the worst of all, for, by dipping down to the subjacent textures, it may pierce through the abdominal integuments to the peritoneum, which it may inflame, and thus cause the patient's death. Buboes, if not healed from within, but when made to cicatrize by external artificial means, may, like chancre when not radically healed but suppressed by cauterization, superinduce a general secondary syphilis, for the reason that buboes constitute, properly speaking, a vicarious manifestation of the syphilitic disease in the place of chancre. As regards the assertions of some authors that the supervention of gangrene causes a complete extinction of the syphilitic process by the destruction of all the affected parts, I confess that, for lack of experience, I have no opinion on this subject; moreover, it is my opinion that it is extremely difficult to collect valid observations on this point, unless we have a chance of watching the patient for years.

Sec. 66.—Treatment of Buboes.

It must be evident from what we have said, that a bubo should, no more than a chancre, be treated with cauterizing or desiccating agents, if we desire to avoid the danger of seeing secondary constitutional syphilis break out in its place. The only external application that can be permitted are warm poultices, in case the pain caused by the inflammation becomes intolerable. Even poultices must only be applied in a case of urgent necessity, after it has become evident that suppuration can no longer be prevented. If applied prematurely, they may hasten the bursting of the tumor, which might perhaps have been prevented by the use of judiciously selected agents. Taking all these points for granted, the following is my mode of treating a bubo:

1) If, during a chancre, glandular swellings in the groin supervene, I leave these unheeded, because I am satisfied that these swellings, if the chancre is healed by truly rational means, always get well of themselves.

2) On the contrary, if, during the treatment of chancre, a real, inflammatory bubo develops itself, or, which occurs much more frequently, if I take charge of a patient who is at the same time afflicted with bubo and chancre, I resort to *Præc. ruber*, unless the patient had had a good deal of Mercury given to him by his allopathic attendant; or, if the precipitate should not be sufficient, I give *Cinnabaris*, both remedies with the same good result.

3) If these remedies are not sufficient to disperse the tumor; if the bubo threatens to suppurate, and the condition of the chancre does not demand any immediate, special treatment (which it seldom does under these circumstances); in such a case, I exhibit *Carbo animalis*, generally with the happiest result. This agent has rendered me more then once excellent service, even in cases where fluctuation had already set in; I prefer *Nitri ac.* to it only when this agent is likewise indicated by the fungous condition of the chancre.

4) If, when the patients come to me for treatment, the breaking of the buboes can no longer be prevented, or if they are already discharging, I institute the treatment which I have indicated for the different forms of chancre in §§ 54 and 55, being guided in the selection of the proper remedy by the character of the ulcer.

5) If the buboes develop themselves protopathically, or do

not make their appearance until the chancre has become cicatrized, I commence the treatment, in case fluctuation is not yet present, and the patient has not yet been drugged with Mercury, with *Merc. sol.*, or *red precipitate*, or *Cinnabaris;* but if the patient has already had Mercury, I give *Aurum*, *Nitri ac.*, or *Hepar sulp.* If fluctuation has already set in when I begin the treatment, I first resort to *Carbo animalis*, and, if this does not effect a speedy improvement, I change to *Nitri ac.*

6) Moreover, I prescribe in most cases: *a*) for *gangrened* buboes, Arsenicum; *b*) for old, *indurated* buboes, *Carbo an.*, *Hepar*, or perhaps *Sulphur; c*) for *suppurating buboes*, if, after the extinction of all syphilitic symptoms, the sore has become converted into a clean ulcer, but the secretion of pus still continues, and the wound does not close: *Silicea*, *Sulphur*, and sometimes *Hepar sulp.*

At the same time, I avoid, under all circumstances and at all times, the artificial opening of fluctuating buboes; I do not even allow the use of emollient poultices except when urgently required, and discontinue them at once as soon as the inflammatory pains have become more tolerable.

NOTE BY DR. HEMPEL.

[I fully agree with Jahr that buboes should not been opened prematurely, but if the abscess is fully matured, and there is no evidence that it will discharge voluntarily, I do not hesitate to make a free incision in order to secure a full and free escape of the pus. It has happened that in cases where the abscess was allowed to take its own course, the pus has burrowed downwards, behind the fascia, in consequence of which untoward circumstance, the patient may remain crippled for life. Whatever Jahr may advise to the contrary, I can affirm from abundant experience that the *Biniodide of Mercury*, first or second decimal trituration, is a very efficacious remedy for chancre and bubo; a solution of thirty grains of the *Iodide of Potassium* in eight ounces of water, to which half an ounce of the tincture of Iodine may be added, will likewise be found very useful; I give a dessert spoonful of this solution three times a day. In obstinate cases, I sometimes paint the bubo with the tincture of Iodine; this will either facilitate resorption, or, if resorption is no longer possible, it will hasten the suppurating process.]

Sec. 67.—Observations by other Physicians.

These are not very numerous, but perhaps so much more important.

1) Hahnemann. Hahnemann likewise, like many other homœopaths, particularly Gross, Hofrichter, and Rosenberg, believes in the existence of idiopathic buboes, that manifest themselves without any previous chancre, but, beside *Mercurius*, he does not propose any other remedy for the treatment of these tumors, although, as I know from himself, he likewise employed *Aurum*, *Nitri ac.*, and *Carbo animalis.*

2) Attomyr (in his essay on the different forms of chancre) is of the same opinion as the above-named physicians; he relates two cases, one of which he cured with *Nitri ac.* and *Sulphur*, and the other with *Nitri ac.* alone. During the inflammatory stage, he proposes *Merc. sol.* and *Nitri ac.*, and for the suppuration, after the bubo has begun to discharge, *Sulphur* and *Silicea.* This practitioner likewise confirms the statement that, if buboes break under homœopathic treatment, they discharge without any untoward circumstances.

3) Buchner (Hygea, vol. 13) pleads against the opening of buboes, either by the knife or cauterizing agents; he likewise asserts that, if the body is kept in a state of quietude, *Acidum nitricum* will almost always prevent suppuration, and induce a dispersion of the tumor.

4) Gaspary (Vehsem. Jahrb. vol. 4) praises *Carbo an.* as one of the most efficient means by which the resorption of the bubo can be effected, even after fluctuation has fairly set in, without, however, affecting either the gonorrhœa or chancre; a cure is generally accomplished in three to five, or at the latest in eight days. I am able to confirm the correctness of these remarks from my own extensive experience.

5) Hofrichter (All. hom. Zeit., vol. 35) has seen buboes arise after the suppression of figwarts by external means. Under certain circumstances, this may undoubtedly be the case. He too, next to the *red precipitate*, regards *Nitri ac.* as the chief remedy;

it seems to me, however, that Hofrichter confounds the fungous, condylomatous chancres with figwarts, since he adds that "latterly the chancres show an uncommon tendency to run into condylomata, that is to say, not to dip down to the subjacent textures, but to grow upwards."

6) SOMMER (All. hom. Zeit., vol. 38) regards *Hepar* as one of the chief remedies, if, after the healing of the chancre (most likely "with *Mercurius*"), the bubo has not yet broke, and no fluctuation is perceived; and, if the bubo has begun to discharge, or heals too slowly, he recommends *Silicea;* in my opinion, however, this agent will only help, if all the signs of a syphilitic taint have entirely disappeared.

7) TRINKS and VEHSEMEYER likewise recommend *Nitric ac.* as the chief remedy for buboes, without, however, stating in what stages or under what circumstances.

8) WAHLE (All. hom. Zeit., vol. 15) is certainly mistaken, as will be admitted by all practitioners who have had any opportunities of treating syphilitic diseases, when he expresses the opinion that buboes are not of a syphilitic but of an *herpetic* or *psoric* nature; that patients of this kind "infect by their breath," and that not *Mercurius*, but *Sulphur* is the specific remedy. It is true that *Sulphur* may have to be given, if, after the complete cure of syphilis, the buboes still continue to suppurate, and cicatrization proceeds too slowly; but, if syphilitic symptoms are still present, Sulphur will never be sufficient.

If my memory does not deceive me, I have read somewhere that Gross (the elder) has been in the habit of recommending *Aurum* and *Carbo an.* for buboes at a very early period, both idiopathic and consecutive; this recommendation had been known to me for years before I became acquainted with Gaspary's recommendation in "Vehsemeyer's Jahrbüchern."

II. MUCOUS TUBERCLES, OR MUCOUS CONDYLOMATA.

Sec. 68.—Description.

This morbid product, first described by French authors as a sign of *primary* syphilis, is to be carefully distinguished from so-called *pustulous* syphilides, but likewise from chancre and figwarts; it is a syphilitic product which generally shows itself from six to eight days, or even a fortnight or four weeks after an impure coït. It consists in a few moist, broad, flat, and rounded tubercles which, though not usually very numerous, originate in a morbid development of the skin or mucous membrane of the affected part. They occur most frequently on the inside of the labia majora, on the glans, in the region of the anus, on the breasts of women who nurse syphilitic infants, and sometimes, if the infection had been communicated by local contact, on the outer side of the labia majora, on the integuments of the penis, scrotum, perineum, and on the inner surface of the thighs. They are generally of a more or less dark-red color, from three to six lines in diameter, of a rounded form, *flat* on their surface, incline to form groups of two or three, without, however, always becoming confluent, and secrete a *glutinous, slimy matter*, having a specific odor that reveals their true nature to any one who has experienced this odor once. Most frequently they are seen on females, and on persons who do not keep themselves clean. Sometimes, however, these tubercles unite by their edges, in which case they form rather broad disks, with borders that rise abruptly over the surrounding skin or mucous membrane to a height of one or two lines. Their surface is generally rough, granular, even deeply furrowed, and not unfrequently, like most other syphilitic products, they are surrounded by a red or more or less copper-colored areola, especially when they are seated on the external skin, in which case the redness is much less distinct, whereas those that are seated on the mucous membrane, exhibit a much more vivid redness. It is only now and then that they are quite dry, without any secretion; sometimes their usually smooth surface may become slightly roughened by ulceration, so that they assume the appearance of chancre, and might readily be confounded with the ulcus elevatum, if their base had not an entirely different look from that of chancre. Not unfrequently they break out on women in the course of gonorrhœa, or some other dubious discharge, or on men while affected with chancre; but in many cases they come all of a sudden, without any sign of previous chancre or other syphilitic symptoms, whereas in other cases they only show themselves months after the first primary signs of infection had been discovered. If badly managed, or when left to themselves, their disappearance from their original locality, or even while they still remain visible, may, as in the case of chancre, give rise to buboes and to all the symptoms of constitutional syphilis.

Sec. 69.—Nature of these Tubercles.

Writers on syphilis have not yet agreed whether these products are manifestations of primary or secondary syphilis. Ricord, who knows of no higher criterion to verify the syphilitic character of a dubious eruption than inoculation, contends that these tubercles belong to the domain of secondary syphilis, for the reason that he has never been able to produce, by means of them, the least symptom of infection; hence he denies their contagious nature. Others, on the contrary, like Baumès and Reynaud, have shown by a number of observations that, even if these tubercles cannot be inoculated, yet they can be communicated by sexual connection, with this difference, that a chancre may indeed communicate a mucous tubercle, but a mucous tubercle can never produce a chancre, but only a tubercle of a like character; this would demonstrate, on the one hand, that they may break out as primary phenomena, and, on the other hand, that their derivation from chancre would be evidence in favor of their character as idiopathic and protopathic products. Whether such tubercles are always *primary*, and not as frequently, or perhaps more frequently, *secondary* products, is another question which it may not always be easy to solve. All existing observations seem to show that they have not only appeared without any previous signs of syphilis, but likewise after a chancre had been healed, and that consequently they may be of a *twofold* order; provided always that, notwithstanding they break out after the appearance of the chancre, and, for this reason, cannot be regarded as absolutely *primary* phenomena, they may, like buboes, continue to appertain to the *primary period* of syphilis; this fact is, indeed, proven by their capacity to transmit the infection. At the same time, the fact that they are of a syphilitic nature, and are not produced by the virus of gonorrhœa but by that of chancre, is not only proven by the circumstance that their violent removal by external means is often succeeded by an outbreak of all the symptoms of constitutional syphilis, but likewise by this other circumstance, that, if these tubercles appear on women together with a discharge, this discharge scarcely ever communicates gonorrhœa to the male, but *mucous tubercles*, at most associated with *balanorrhœa.* These discharges which, in females, are so easily confounded with gonorrhœa, but result altogether from the contact with syphilitic secretions, most likely constitute the larger number of the cases where a supposed so-called simple gonorrhœa has not only produced on males chancre-like products, but likewise, in the case of women, all sorts of phenomena of secondary syphilis after a shorter or longer period. According to some authors, these mucous tubercles are even more contagious than chancre. Reynaud asserts that they occasion exceedingly chronic blennorrhœas from the sexual organs of females, which continue even after the tubercles have disappeared, and constitute the larger number of those infectious blennorrhœas and balanorrhœas where a careful inquiry into the history of the case, and an examination of the sexual organs, does not reveal the least trace of gonorrhœal or syphilitic infection. (Compare §§ 14, 15, 16, 17). It is probably from such like gonorrhœas that the phenomena, by means of which Ritter has constructed his *lues* gonorrhœica, have resulted.

Sec. 70.—Differences between the tubercles according to their locality.

We have already stated above that these tubercles occur more frequently among females than males. Among tubercles which occur on other parts than the sexual organs, there prevail different forms, so that, in order to facilitate a knowledge and recognition thereof, we deem it proper to add a few remarks. According to the observations instituted by Dr. Davasse, of Paris, they exhibit the following different shapes:

1. *In the Mouth.*—In the mouth they are seen most frequently on the inside of the borders of the lips, or on the inside of the cheeks. On the borders of the lips they generally assume the shape of projecting, somewhat flattened elevations, are almost always oval, rather small, more or less numerous, always single,

grayish or rose-colored, rarely moist, sometimes covered with thin scurfs, and exhibiting trifling, ulcerated cracks. They are not very persistent, frequently disappear as rapidly as they return, and are very often associated with similar symptoms in the throat or on the sexual organs. In the corners of the mouth they generally exhibit the same characteristics; here they are frequently mistaken for ordinary rhagades. On the inside of the cheeks they likewise have the same appearance; but on the tongue, where they break out at one time at the tip, at another at the edges, and then again at the root of this organ, they most frequently resemble the tubercles that break out on the pudendum, are oval or rounded, rather large, of a grayish or dirty-red color, frequently ulcerate, and in general exhibit all the symptoms that we have described (§ 68).

2. *In the Throat.*—Here they are most frequently seated on the velum or tonsils, in which case they frequently constitute an affection described under the name of *syphilitic angina.* In the throat they generally appear in the shape of small, round elevations, which are at times broad, at other times small, and sometimes very numerous or even confluent, having a whitish-gray color. At the same time the tonsils may be somewhat swollen or red, the tubercles may be eaten into, giving rise to deep syphilitic ulcers, whereas in other cases all signs of ulceration may be wanting. At the same time the throat is generally affected in other ways; for instance, there is pain during deglutition, and more particularly a peculiar huskiness or loss of voice, known as syphilitic. These tubercles in the throat are very frequently accompanied by chancres on the sexual organs, more particularly indurated chancres.

3. *On the Nose.*—Here they may be seated on the nose as well as in the interior of this organ, at the entrance of the nostrils. In the former case they generally break out in the outer angle of the alæ nasi, where they exhibit almost the same characteristics as when seated on the lips, except that they are smaller and frequently not much larger than a pin's head. Most generally they appear in clusters of two or three, of a granular surface, and frequently forming an excoriation in the angle between the cheek and ala nasi. When located in the nostrils, they generally occupy

the entrance, where they form an annular crust, which, when falling off, exhibits a grayish-red base that soon after is covered again with new crusts. These nasal tubercles are always accompanied by syphilitic appearances on the sexual organs; very frequently they break out simultaneously with these latter as primary phenomena.

4. *On the Toes.*—Here they may show themselves at the commencement of the toes as well as on the nails. Being almost always ulcerated, they resemble most frequently the rhagades at the anus. Their elevated portion is of a violet-red color; between the toes they are rounded, on the nails oblong, surrounding the root of the nail and forming irregular cracks, whose fungous borders cover the nail more or less, while the livid, grayish-red base secretes a profuse quantity of a very fetid, purulent ichor. As a rule these ulcers likewise break out while the sexual organs are still affected by disease.

5. *Upon the Skin.*—Here they are principally seen on the nipples of the mammæ, on the ears, cheeks, chin, the inguinal region, and the umbilicus; in the case of infants with congenital syphilis, they are spread over the whole body.

Sec. 71.—Diagnosis.

This is generally not very difficult, especially if other syphilitic symptoms are present on the sexual organs. The only appearances with which they might possibly be confounded, are the elevated chancre, figwarts, mercurial ulcers, and, at the anus, with ulcerated hæmorrhoids or hæmorrhoidal rhagades. From the elevated chancre, and from figwarts, they will readily be distinguished by any one who has read our description of both these appearances in §§ 37, 68, and 73. It is likewise impossible to confound them with mercurial ulcers, even when these are seated in the mouth and fauces; for these ulcers are never raised, but always flat, generally spreading over an extensive surface, and always of a milky-white appearance. As regards hæmorrhoidal ulcers or rhagades, they are always of a more or less violet-red color, never flattened, but always globular, elastic and not resisting to the feel. But it is more difficult to distinguish these tubercles from an old, neglected or mismanaged, ordinary, simple chancre, for the reason that a mucous tubercle, if it occurs singly, very frequently resembles a chancre in the stage of fungous growth. It is true that, in most of these cases, the remnants of the sharply-circumscribed edges of the chancre can be readily distinguished from the less sharply-circumscribed border and base of these tubercles; but chancres which, like syphilitic erosions, have remained superficial, and which afterwards become suddenly raised, or exhibit marked granulations, very frequently bear a very close external resemblance to these tubercles. Ricord's assertion that we may always be sure of having to deal with an old chancre, if a patient who had no previous syphilitic symptoms about him, presents himself for treatment after having become infected with one or two such tubercles that had broken out at the spot where chancres are in the habit of making their appearance, may be perfectly correct in most instances, but not by any means in all. I have seen two such tubercles on a young mechanic—one on the frænulum, the other on the inner surface of the prepuce—three days after they had broken out all at once, which I certainly should have mistaken for old chancres in the period of fungous reproduction, if I had not been well acquainted with the patient, who was in the habit of consulting me for the smallest trifles, and would not have allowed a chancre to reach this period without coming to me for treatment. No other symptoms of either primary or secondary syphilis could be discovered in this case; but the girl who had infected him, and who did not keep herself very clean, had a number of such tubercles on the inside of the labia majora and at the anus. On the other hand, it is undoubtedly correct that these mucous tubercles generally break out on different parts at once, in greater or less quantity; in a case of chancre this never takes place in the same manner.

Sec. 72.—Treatment.

If old-school physicians assert that nothing is easier than to cure these tubercles, since they yield very readily to appropriate external applications, their assertion is undoubtedly correct, provided we understand by the term "cure," a simple removal of these tubercles from the skin by external means. But if we consider that a mere external suppression may superinduce all the symptoms of constitutional syphilis, and that a cure implies not only their suppression, but a complete annihilation of the internal syphilitic disease, we may be willing to admit that the healing of such tubercles is attended with the same greater or less difficulties as that of any other form of primary syphilis. If there ever was a case of syphilis, where it is of the utmost importance to heal the disease with internal means, it is mucous tubercles. These tubercles, like buboes, appertain to a period of development of the syphilitic disease (as we shall show in the second division of this work, § 79, etc.) where they still constitute a primary form of syphilis, although the whole organism may already be tainted, and where they may lead to *consecutive*, but not strictly speaking *secondary*, phenomena; inasmuch as the contagious virus is not yet, as in the secondary period, chemically combined with the fluids of the body (for this is evident from the fact that its products are still possessed of a capacity to transmit the disease), but still exists in a state of freedom, and hence is much more readily excreted than at a later period. However, inasmuch as the period when tubercles make their appearance already constitutes a transition-period, *Mercurius*, which is a chief remedy even in this period, particularly *Merc. subl.* and *Cinnabaris*, may not always be sufficient, but has frequently to be replaced, or assisted in its action, by other agents, such as *Nitri. ac.* and *Thuja*, which will always prove curative, as I have seen in a number of cases, as long as no real symptoms of secondary syphilis have yet made their appearance. In these last-mentioned cases, of which, until now, I have only seen one with simultaneous Corona veneris, and where the tubercles were seated on the tonsils, inducing a sort of angina syphilitica, other remedies may have to be resorted to. In the case I have just alluded to, neither *Merc.*, nor *Nitri. ac.*, nor *Thuja* proved of any avail; *Lycopodium* effected a cure. It is strange that, in our own literature, not a single case of these tubercles should as yet be mentioned. Have they been confounded with chancres; or, as in Hartmann's Therapeutics, with figwarts; or do they occur less frequently in Germany than in France? Attomyr's description of his second form of chancre, which he cures with Nitri. ac. (see his "Venerische Krankheiten," page 23), leads me to suspect the former; for his statements: "Ulcers *flat* and *raised; clean, flesh-colored*, almost *fungous* appearance, and simultaneous breaking out of several ulcers," may refer to numerous tubercles, rather than to the elevated ulcer. As for the rest, these tubercles occur much less frequently than chancre, buboes, and figwarts, perhaps, only in hospitals, where chancres are generally removed by ointments and cauterization. Indeed, most of those who come to me for treatment, when afflicted with such tubercles, are poor servant-girls, who leave the hospitals with all the symptoms of a badly-healed chancre still upon them. Thorer's cases (Arch. vol. XIII., part 3, pages 80–86) most likely belong to this same class of mucous tubercles.

III. SYCOSIC EXCRESCENCES.

Sec. 73.—Description.

Almost all recent French authors distinguish, after the fashion of Lagneau, two kinds of sycosic excrescences:

1) The *grafted* or *implanted* excrescences of greater density than that of the skin, to which they adhere by their base, a sort of pedicle; most of the sycosic products belong in this class under the name of *figwarts.*

2) *Hypertrophic excrescences:* these arise by a simples welling of the cellular tissue of a fold of the skin or mucous membrane, and ulcerate readily, after which they secrete a fetid, slimy pus.

The former of these two kinds occurs most frequently, has the most varied forms, and is much more numerous than the humid excrescences. As a general rule, they are seen on the mucous membrane of the genital organs, for instance, on the prepuce, glans, behind the corona, or on the side of the frenulum; sometimes in the orifice of the urethra; among females, we see them on the inside of the labia majora and minora, on the clitoris, around the orifice of the urethra, at the inferior commissure, on the lesser papillæ, and even around the os tincæ. They are even not unfrequently seen on the margin of the anus, even in the rectum; in some cases they are even seen on the nipples of women, who have been infected by nursing syphilitic infants, on the perineum, on the outer side of the labia majora, on the mons veneris, the inside of the thighs, in the groin, and on the navel of new-born infants. They may even break out on the tongue, velum palati, and eyelids. Generally they are much smaller than the humid excrescences, but occur very frequently in large quantities on the same spot, forming considerable fungous masses. As regards their forms, they sometimes are shaped like *cauliflowers*, sometimes like *warts*, sometimes like long *stems* (they have been known to shoot up from behind the corona glandis to the height of two inches, like goose-quills, becoming erect when the prepuce is drawn back, and, when the prepuce is brought forward again, reclining over the glans like flexible, vegetable stems); and sometimes like *raspberries*, more especially among women, on the clitoris, or round the orifice of the urethra, etc. Their color likewise varies. The wart-shaped excrescences are generally paler than the surrounding skin; those with long pedicles are generally a little redder; the cauliflower and raspberry-shaped excrescences, having frequently a good deal of blood, have likewise the most redness. In general, all these varieties are very dry, except the cauliflower variety, which generally excrete an exceedingly copious, yellowish, and sometimes bloody moisture. If neither irritated by friction nor by acrid substances, all these varieties are very seldom painful; the cauliflower and raspberry-shaped excrescences are the most sensitive.

The excrescences of the second class, which, as has already been stated, arise from a tumefaction of the cellular tissue of a fold of the skin, and among which we number the fig-shaped condylomata, and those that are shaped like the articular head of a bone, occur most frequently in the region of the anus, but often likewise at the entrance of the vagina, on the labia majora or minora, on the penis between the prepuce and glans, sometimes even on the perineum, and on the inner surface of the thighs. These condylomata are generally more or less oblong, flattened tubercles, whose free margin is rounded, except when these excrescences are already seated upon an already round elevation, such as old piles, in which case they are attached to a more or less elongated pedicle. They are very seldom of a large size, although some authors assert that they have seen condylomata of the size of a hand, weighing several pounds. From these condylomata, those that are shaped like a cock's crest are distinguished by this circumstance, that the latter are elevated on the skin with an indented border, and flat like the blade of a knife. Both forms are generally of a hard, almost cartilaginous consistence, and not very painful; at the same time they are very red, easily excoriated, in which case they excrete a very fetid, slimy, more or less acrid matter of a yellowish color.

Sec. 74.—Nature of these Excrescences.

Among all venereal phenomena there is scarcely any whose nosological nature has given rise to so many arguments, and has, nevertheless, been explained with so little satisfaction, as these excrescences. For, while Hahnemann and several authors of the Old School contend that these excrescences arise from a miasm that is neither the miasm of gonorrhœa nor that of chancre, other authors, on the contrary, regard them either as products of the virus of gonorrhœa or that of chancre, without, however, agreeing whether they ought to be attributed to the former or to the latter, or whether they constitute primary or secondary symptoms of syphilis. In view of these differences of opinion, our reasonable readers will not expect at our hands an authoritative settlement of the dispute. All we can do is to exhibit in the clearest light all the facts that have been well substantiated so far, namely:—

1) Whatever may be said concerning the *syphilitic* or *idiopathically sycosic* nature of these excrescences, they are at all events *venereal*, that is, products arising sooner or later from venereal infection, either as *protopathic* or *consecutive* phenomena, and capable of transmitting a similar disease during the act of coït.

2) They may occur during, or at the termination of a gonorrhœa, or they may break out before any symptoms of gonorrhœa have set in; in the same way as we see them appear during or after a chancre, even a long time after the chancre has disappeared, in company with a variety of other consecutive affections.

The form of these growths is immaterial, although those which occur during the fungous period of a chancre, generally belong to the second variety, the *hypertrophic*. This might lead us to regard this form as a positively *syphilitic* product, resulting from the action of chancre-virus, so much more as in more that one respect they resemble mucous tubercles, from which they are often distinguished only, especially when in a state of ulceration, by their greater, characteristic, *cartilaginous hardness*, which reminds one of the Hunterian chancre. Be this as it may, these excrescences occur after chancres as well as after gonorrhœas; if they communicate the infection, this never develops chancre but either similar excrescences or gonorrhœa, in which case the only question is whether this gonorrhœa is to be considered as an idiopathic, sycosic discharge, or whether this discharge is identical with one of the two classes of gonorrhœa that have been mentioned, §§ 15 to 17, the *common clap* or the *syphilitic gonorrhœa*. If we consider that both the chancre-virus as well as the gonorrhœal poison can produce excrescences, and that, where gonorrhœa is followed by this phenomenon, it, as frequently as chancre, is followed by all the symptoms of secondary syphilis, we are inclined to believe that a gonorrhœa resulting from such a cause is nothing else than the syphilitic gonorrhœa, described §§ 15 to 17, differing greatly from the common clap, and where the chancre-virus appears indeed modified, but ought nevertheless to be regarded as the source of these phenomena.

Sec. 75.—Diagnosis.

Upon the whole this is not very difficult, particularly as regards a differential diagnosis of the two kinds of excrescences mentioned in § 73. They are likewise readily distinguished from other syphilitic products, inasmuch as the only phenomena with which they might be confounded, and indeed have been confounded by some (by Hartmann in his Therapeutics), or have been ranged in the same class, are *mucous tubercles*, whose want of cartilaginous hardness, however, distinguishes this product as one that does not belong to the class of which we are speaking. There might perhaps be some difficulty in distinguishing these from non-syphilitic, so to say, purely mechanical formations. Lagneau is perfectly correct in observing that on the same spots which are generally the seat of these excrescences, similar growths may make their appearance that cannot be attributed to venereal infection. This may happen in the case of pregnant females, for instance, upon whose sexual organs small wart-shaped elevations are sometimes noticed, that arise from no other cause than from the pressure of the child upon the rim of the pelvis, and from the varices which this pressure gives rise to in the capillary system; or which varices may likewise arise after forced marches, frequent frictions during sexual intercourse, or any other more or less continued pressure upon the sexual organs. These last-mentioned appearances, however, occur very rarely, but had to be mentioned, in order not to omit any thing that might possibly resemble, and be mistaken for, sycosic growths; on which account the physician will do well, if other syphilitic symptoms should be present, or venereal affections have existed some time previous, or in all cases where venereal taint may be suspected, not to allow himself to be led into error by the supposition that the suspected products may possibly have been occasioned by some harmless cause, and not to entertain any doubt, except in cases where the previous history of the case, and the present circumstances surrounding it, do not reveal the least sign of a syphilitic taint, and where the whole aspect of these growths is entirely different from what it would be, if they had originated in venereal poisoning. Another circumstance which cannot be sufficiently impressed upon the attention of the physician, is the shape that these growths assume when they are neglected and continue to spread. In such a case they sometimes cover the whole glans; if, at the same time, they should become ulcerated, the whole mass contracts such a horridly-repulsive appearance that one might be tempted to regard them as carcinoma of the glans or prepuce. Nevertheless all doubt regarding the sycosic nature of the excrescence may be removed in a case of this kind, not only by an inquiry into the history of the case and by the accompanying circumstances, but likewise by a consideration of the fact that carcinoma of the glans and prepuce are very rare occurrences that generally befal only old people. Of course, our conclusions will undoubtedly be corroborated by a more particular examination of the phenomena exhibited to our view.

Sec. 76.—Prognosis.

If these excrescences are considered by themselves, independently of their primary cause, we shall very readily be led to the conclusion that their cure is comparatively easy; for in many cases they are even removed by the scissors, and yet do not break out again so very readily. On the other hand, there are many cases of such excrescences, where, if left to themselves, they remain unchanged for years, or, if removed by artificial means, break out again, except that they increase in volume, especially on the penis and at the anus, where they often attain a considerable size, and sometimes form the most hideous ulcers; in addition to which, by virtue of their inherent faculty of growth, they repair the waste of substance consequent upon the ulcerative process, and by this means frequently occasion the destruction of a considerable portion of the penis. Even with regard to the accessory affections which these excrescences may engender, their prognosis is not very dubious, inasmuch as they may sometimes, when no other syphilitic ulcers are present, and they are otherwise accompanied by violent inflammation, occasion a slight sympathetic swelling of the inguinal glands, but never true buboes in the more rigorous meaning of the term, neither phimosis nor paraphimosis. It is only when the figwarts are very large and numerous, suppurate profusely, and the patient's mind is very much depressed, the vital functions may become disturbed, and the patient may lapse into a sort of marasmus, such as takes place in consequence of cancerous ulcers, and which, unless the excrescences are healed, must render the prognosis more dubious. At the same time, we should never forget that these excrescences, no matter whether they occur primarily or secondarily, never constitute the disease itself, but that they are always symptoms of a more general constitutional diathesis, superinduced by the action of some infectious virus (gonorrhœa, chancre, or sycosis), and which has to be extirpated. With reference to this task, we have a right to declare that there is probably no form of syphilis which is more difficult to reach by internal treatment than these excrescences, which sometimes remain, even after all other syphilitic symptoms have been removed, with all the obstinacy of indolent cicatrices of chancres that had been healed long ago. In such cases, these remaining figwarts may be nothing more than remnants of the disorganizations caused by the action of the syphilitic virus, which no internal remedy can heal, any more than the cicatrices of old wounds can be wiped away by internal treatment. Admitting, however, that these remnants can be healed, it can only be done where, after the extinction of every syphilitic symptom, the figwarts themselves are deprived of every sign of morbid activity.

Sec. 77.—Treatment.

It must be evident from what has been said, that, where figwarts are to be radically cured, a mere external treatment will prove insufficient, as long as other symptoms of the syphilitic disease are still present, or the excrescences are still painful, continue to grow, spread, and suppurate, in one word, still continue to manifest symptoms of morbid activity. When Hahnemann advised, even in the most inveterate and long-standing cases, to touch the figwarts with the extract of *Thuja*, he undoubtedly meant no other cases than those which we have described; with the exception of these obdurate cases, the cure of figwarts, by homœopathic remedies, is not by any means as difficult as those, who do not keep in view the difference between active figwarts and the remnants of a defunct syphilis, imagine. In my own practice, I have derived the greatest advantage, in cases where the figwarts were complicated with chancre, from the use of *Cinnabaris* and *Nitri ac.*, and sometimes from the use of *Phosph. ac.*, or *Staphysagria;* whereas, when these excrescences were complicated with gonorrhœa, I have derived the most benefit from *Thuja*, sometimes from *Merc. corr.*, likewise from *Cinnabaris* and *Nitri ac.*, even from *Sulphur* and *Lycopodium*. In a case of humid condylomata, I prefer commencing the treatment with *Nitri ac.*, after which, if this remedy should not prove sufficient, I resort to *Thuja*. For *dry* excrescences, especially when of the cauliflower, mulberry-shaped variety, I at once administer *Thuja* or *Staphysagria;* for pedunculate condylomata, I first employ *Lycopodium*. In my experience, the locality of the ulcers has never seemed to have much to do with the selection of a remedy.

Other practitioners have employed the following remedies:

a) Acording to their forms:

for *broad*, flat, bean-shaped condylomata: Thuja, Nitri ac.;
for *elevated*, cauliflower, raspberry, mulberry-shaped: Thuja;
for *fan-shaped:* Cinnabaris;
for *pedunculate:* Lycop., Nitri ac.;
for *cone-shaped:* Merc. sol.;
for *dry:* Thuja, Merc. sol.; Corr. subl., Nitri ac., Lycop.;
for *moist*, suppurating: Nitri ac., Thuja, Sulphur, Euphrasia;
for *soft*, spongy: Sulphur.

b) According to their locality, when first manifesting themselves:

on the *glans*, or corona glandis: Nitri ac., Thuja, Cinnab., Lyc., Sulphur;

on the *prepuce:* Thuja, Nitri. ac., Lyc., Corr. subl.;
on the *scrotum:* Thuja.
at the *anus:* Thuja, Euphrasia, Corr. subl.
c) According to their origin, when first appearing:
after *chancres:* Thuja, Merc. sol., Staphys.;
after *gonorrhœa:* Thuja, Lycop., Cinnabaris.

Sec. 78.—Practical Observations by other Practitioners.

These are mixed up with a good many hypothetical speculations, to which we shall add our own observations.

1. HAHNEMANN.—If Hahnemann states in his "Chronic Diseases," that the suppression of the local symptom, the original figwart, is followed by other similar excrescences in other parts of the body—for instance, by "*whitish*, spongy, sensitive, *flat elevations* in the buccal cavity, on the tongue, palate, lips," etc.—he evidently means the *mucous tubercles*, which have been recently observed after chancres (see § 70); it would be interesting to know whether he had seen these tubercles, that are at the present time so frequently seen after chancres, break out in consequence of a sycosic gonorrhœa; if so, this would demonstrate the original identity of syphilis and sycosis in an almost irrefutable manner.

2. ATTOMYR (in his "Venereal Diseases") recommends *Thuja* for cauliflower-excrescences which at first are dry, and afterwards become humid. This distinction, between "*at first* and *afterwards*," affords, however, no indication for the selection of a remedy, inasmuch as Thuja cures both dry and moist figwarts.

3. HARTMANN (Therapeutics) is of opinion, and very correctly, that sycosis, although presenting peculiar characteristics, yet has its root in the syphilitic disease (see § 74). But if, in vol. II., page 167, he recommends *Nitri ac.* for a fungous, crusty "ulcer, with a dark-blue, greasy base, and having the appearance as if it had sprung from a boil," such an ulcer is more likely a chancre in the period of fungous reproduction, than a purely sycosic growth. As regards his statement concerning the curative power of *Sabina* for condylomata with intolerable burning and itching, or with abnormal granulations; concerning *Cinnabaris* and *Thuja* for condy-

lomata that had grown up from chancre; and concerning *Nitri ac.* for pin's-head-shaped condylomata (which are most likely the *mucous tubercles* described § 70), I am prepared to confirm all such statements from personal experience.

4. Hofrichter (All. hom. Zeit., vol. 35) is of opinion that chancre and figwarts spring from the same root, and in so far are identical; but, if he infers this identity from the circumstance that "chancres at the present period tend more to fungous growth than to dip down to the subjacent textures," he evidently commits an error in classing fungous chancres and sycosic excrescences, with which the former are not absolutely identical, in one and the same category; considering their structural differences, however, this is not admissible.

5. Rummel (All. hom. Zeit., vol. 18) very justly observes that *Thuja* heals most reliably the thick, red, humid, raspberry-shaped, but never the thread-like excrescences; he relates an important case, where, after a chancre had been treated by a homœopath for several weeks with large doses of Mercury, large figwarts made their appearance with suspicious-looking suppurating surfaces at the anus, for which *Staphysagria* proved speedily curative; at the same time it removed the burning, twitching, stinging pains that became intolerable during an alvine evacuation. On this occasion he warns against the obstinate use of mercurial preparations, especially in increased doses, if it has become evident, after using them for ten days or a fortnight, that they will not improve the case; for the aggravations resulting from such abuse he advises *Nitri ac.*, and sometimes *Sulphur*, as appropriate remedies.

6. Lobethal (All. hom. Zeit., vol. 13) considers sycosis and syphilis as identical; but he is mistaken in his assertion that figwarts can never break out without a previous chancre; this statement is refuted most positively by the observations of a number of writers on syphilis.

7. Thorer (Arch. 19) does not think that sycosis is identical with syphilis, for the reason that he has seen figwarts break out after chancres that had been cured with *Mercurius.* I have met with similar cases, but in all of them, as in the cases related by

Thorer, the chancre had already continued for several weeks, and the breaking out of the sycosic excrescences, which had been preparing all this time, could no longer be prevented in spite of the *Mercurius*, that does not heal every kind of chancre any more than it cures every form of figwarts. Moreover, according to what we have said before (§§ 68–71), it is not by any means sure whether the numerous ulcers on the female organs, of which the author makes mention in those cases, were not ulcerated tubercles rather than chancres, in which case it seems quite natural that *Mercurius* alone was not sufficient to remove products that had already the character of consecutive symptoms; but that other remedies were required to extirpate the syphilitic disease at this stage, as we have shown § 72.

8. Wahle (All. hom. Zeit., 15) admits that figwarts may partake of the nature of syphilis; but if he imagines that all chancres which, after having been unsuccessfully treated with *Mercurius*, pass into the period of fungous growth are no longer syphilitic, but of an herpetic, or scrofulous character—this theory has been refuted in thousands of cases by the fact that such chancres may be succeeded by the most loathsome and terrible destructions of the organic tissues.

NOTE BY DR. HEMPEL.

[One of the most important remedies in the treatment of sycosic excrescences, is *Tartar emetic.* The following case affords a remarkable illustration of the curative virtues of this agent in sycosis. The patient was a fine-looking young man, 25 years old. The first two-thirds of the penis, including the glans, were covered with an almost countless number of figwarts, of various shapes and sizes. After trying in vain all the usual remedies for figwarts, I prepared a solution of ten grains of Tartar emetic in four ounces of water, and directed him to bathe the figwarts with it, and to keep a compress, moistened with the solution, applied to the penis. At the same time I gave him the one-hundredth part of a grain of Tartar emetic, dissolved in eight ounces of water, to take internally, in tablespoonful doses every four hours. In two days the young man returned, and to my amazement this whole mass of figwarts, which had been treated by several allopathic physicians for over six months, had been completely melted, as it were. There was nothing left but a small quantity of moisture where each condyloma had stood, to which lint was applied for a few days, when the skin looked dry and healthy. Only one of these warts did not yield to Tartar emetic. It was removed without difficulty by means of Sabina, used externally and internally. I saw this patient about nine months after, when he still enjoyed the most perfect health.

In the case of female patients, the greatest care must be had when applying Tartar emetic to the sexual organs externally. Otherwise we may see the labia studded with vesicles, even after one application. What would a one-hundred-thousandth potentialist have done in the case of my young gentleman? Most likely he would have driven him to suicide. When this young man came to me, his spirits were profoundly depressed, and he told me that he could not bear life any longer.

A year ago I treated one of our young merchants for chancre, Hunterian variety. The cure seemed perfect. Six months after this event, he married a very excellent and refined young lady. About four months after his marriage, he came to me with his wife, informing me that she was diseased. An examination revealed three condylomata; two of them, mucous tubercles, seated on the edge of one of the labia majora, near the inferior commissure; and one, of the pedunculate variety, situated within the vulva. He pledged his word to me that, since his last mishap, he had kept clear of women, and that, when he married his wife, she was as pure as an angel in heaven. I examined him, and discovered a small condyloma under the head of the penis. He brushed it away with his fingers, after which it bled furiously. He could not tell me how long it had been there. Feeling confident that Thuja and Nitri ac. would cure the lady, I gave her these remedies in small doses, but without any effect whatsoever. I tried other remedies, without results. I then gave her *ten drops* of the extract, three times a day, and a cure was speedily accomplished.]

SECOND DIVISION.

THE SECONDARY FORMS

OF

SYPHILIS.

FIRST CHAPTER.

OF SECONDARY SYPHILIS GENERALLY.

I. GENERAL DEFINITION OF SECONDARY PHENOMENA.

Sec. 79.—Various Definitions.

On perusing the works of those who have written on the treatment and nature of venereal diseases, and upon examining the expressions of which most practitioners make use in designating the nature of single cases, we cannot help being amazed at the confusion which prevails, even to this day, in regard to the terms: *general, constitutional, and secondary phenomena*, etc. Not a few regard all these terms as *synonymous;* according to them, secondary syphilis begins at the moment when, after the appearance of the primary *protopathic* symptom (gonorrhœa, chancre, or figwart), some other consecutive phenomenon is superinduced as a pathological consequence of the former; whereas others maintain that the *consecutive* phenomena do not always, by any means, belong to the *secondary* period, since even general *constitutional* symptoms may really and truly constitute a *primary* malady. Hence the dispute what symptoms constitute *primary*, and what *secondary;* some even contending that not one syphilitic phenomenon is in truth either primary or secondary, but that everything depends upon the chronological order in which the symptoms appear, whether protopathically or consecutively, so that we may not only have *secondary buboes, mucous tubercles*, and *figwarts*, but likewise *secondary chancres* and *gonorrhœa.* This theoretic confusion may not deserve any consideration at the hands of homœopathic physicians, who are never guided in the selection of remedies by speculative categories, but by the totality of the existing symptoms; but since, in many cases, where the outlines of the symptoms are not delineated with sufficient clearness, we have to consider *the cause* in which an existing malady originates; and since all previous experience shows that one of us will reject remedies for secondary syphilis which another praises for the same malady; it is evidently of the utmost importance that we should, in the first place, clearly define our understanding of the term *secondary phenomena*. Hence, before we enumerate and describe secondary phenomena, we will endeavor to furnish a precise definition of this term, in order that our readers may be enabled to distinguish between symptoms that really deserve the appellation of secondary, and such as are improperly classed in this category.

Sec. 80.—Truly Secondary Phenomena.

If we survey the phenomena which, during the course of the gradually unfolding and progressing malady, may manifest themselves as consequences of the primary manifestation, from the first *protopathic* symptom (chancre, gonorrhœa, figwarts) to the remotest affections of bones, which sometimes do not break out till years after the first appearance of the disease; an attentive observer must become aware that, no matter at what period the secondary symptoms follow this first manifestation of the syphilitic disease, they can be ranged in two classes which, in a *nosological* point of view, are essentially distinct from each other. For while many of these symptoms show themselves already a few days after the suppression, or even during the presence of a chancre, or of some other protopathic product, without, however, being able to transmit themselves by infection or inoculation to other individuals; on the other hand, there are other symptoms belonging to this order, which, in spite of their apparently much more retarded appearance, still possess this faculty of transmitting their own virus, in an extraordinary degree, such as: *consecutive buboes*, *mucous tubercles*, and *figwarts*, which are just as contagious as protopathic products of the same kind. From these facts it is furthermore evident that, during the unfolding of the consequences of a protopathic symptom, a period must necessarily arise when the virus undergoes an essential modification in the organism, passing, as it does, from its original primary condition into a subsequent modified condition, which, occurring subsequently to the former, may be justly regarded as *secondary*. It is not only with regard to single phenomena (such as ulcerated and fungoid chancres, etc.), but likewise with regard to the course of the whole *syphilitic disease*, that we distinguish a first or primary, and a second or secondary stage, whose respective phenomena, the products of two essentially distinct modes of action of the infectious virus, must not be confounded with each other. If, in accordance with what a rigorous scientific logic would seem to demand, we limit the term "*secondary* phenomena" to those sequelæ of the original symptom which appertain exclusively to the *second* of those two periods; and if, from a similar reason, we designate as "*primary*" phenomena, those that exhibit the characteristic signs of the former of those periods; it is evident that a phenomenon may be *consecutive*, without being on that account *secondary*, and that these two series of phenomena may differ from each other in all their essential properties. For this reason, and in order to avoid all confusion of ideas, all deep-thinking, and logically-discriminating physicians have limited the term "consecutive" phenomena to the designation of products which, although occurring subsequently to the protopathic manifestations of the syphilitic disease, yet continue to show all the diagnostic signs of the *primary* period of this disease. In the third division of this work, where we shall enter upon a survey of the whole course of syphilis, we shall see that this division is founded in the nature of things, and rigorously justifiable from a scientific point of view; for the present it may suffice, that we should declare our adhesion to this general classification into *primary* and *secondary* phenomena, and that, by "secondary," we never understand the simply consecutive symptoms of the primary period, but always the phenomena of the *second* period, which are no longer capable, owing to some essential modification of the nature of the contagium, of transmitting the syphilitic disease by direct infection of the individual.

Sec. 81.—Boundaries of the Secondary Phenomena.

When asking the question what constitute more particularly secondary phenomena, it is at once evident that *buboes*, *mucous tubercles*, and *sycosic condylomata*, being still endowed with the faculty of communicating the primary disease, cannot be classed among secondary phenomena. This point being conceded, another no less important question arises for our consideration; by what specific signs do we recognize the *secondary* character of a syphilitic product, and its consequent inability to transmit the disease, independently of all sexual connection and experiments by inoculation? Some have sought to determine this question by the greater or less extent of the simultaneous manifestations of syphilitic phenomena, and, for this reason, have seen secondary syphilis wherever these phenomena did no longer show themselves at the original site of the malady, but appeared more or less diffused in other localities, in consequence of which the terms "general" and "secondary" were considered synonymous. That they are not always synonymous, is evident from the fact that among the syphilitic phenomena, more particularly among the mucous tubercles and figwarts, many of them, even when protopathic manifestations, show themselves in localities more or less remote from the original site of infection, without having ceased, on that account, to be any thing else than products of the primary period of syphilis, and without having lost their power of transmitting the original disease. It is true that such general phenomena, appertaining as they do to the second stage of the primary period, constitute a sort of transition-stage to the secondary morbid process, where the virus no longer produces chancres, but transition-forms; but inasmuch as these forms, more especially buboes, tubercles, and figwarts, are still capable of pepetuating themselves by the act of coïtion, they cannot, even if scattered over the whole surface of the body, properly be considered as *secondary*, and hence the terms "*general*" and "*secondary*" syphilis cannot be considered as synonymous. The fact, however, is, that where there are secondary phenomena, the affection is always general; but not the reverse, that, where the affection is general, there are always secondary phenomena. A similar, only opposite difference takes place with reference to *constitutional* syphilis. Where the syphilis is constitutional, secondary phenomena will always be present; but the first manifestation of secondary phenomena is not necessarily always accompanied by a complete infection of the whole constitution with the syphilitic disease. Thus it is that secondary phenomena are not only distinguished from the simple consecutive phenomena of the second stage of the primary period, but likewise, to a certain extent, from those which constitute the general and constitutional syphilis; hence again, we class among secondary phenomena those that NEVER occur as primary PROTOPATHIC symptoms after an infectious connection, and, for this reason, do not communicate the disease, but always manifest themselves as remote consequences of previously-existing primary syphilitic products.

II. SPECIAL CAUSES AND PERIODS OF MANIFESTATION OF SECONDARY PHENOMENA.

Sec. 82.—Chancres and gonorrhœa as causes.

The fact that secondary phenomena are the remote sequelæ of an infection caused by a specific virus, is no longer doubted at the present time either by the former adherents of Broussais' Physiological School in France, nor even by the adherents of the same school in Germany, where it still flourishes, even after it had been almost universally abandoned in the country of its nativity some ten or fifteen years ago. Whereas all modern practitioners agree that the symptoms of syphilis originate in some previous chancre or bubo, this unanimity disappears again when we are to decide whether the legion of secondary phenomena can only be superinduced by chancre and buboes, both being equally primary phenomena; or likewise by simple gonorrhœa. A superficial glance at the annals of medicine would seem sufficient to at once decide the matter in favor of gonorrhœa, since in the Paris hospitals alone the secondary syphilis of fifty among every hundred patients is distinctly traceable to gonorrhœal infection. However, upon examining these irrefutable and striking proofs more carefully, we shall stumble upon various circumstances that lead us to doubt the correctness of that evidence. In the first place who knows whether these patients who, when entering the hospital, were seemingly infected with nothing but gonorrhœa, had not contracted the syphilitic disease by some prior connection, but whose manifestation had been mistaken for a simple excoriation caused by the act of coïtion, and had been suppressed by an astringent wash? Who knows whether this suppression was not the real cause of the secondary phenomena, instead of the gonorrhœa which, happening to be the most recent and most ostensible infection, had the honor of having the secondary appearances attributed to it? Adding to this that the French, who have furnished the most circumstantial statistics, designate as *blennorrhœa*, more particularly among females, every infectious discharge from the vagina, no matter whether the discharge is *idiopathic* or *symptomatic*, caused by chancre or syphilitic ulcerations; and that, among the Germans, the terms blennorrhœa and gonorrhœa by no means refer to the same pathological condition; we may regard this as sufficient evidence that the French statistics are not applicable to what we Germans call simple gonorrhœa, which is indeed a venereal but not, by any means, a syphilitic disease. It is indeed beyond doubt that syphilitic gonorrhœa, more especially when originating in sycosis, has power to superinduce secondary phenomena; but whether *simple*, non-syphilitic gonorrhœa can have the same effect, remains to this day a matter of great doubt, owing to the fact that a discriminating diagnosis of these two forms of gonorrhœa has been too sadly neglected. All that can be said on this subject is, that there is a kind of gonorrhœa that may cause secondary symptoms, and that there is another kind that will have no such effect; at any rate, this point is so far involved in the greatest doubt. In my own practice I have never yet had an opportunity of witnessing such a result.

Sec. 83.—Causative conditions.

Omitting for the present all considerations of the question about simple and syphilitic gonorrhœa, and taking it for granted that secondary syphilitic phenomena always originate in some manifest or concealed chancre, or in something equivalent, such as buboes or mucous tubercles, as their remote cause, an equally important question will then arise: Under what conditions will primary syphilis be capable of causing secondary phenomena? It is an admitted fact that secondary phenomena always arise when the primary symptoms are either neglected or removed by external applications alone; another question is, whether secondary phenomena can develop themselves even after the primary infection had been apparently eradicated from the system by means of the most appropriate specific internal treatment, in consequence of which, all external manifestations of the internal disease had been completely removed and extinguished. Concerning this question we have no reliable records, for the reason that authors have not paid the least attention to the important distinction between a real chancre-cure effected by the internal administration of specific antidotes, and a mere cicatrization of the chancre by external applications; or for this additional reason that, even where the cure had been effected by internal means, the patient had taken such large quantities of Mercury that it would be difficult or even impossible to decide whether the secondary phenomena, manifesting themselves subsequently to the supposed cure, were really of a syphilitic character, or rather the result of excessive mercurial action. On this account I have only my own experience to refer to, and am enabled to assert that, among all the patients whom I have treated for the last thirty years for primary syphilis, I have never seen a single sign of the syphilitic disease manifesting itself even ten or twenty years after the internal use of specific antidotes; the only untoward symptom that may have occasionally shown itself was, perhaps, an evanescent manifestation of excessive mercurial action, which, owing to the smallness of the doses administered, soon passed away again forever. What I am able to assert of the cure of chancre while yet in the stage of primary ulceration, I am unfortunately not able to assert of the cure of chancre after it had passed into the stage of fungoid growth, or had become complicated with buboes, tubercles, or figwarts, and hence was on the point of entering into the *secondary* period. In such cases, even after the primary symptoms had been completely and apparently radically removed by the use of *Merc. sol.*, *Nitri ac.*, or *Thuja*, I have often, even after the lapse of three, eight, or even eighteen months, seen syphilitic phenomena still make their appearance, consisting almost without an exception of unimportant cutaneous affections that never assumed the form of extensive syphilidæ, and yielded very speedily to proper treatment without ever returning; but, if neglected by the patient, became very obstinate and remained visible for a long period; all of which shows in the most indubitable manner that, if the primary symptoms have left their first stage of primary ulceration, their removal, even by the best internal treatment, may not constitute a perfectly complete cure of the syphilitic disease, and not *all* danger may as yet be obviated.

Sec. 84.—Period of Manifestation of the Secondary Phenomena.

Here two questions arise: 1) What is the *shortest* period when they may manifest themselves subsequently to the breaking out of the primary, protopathic symptoms? and 2) What is the *longest* period when the danger of secondary symptoms breaking out may still exist, even after the primary disease seemed to have been thoroughly eradicated? As regards the *first* question, when secondary phenomena may arise in the shortest time, it is certain, not only according to my own observations, but likewise those of all other physicians who have had opportunities of observing the course of the syphilitic disease, that they not only arise after the disappearance of the primary protopathic phenomena, but likewise while these phenomena are still running their course. Whatever may be said of the protection which a chancre or a vicarious bubo affords against the breaking out of constitutional syphilis, there is unimpeachable testimony that this protection does not always exist. It is positively certain that, even if secondary symptoms very seldom manifest themselves during the primary ulcerative stage of chancre, yet, if a chancre, without being treated with external ointments or astringents, is left to itself for six or even only four weeks, or up to the period when it passes from the stage of primary ulceration into the state of fungoid growth, this transition period is simultaneously ushered in by the appearance of some cutaneous eruption, most generally syphilitic maculæ, and that such an event may take place, both when vicarious buboes are present or absent. Inasmuch as *buboes*, *mucous tubercles*, and *figwarts*, although in some rare cases they may occur as protopathic symptoms appertaining to the primary period of syphilis, in most cases do not make their appearance until the second term of the primary chancre, that of fungoid growth, has set in; and inasmuch as truly secondary phenomena may develop themselves during this term, we cannot wonder if these consecutive products of the primary period, even at the very time when they first break out, superinduce, as immediate consequences, or are even accompanied by *secondary* cutaneous affections, or even affections of the mucous membranes. Moreover, inasmuch as more particularly mucous tubercles and figwarts, in spite of their inherent capacity to reproduce *their like* by infection, nevertheless, in consequence of the changes which their reproductive energies had undergone, belong to a stage where the original chancre-virus had become pathologically altered, it must be evident that these last-mentioned phenomena, even when they seemingly occur as protopathic products, in many cases are followed by *secondary phenomena* more rapidly than the chancre itself, and may even be accompanied by them at the outset. The same remarks apply to syphilitic gonorrhœa, whether occasioned by the virus of chancre, tubercles, or figwarts; this kind of gonorrhœa is likewise very frequently and very speedily associated with *secondary cutaneous affections*, by which it can easily and safely be distinguished from common gonorrhœa, as a disease of much more dangerous consequences.

Sec. 85.—Sequelæ breaking out after the Lapse of Years.

Having seen that *secondary* phenomena generally may set in in four or six weeks, or even at a much earlier period, after the breaking out of the first protopathic symptoms, or at any rate, prior to their complete disappearance; the other not less important question now presents itself, how long a period may elapse, after the disappearance of the primary product, before all danger of further developments of the syphilitic disease shall have passed away entirely? If we would believe every thing that writers on syphilis have related on this subject as authentic, it would seem as though this danger continued during the whole lifetime of the patient; so that, if he had been afflicted years ago with a chancre, or even a simple gonorrhœa, and had enjoyed the most perfect health ever since, even for the period of twenty or more years, he may, nevertheless, wake one fine morning with one or the other suspicious-looking symptom, or even, according to circumstances, with a whole legion of the most horrid syphilitic products, from the most disgusting cutaneous ulcerations to the most destructive chancres in the throat, and the most painful affections of the bones! Fortunately, in spite of what some authors may write, things are not quite so terribly bad. It is indeed true, that if secondary syphilis has once set in, and is not treated with proper specific means, the disease may break out again, every now and then, in five, seven, ten, or even fifteen and twenty years; but experience has likewise shown that, where traces of a prior infection still continue to show themselves, after the lapse of so many years, a careful examination of the case leads to the conviction, that a continual series of syphilitic phenomena had existed from the first outbreak of the disease, to the very day when the patient afterward presented himself for treatment. We admit that the phenomena of such a series must have been inconsiderable; but they certainly existed, and must have been overlooked by the patient, or not properly recognized by the physician, and treated for something else. If patients tell us that five, ten, or fifteen years after a period of perfect health, they were all at once attacked with symptoms of a previous gonorrhœa or chancre, we feel satisfied that the original disease must have either been badly managed, or that the patient is trying to deceive. What physician does not know that men, who feel interested in concealing former transgressions, are disposed stoutly to deny the suspicious character of existing discharges or ulcerations, even when of recent origin, and undertake to impose upon the physician by the bold assertion, that these symptoms are nothing else than the reappearance of a former infection contracted years ago! Secondary affections, if neglected, may indeed continue for years; but a careful inquiry will show that their first appearance can be traced to a primary infection that had occurred six months, or, at the latest, one or two years previous to that time.

III. VARIETIES AND CLASSIFICATION OF THE SECONDARY FORMS.

Sec. 86.—Essential Differences of these Forms.

Our previous statement, that secondary forms are incapable of transmitting the disease by infection, must not be understood to imply that this transmission cannot take place by the act of coition. On the contrary, it is a well-known fact, that secondary syphilis can be inherited by children. In my own practice, I have met with more than one case, where the father, who, in consequence of a suppressed chancre, had become afflicted with *masked constitutional* syphilis, transmitted unmistakable signs of the secondary disease, not only to his offspring, but likewise to the mother, even after they had cohabited together as man and wife for several years previous to the birth of the infant, during which period no sign of secondary syphilis had been perceived. We shall revert to this case, which we mention in this place simply for the purpose of adverting to the fact, that secondary syphilis may be transmitted from the parent to the offspring, although never by direct infection. By the side of such secondary forms as can be inherited (more especially the syphilidæ) there exist other forms, such as syphilitic affections of the bones, that seem to be exempt from the liability to hereditary transmission; on which account writers on syphilis have adopted two distinct varieties of secondary syphilis: *a*) a variety where the infectious virus, although latent, can still be transmitted to the offspring; and *b*) another variety, where this is no longer possible. It has been supposed, moreover, that the symptoms of the last-named variety manifest themselves at a later period than those of the former. Hence, a *third* period has been constructed with the phenomena of the second variety, under the denomination of *tertiary symptoms*. This classification, to which some writers have even added a *fourth* or *quaternary period*, has been taught for a long time in our therapeutic manuals with the most rigorous scholastic dogmatism, without our authors having, perhaps, examined the matter for themselves, or having even had an opportunity of learning any thing about the subject except from books. In this manner, this purely theoretical classification has been successively adopted by one author after the other, without any of them troubling himself in the least whether it is founded upon actual fact. So far from observing a definite order of succession, secondary phenomena sometimes appear mixed up with tertiary, and even subsequently to the latter. I have treated a woman in whom, after the suppression of chancre by an allopathic physician, an affection of the tibia first broke out, together with cutaneous pustules, after which the throat became affected. Regarding the non-hereditary character of tertiary phenomena, I have treated a child born of very poor parents, that was not only covered with syphilitic, cutaneous ulcerations, but likewise with exostoses of the skull. Not long before, the mother of this child had likewise been affected with similar ulcerations, the characteristic spots of which were still visible. Exostoses on her tibia were likewise still visible.

Sec. 87.—Classification of the Secondary Phenomena.

However tenaciously we may still adhere to the old-fashioned and customary division of constitutional syphilis in secondary and tertiary phenomena, we cannot, for the reasons already stated, and for other reasons that will be explained in subsequent paragraphs, accept this arrangement, but prefer following the arrangement which has been adopted by modern writers on syphilis as the most convenient, since it ignores all unprofitable discussions concerning the pathogenetic differences between these phenomena, and otherwise facilitates their diagnosis to a great extent. Modern writers arrange the secondary phenomena in accordance with the tissues where they are located, and where we have the *epidermis*, the *mucous membranes*, the *bones*, *muscles*, and still other anatomical systems. Considering the degree of predilection which the syphilitic virus seems to manifest for each of these different systems, we shall find that the skin is most frequently affected by the poison, as if, pressed onward from the centre to the periphery, it sought to obtain an outlet from the organism. Once located upon the skin, the syphilitic disease assumes the most varied forms, from the simplest maculæ to the most hideous ulcerations. Inasmuch as syphilis at its first appearance was, properly speaking, nothing else than an exanthematic disease: the phenomena by which the disease manifests its endeavour to approximate again to its original form, are necessarily the most important, constituting one whole side of secondary syphilis; whereas all the other phenomena occurring in the mucous membranes, bones and other tissues, together constitute the other side of this disease as so many manifestations of an excretory process through the skin, that is either not yet completed or had been interrupted in its course; so that all the secondary syphilitic phenomena together may be ranged in two great, pathologically essentially distinct categories: A) those where the excretory process has been completed, (cutaneous diseases;) and B) those where this process has not yet been terminated, (secondary syphilis of other tissues.) In §§ 124, 125 we shall see what these two categories have in common in pathological respects, and how evidently it follows from a relative contrast of their respective phenomena that there is only a *secondary*, but that there cannot be a *tertiary* syphilis; for the present we will simply state that, in accordance with these views, we shall first consider, 1) the *cutaneous eruptions*, being of most frequent occurrence and deserving our first attention; and 2) under the general denomination of secondary *intermediate forms*, the secondary ulcers, affections of the mucous membranes, bones, and other phenomena; premising, however, in the first place some general remarks on the diagnosis, prognosis, and treatment of secondary syphilitic diseases.

IV. GENERAL DIAGNOSIS, PROGNOSIS, AND TREATMENT OF SECONDARY SYPHILIS.

Sec. 88.—Diagnosis.

In most cases, if the question is merely to distinguish syphilitic products from similar products of non-syphilitic diseases, such a diagnosis is comparatively easy. All syphilitic products are so characteristic in their appearance that any one who has seen them only once, and has read our description of these products in the following paragraphs, can scarcely ever remain in doubt concerning their true nature, so much more as, besides the anamnestic influences bearing upon the case, the diagnosis is facilitated by this other circumstance, that these secondary forms or products never occur singly, but always in company with others; for instance, ulcerations of the mucous membranes, or affections of bones, in company with suspicious cutaneous eruptions, or several kinds of the different syphilidæ, such as pustules, maculæ, herpes, etc., at one and the same time. At the same time, a close examination will very frequently reveal the existence of old chancres in the period of reproduction, or remnants of badly healed cicatrices, even mucous tubercles, or other remnants of the second or transition-stage of the primary period; for the reason that the secondary period does not set in after the completion of the primary period, but while the transition-stage is still running its course, or even simultaneously with its commencement. This takes place likewise with other diseases, where the different stages are not always sharply circumscribed. This simultaneity, in the manifestation of different forms, likewise distinguishes the secondary period of syphilis with great definiteness from the primary. If, in the course of a neglected chancre, sycosic gonorrhœa, or other primary appearances, pustules or other syphilitic manifestations on the skin supervene, we may rest assured that the secondary period has already commenced, and that the existence of a general constitutional infection will very soon become manifest by the supervention of other symptoms. If the diagnosis of true syphilis is in all cases unattended with any marked difficulties, on the other hand, it is not always equally easy to diagnose the true character of similar appearances in case they appertain to non-syphilitic diseases; the probability is, therefore, that phenomena which have not the remotest connection with syphilis may be mistaken for syphilitic symptoms much more frequently, than that a somewhat practised physician should misapprehend truly syphilitic phenomena for manifestations of a non-syphilitic disease. Such misapprehensions are more apt to occur in regard to mercurial symptoms, which, after the effects of mercury have reached a certain point, share with secondary syphilis the faculty of not only producing local phenomena that are readily mistaken for syphilitic appearances, but of producing several of them at once and at the same time. There is no other way of avoiding such misapprehensions than to become perfectly familiar with the analogous effects of Mercury. In order to facilitate this study, I have added at the close of this work an article on the so-called *mercurial syphilis*, which the practitioner will do well to compare with the symptoms in the case of patients who, some time previous, had been treated with large quantities of Mercury for real or supposed syphilis, or who had been much exposed to the influence of Mercury in their business. Many of these mercurial symptoms I have seen breaking out even after a persistent homœopathic treatment with large doses, not only ulcers and aphthæ in the buccal cavity, but likewise papulæ and flat ulcers on the skin, of a very suspicious look, but distinguished from syphilitic ulcers by the pruritus which is never present with the last-named products of disease.

Sec. 89.—Prognosis.

If the syphilitic disease has left the primary stage, and has passed into the second stage, the prognosis is, in so far, somewhat unfavorable, as the symptoms of the second stage are rather changeable, sometimes disappearing suddenly in order to reappear again in other localities, and in different forms, so that the physician can scarcely ever be certain whether, after the existing phenomena have apparently been cured, other phenomena may not break out in their place. What has been said of the greater or less curability of some of the above-mentioned forms—such as that cutaneous affections generally admit of a more favorable prognosis than affections of the mucous membranes, and these again of a more favorable prognosis than the affections of the osseous system—can only refer to the more or less accelerated, or retarded disappearance of these forms, but not to the morbid process in the interior of the organism in which these forms originate. To eradicate this process, and not merely to suppress a few isolated manifestations thereof, should be the task of the true healing art. If we keep this task in view, there is no doubt that the solution of this problem is infinitely more difficult than the removal of primary, and more particularly of protopathic symptoms, which, if accomplished by means of a rational internal treatment, always results in a simultaneous annihilation of the whole morbid process. Even during the transition-period, when no other than primary symptoms are as yet in evidence, it may happen, as in Dr. Thorer's cases, quoted in § 78, that, after the cure of the existing form, another form may break out, for the reason that one single remedy is scarcely ever sufficient, in the secondary period, to overcome and excrete the contagium after its nature had become modified by the most diversified combinations. Nevertheless, a radical cure is still possible even in these cases, provided the physician knows what remedies will surely lead to this result; although we should never expect to accomplish such a cure as rapidly as we cure primary ulcers; notwithstanding that, even after curing them, we still have to keep a watchful eye on that which may yet happen to come afterwards. That the probability of the supervention of subsequent symptoms is the greater, the more remotely from the primary symptoms the manifestation of secondary phenomena takes place, and the more complete the disappearance of the earlier symptoms appertaining to this period, is self-evident. If the physician, while the primary signs of the disease are still visible upon the sexual organs, should be very cautious in his promises concerning the possible supervention of subsequent phenomena; he will have to push this caution to the highest degree if, when taking charge of his patient, every symptom of the primary disease has already vanished from the sphere of ocular observation. However, under a truly rational treatment, the symptoms will gradually become weaker at every successive outbreak, so that even in the worst cases, the patient may be dismissed as cured, after the lapse of two or three years, provided no new symptoms have appeared for the last year. But, if the patient had been treated with large doses of Mercury, and if the syphilitic symptoms had become mixed up with the effects of Mercury, the final radical treatment may have to be conducted for a much longer period, for the reason that the mercurial symptoms, like the syphilitic, may reappear at intervals, and, unless overcome from their very foundation, may, if left to themselves, continue their assaults for a period of ten, and even twenty years.

Sec. 90.—General Treatment of Secondary Phenomena.

Howsoever indispensable the mercurial preparations may be to the cure of syphilis, more especially during the primary period, or the period of protopathic phenomena, and even to some extent during the second stage of these phenomena, yet in treating secondary symptoms, we shall most generally have to employ more than one remedy, in order to meet the diversified combinations which the infectious virus has entered into during this stage with the other tissues of the organism. Even during the transition-stage, when the chancre is on the point of passing into the secondary stage, it frequently happens that in spite of the cure which *Mercurius* had achieved, other symptoms, such as figwarts, against which Mercurius was unable to exert either a prophylactic, or a curative action, make their appearance. Nevertheless, mercurial preparations may continue to prove curative as long as the symptoms of the primary period, namely, the original ulcers are still existing, or have not yet commenced to pass into the stage of fungoid growth. I have witnessed this more than once in the case of chancres, where initial symptoms of the secondary period had already broken out upon the skin; where the chancre had already become converted into a red surface without having become fungoid, and where *Merc. sol.* healed this chancre together with the attending maculæ, without any secondary symptoms appearing at a subsequent period. If, in the second stage of the primary period, or the period of fungoid growth, or in treating the products peculiar to this stage, such as buboes, mucous tubercles and figwarts, *Merc. sol.* has frequently to be replaced by other remedies, such as *Nitri ac.*, *Thuja*, *Lycopodium*, *Sabina*, etc., this necessity occurs so much more frequently in purely secondary affections, where *Mercurius*, especially if no primary phenomena are any more to be seen, is not only without any curative effect, but, when given in large and continued doses, frequently produces the utmost ominous aggravations. At any rate, if secondary symptoms become manifest while the primary ulcers are still existing, *Merc. sol.* should be employed with great caution, and should at once be replaced by some other remedy, such as *Nitri ac.*, *Thuja*, *Phosphori ac.*, *Sulphur*, *Lycopodium*, etc., if its use superinduces the least appearance of aggravation. In the ulceration of the secondary period, especially in ulcers of the throat and mouth, *Merc.* may be of great use (though *Nitri ac.* is no less efficient for these phenomena); but in such a case, it has to be given in smaller and less frequent doses. In ulcerations of the transition-period, and even in decided cases of secondary ulcers, I always commence the treatment, provided the patient has not yet taken any Mercury, with a suitable mercurial preparation, of which, in case the products of the primary period are still existing, I give half a grain of the first or second centesimal trituration, at least once a day; and, if the secondary phenomena have already made their appearance, the same dose every two, three, or four days, according to circumstances, when it soon becomes evident whether this agent will be of any use in the present case or not. If *Merc.* improves the symptoms, I continue it as long as the symptoms continue to improve; but discontinue it at once, and select some other remedy in its stead, as soon as the improvement ceases. What remedies are chiefly required in all such cases will be stated when the different forms are treated of; we subjoin hereafter a list of the different remedies, with a reference to the different stages for which they are most adapted.

1. Primary Period.

a) *First stage* (*recent* chancres, *protopathic*, buboes, or tubercles): Merc. sol., Sublim. corr., Præcipitatus ruber, or other mercurial preparations.

b) *Second*, or transition-stage (fungoid chancres, or *deuteropathic*, consecutive buboes, mucous tubercles, figwarts): Nitri ac., Cinnabaris, Thuja, Staphysagria, Lycopodium, Sulphur, and occasionally only mercurial preparations.

2. Secondary Period.

a) *First* stage (remnants of the original primary symptoms being still present): As a general rule, the same remedies that have been indicated in 1), *b*, for the symptoms of the transition period.

b) *Second* stage (the primary symptoms having disappeared or become cicatrized): Mercurial preparations only, in case no mercury had as yet been given, and always in diminished and less frequent doses. Beside these, the most frequently indicated remedies are: Lycopodium, Kali jodatum, Staphysagria, Aurum, Sulphur, Sarsaparilla, Lachesis, and other remedies pointed out in subsequent chapters. [Also Mercurius jodatus, and Kali bichromicum.—Ed.]

These general indications may serve as a practical hint to physicians. In the following chapters, we shall furnish more definite statements concerning the use of these agents, premising in this place that, where other remedies are mentioned instead of the mercurial preparations, it will have to be understood that we always employ them in the 18th to 30th attenuation.

SECOND CHAPTER.

SYPHILITIC CUTANEOUS AFFECTIONS.

I. THEIR COMMON CHARACTERISTICS.

Sec. 91.—External Appearances.

THESE phenomena, which have been described by modern writers under the name of *syphilidæ*, are generally the first sign by which the second period of syphilis announces itself. In very many cases they already show themselves during the second stage of the primary period, that is to say, about the time when the protopathic chancre, bubo, or tubercle, commences to lose its primary syphilitic appearance, to exhibit a dark-red surface instead of its characteristic lardy-looking base, and to pass into the stage of fungoid growth. If the commonly consecutive signs of the primary period (such as buboes, tubercles, etc.) do not appear protopathically, but deuteropathically, or, which is the same thing, as truly consecutive symptoms, they may likewise, in such cases, be at once accompanied by a syphiloid eruption. But they never break out during the first stage of the primary period, and still less as protopathic signs of a syphilitic infection. Only in the case of children, who are affected with hereditary syphilis, they sometimes constitute the first sign by which the hereditary disease manifests itself. In this form, this disease has been noticed on mothers who had inherited it during their pregnancy from the father of their offspring. In by far the larger number of cases, these syphilidæ do not break out until the original protopathic phenomena have entirely disappeared, sometimes only after the lapse of two or three months, or even years. All of them, without an exception, run a chronic course in spite of the violence with which they sometimes make their first appearance. Above all things, their whole look is exceedingly characteristic and peculiar; whether they appear in the shape of vesicles, papulæ, tubercles, or maculæ, their whole look is so peculiar and characteristic that it at once betrays their nature and origin. Among their characteristic peculiarities, we notice, in the first place, their peculiar *color:* nobody who has observed this once will ever fail, howsoever difficult it may be to describe it, to recognize it again. It has been described as *copper-brown.* However, although this color is the most common, yet it cannot be said that it constitutes the peculiar shade of syphiloid eruptions. In some cases, this copper-color is not very distinct, but seems to be an intermediate shade between copper-red and brown-gray, like the color of venison, but always exhibits between these two shades a *faint, dark brownish-gray,* which, after all, seems to constitute the specific color of the syphilidæ. We should not forget, however, that the more recent the eruption, the darker the color, and the longer it has been out on the skin, the more the color will approximate the gray. As regards their common shape, all of them, without an exception, show a disposition to form *circular* spots or papules; even where they come out in groups, the whole group has a rounded form, which, if not a perfect circle, forms at least a segment of a circle, or a ring. This peculiarity becomes particularly striking, if the eruption is viewed at a distance, in which case we often notice that even if the single groups deviate from the circular form, the whole mass of these groups together, forms the most perfect, exactly-delineated ring. Another characteristic which all these eruptions have in common, is the almost total *absence of pruritus,* at least in older eruptions; for, during the first days of their appearance, in the case of *tuberculoid* eruptions, for instance, a tolerably violent itching may be felt, which, however, always disappears again in three or four days, without ever reappearing during the whole course of the eruption.

Sec. 92.—Course of the Syphilidæ.

It has already been stated that syphiloid eruptions always run a chronic course; this is indeed one of their characteristic peculiarities. It is only when they show themselves already during the transition-stage of the primary period that their appearance is sometimes ushered in by constitutional disturbances, with, or without fever, that might lead us to suspect the approach of an acute eruption, but disappears again as soon as the syphiloid has broken out. A similar disproportionate announcement of a product of little magnitude ushers in the eruptions themselves, which sometimes set in with a broad, red base, and tolerable hardness, that might lead us to expect an abscess, but finally run into a small purulent point that does not increase in size; or a vesicle of tolerable size may arise, with a large red areola, which remains for several days without bursting, during which the red areola becomes paler and loses the appearance of inflammation, which latter, indeed, never existed. Some of these syphiloids, not only the pustulous and tuberculoid forms, but, under certain circumstances the maculæ, may terminate in long-lasting *ulcers*, which assume a rounded shape, with somewhat raised, red, abruptly rising edges and ash-colored base, which, if the ulcers are located on the lower extremities, may assume a bloody appearance. If the ulcer is isolated, it spreads at first in every direction until it has attained a certain size, after which it spontaneously commences to cicatrize. If, on the contrary, two or three ulcers have arisen from a number of neighboring pustules, they generally run into one large ulcer of two or three inches in diameter, which betrays its threefold origin by the three rounded segments of its edges. Sometimes the little ulcers may become gangrenous and serpiginous; but in every case they become very shortly covered with crusts of a grayish-yellow color, with a brownish tint, arranged in layers, arched above, and not unlike oyster-shells, generally adhering very firmly, and not falling off until the ulcers have become completely cicatrized. Moreover, they greatly incline to spontaneous cicatrization. Nevertheless, after an ulcer has become cicatrized, or even while the process of cicatrization is still going on, new pustules may break out, so that, as might be inferred in the case of many patients from their numerous cicatrices, a multitude of ulcers may co-exist simultaneously with the pustulous eruption, even after it had spread over localities that had not been implicated heretofore. The cicatrices, like the syphiloids and ulcers from which the former had arisen, bear unmistakable signs of their syphilitic character. Like the original chancres, they are round, or, in case several ulcers had coalesced, the combined ulcer is, at any rate, provided with arc-shaped edges, and more or less depressed. Recent ulcers are generally quite round, of a more or less violet-red color, and provided with a bronze-colored border, which sometimes, however, may seem quite colorless; in *older* ulcers, the centre is white, and shows no sign of vascularity, while the bronze-colored border continues. If the ulcers are several years old, their surface becomes depressed, of a pale-white, without any border, and very similar to the crusts arising from vaccination. In addition, all syphiloid forms show a marked tendency to break out again, so that the course of such an eruption is scarcely ever entirely closed, so that, even before the first pustules, maculæ, tubercles, etc., have become cicatrized, dried up, or have otherwise disappeared, yea, even before they are fully formed, a new eruption may become manifest, which, in its turn, runs through all the different stages to the end, and so on indefinitely.

Sec. 93.—Distinctive Characteristics of Syphiloid Eruptions.

So far we have indicated the diagnostic signs which characterize syphiloid eruptions whenever they show themselves; but circumstances may arise in consequence of which some of these signs become more or less obscured, and slight deviations from the main rule may take place. They may be owing to the age of the eruption, to its particular shape, and to the stage of development, when the physician is first consulted. In order to be sure of our diagnosis, it becomes indispensable that these differences, in the color, shape, and course of the syphiloid, should be carefully considered; previously, however, we have to consider more particularly the different forms under which the syphilidæ may appear. We have already stated that they may assume all the different forms of ordinary cutaneous diseases, from the simplest spots to the most hideous ulcers; on which account modern syphilographic writers have attempted to classify them in accordance with Willan's and Bateman's anatomical system as maculæ, papulæ, eczema, tubercles, etc. There could be no objection to such a classification, if these anatomical forms appeared in practice as rigorously delineated as they do in books, and did not occur more or less mixed, especially the higher, more perfectly developed forms; or, in other words, if several syphilidæ did not appear upon the skin at one and the same time. Far from constituting as many *idiopathic* syphilitic diseases as they adopt various anatomical forms, these pretended varieties of syphiloid eruptions are in reality nothing but diversified manifestations of one and the same cutaneous action of the syphilitic disease, originating in a variety of unknown, accidental circumstances, or perhaps in different degrees of an inherent tendency towards outward growth: the differences being simply *apparent*, of an external nature, not, by any means, founded in any *essential* distinction. This classification has this great and sole advantage, to place before us a lucid and compact view of all the forms of cutaneous syphilis, and greatly to facilitate a correct appreciation of these forms in all possible cases. Viewed from this point of view, such a systematic arrangement, being a classification of the different symptoms of one and the same malady, has indeed a real value. Accepting this classification in this light, and in no other, we propose in the following chapters to consider the different syphilidæ, so far as may be necessary for a correct diagnosis of these affections, under the following categories: 1) Maculæ; 2) eczema; 3) pemphigus; 4) pustulous; 5) papulous; 6) scaly; and 7) tuberculoid forms.

II. THE DIFFERENT FORMS OF SYPHILITIC ERUPTIONS.

Sec. 94.—Maculæ.

The form which is described under the name of *syphilitic roseola*, consists of irregular, circular, more or less confluent, measle-shaped spots, raised but little above the skin; at first of a copper color, after a while changing to a yellowish red-gray appearance, and but slowly, and finally only imperfectly paling under the pressure of the finger. The outbreak of the spots is sometimes preceded by, and sometimes attended with, fever and a general feeling of indisposition. They run a *chronic* course, sometimes disappearing after a while spontaneously, either by scattering or after a bran-like desquamation, but always without ulceration or cicatrization; however, after disappearing in one locality, they are very apt to re-appear in another. They are generally located on the neck, in the posterior cervical region, on the shoulders, breast, upper extremities, very frequently in the face, and sometimes around the sexual organs and on the inner surface of the thighs. Very frequently these spots break out during the second stage of the primary period, after the chancre has passed into the stage of fungoid growth; and it is at this period that their breaking out is attended with a general malaise, a feeling of weariness and lameness, headache, and pains in all the limbs. Sometimes these accessory affections are associated with pain in the throat, violet redness of the mucous membrane of the mouth, the velum palati, and fauces, together with great dryness of the affected parts, an unusual sensation of heat and difficulty of deglutition; even superficial ulcers in the throat may be seen in some cases. This measle-shaped eruption may remain unchanged for days in the same locality; at times only its peculiar red color may seem more intense without ever being accompanied by pruritus or a feeling of heat. After a while this redness changes more and more to a light-brown, and afterwards to a gray color, until finally it becomes so imperceptible that it can only be seen when the parts are held against the light, when the skin has the appearance of being dirty and might easily be cleansed. This tint may remain unchanged for months, and even years; only in cold weather, and after washing, the color may sometimes become more marked.

Beside these smooth maculæ, others describe a *papulous redness* (*erythema papulosum*). This eruption is distinguished from the former by its small spots, at most of the size of a dime, not very red, papulous, and supposed to break out only subsequent to gonorrhœa. But, inasmuch as the first observer of this eruption, Dr. Cazenave of Paris, admits that he has only seen it on persons who had suppressed their gonorrhœa with large doses of Copaiva, and it is a well-known fact that Copaiva produces such an eruption, it is questionable whether this is justly chargeable to the disease, or ought not rather to be attributed to the action of the Copaiva. I have seen this eruption a number of times on individuals who had been dosing themselves with large quantities of Copaiva for gonorrhœa; but I have never seen it after gonorrhœa for which no Copaiva had been taken, notwithstanding that there has not been a week for the last ten years when two or three new cases of gonorrhœa have not presented themselves for treatment in my office, from every condition and class of society.

Sec. 95.—Syphilitic Eczema.

2) *a.* This eruption, which, until recently, has been described only by Dr. Cazenave, according to some is very rare; according to others, on the contrary, occurs much more frequently, and remains unnoticed by most physicians for no other reason than because every vesicle is not surrounded by the characteristic bronze-colored areola, which is improperly regarded by many as the sole truly diagnostic sign of syphilitic eruptions. For a long time it has likewise been my opinion that this eczema had been seen only here and there by some of our hospital-physicians, until I met with a suspicious-looking eruption in one of our homœopathic dispensaries. The spots were more or less rounded, scattered over the thighs, pubes, abdomen, chest, and upper arm, some of them of the size of a hand, some of the size of a dime. They were covered with little vesicles, did not cause the least itching, but did not seem to be of a syphilitic character, for the reason that the copper or bronze redness was wanting, and the spots had a dirty pale-yellow look. The history of the case, however, and the still-existing primary phenomena of the second stage on the sexual organs, showed that this eruption might very properly be classed among the syphiloids. My attention having been once excited by this case, I did not fail afterwards to notice other similar cases. According to Cazenave this category not only comprehends the syphilitic eczema, but likewise the so-called syphilitic pustules and a sort of syphilitic vesicular herpes. These two last-named forms, however, will be described more minutely each in a separate paragraph; in this paragraph we confine ourselves to the syphilitic eczema. This syphiloid consists of small, transparent vesicles showing themselves in irregular, scattered groups more prominently than the common eczema, each of which vesicles, if examined through a glass, will be found surrounded with a red areola; sometimes the whole spot upon which they are seated, exhibits a faint redness, in which case the vesicles are somewhat larger, and feel harder and denser. They always persevere for a long time in the same condition; the fluid which they contain, remains transparent, scarcely ever becoming turbid; at last the vesicles appear wilted and shrivelled, the areola, or the whole spot upon which the group is located, becomes fainter, exhibiting a grayish tint, the raised epidermis becomes depressed,

and in the place of the vesicle there remains nothing but a slight desquamation of the skin with a border that is generally more blanched than the original site of the vesicle. In some cases the eczema appears somewhat altered, in consequence of the vesicles becoming lacerated by the friction of the clothes, after which they appear covered with small, furrowed, lacerated crusts, of a tolerable degree of density, which are formed out of the sero-purulent fluid of several vesicles, among which ulcers are never found. In this case the specific copper-redness is more marked, and the whole eruption, whose true pathological nature can no longer be doubted, exhibits a mingling of the above-described original vesicles and crusts scattered here and there. In other cases the eruption may assume the form of *impetigo*, when spots of different sizes, of a tolerably vivid redness and covered with vesicles, are seen; these vesicles, which are at first transparent, and afterwards become turbid and filled with a purulent serum, are soon replaced by crusts, and finally cicatrize at the same time that new vesicles start up, so that here, likewise, the different stages of the syphiloid may be witnessed at one and the same time. These crusts are much thicker than those of a non-syphilitic impetigo, and, like other syphilitic crusts, look black, coniform, furrowed, *in superincumbent layers* and firmly adhering; in a few rare cases, these crusts hide cup-shaped ulcers, which always leave a depressed cicatrix that remains visible for a long time. This syphiloid occurs very frequently during the existence of chancre or buboes.

Sec. 96.—Syphilitic Herpes.

This form is not very rare; it is even more frequent than many suppose, but is more apt to be misjudged than any other syphiloid eruption, so much the more easily as it resembles herpes circinnatus. This syphilitic herpes generally breaks out in round, ring-shaped, elevated spots, of the size of a three-cent piece to that of a dime, and is distinguished from the non-syphilitic herpes circinnatus by the well-known syphilitic color, which from a copper-colored hue afterwards passes into the yellowish-gray or pale brownish-gray tint. This form never terminates in ulceration, and hence never makes any scars. Usually this herpes is not very numerous; it seldom breaks out more than two or three at a time; the tettery spots are generally very distant from each other, frequently breaking out simultaneously on opposite sides, for instance on the neck and thighs, etc. These herpetic eruptions seldom break out alone, but almost always mingled with other syphiloids, on which account it may be comparatively easier to diagnose them correctly.

Beside this herpes, there is another variety that might be designated as *herpes furfuraceus* or bran-shaped herpes; this variety is scarcely ever properly diagnosed, being confounded either with the common non-syphilitic eczema, or with pityriasis. Like the simple squamous herpes circinnatus, the sypilitic herpes circinnatus likewise appears in the shape of extremely small, numerous scales, which generally are chiefly spread over the breast and extremities, and which, always perfectly circular, are at first no bigger than a pea, but may increase in size to that of a dime. The vesicles covering the herpes have very thin membranes, and shrink away so rapidly that there is scarcely time left for observation, so that these spots might be mistaken for pityriasis, if a closer inspection with a glass, during the first period of their existence, did not reveal on their border a multitude of small little points arranged in circles and surrounded by remnants of epidermis, which points remain until they coalesce in one general border that is more especially perceptible when the rings are of a larger size. The centre of this herpes is generally inflamed, and looks as if it had become raised by a rapidly absorbed and dried-up fluid, having become the seat of a small scale which is sometimes sufficiently large to cover the whole surface of the herpes. This herpes, which is distinguished from ordinary pityriasis only by its marked copper-color, as well as by its almost *horny* central scale, which resembles the scales of psoriasis, is one of the most frequently-occurring vesicular syphiloids, frequently mingled with other eruptions and even accompanied by bone-pains. It may likewise break out in various localities, even on the glans, where I have seen it, as a genuinely secondary symptom, show itself subsequent to the cure of a chancre which was effected years ago without a trace of a scar remaining behind. Hofrichter's case (Allg. hom. Zeit., 35, p. 135), of small brown spots at the anus, of the size of small split peas, which were accompanied by tubercles and disappeared after the detaching of small particles of epidermis, most likely belongs to this category, and, likewise, the spots described by Rummel (Allg. hom. Zeit., vol. 18, p. 292), and resembling psoriasis, of which

Rummel observes that they occur quite frequently in Magdeburg. This would seem to confirm my suspicion that the syphiloid in question is not so very rare, only it remains unnoticed in most cases.

Sec. 97.—Varicella Syphilitica.

This form exhibits tolerably large, transparent vesicles, which afterwards become torpid, and may either scatter or terminate in the formation of a blackish crust surrounded by a red areola. Generally for some time after the crust has become detached, the affected locality continues to exhibit a dirty-gray color. Very often, their breaking out is preceded for two or three days by a general feeling of malaise, with a sensation of weariness and lameness in the limbs and even febrile symptoms, after which the surface of the body becomes covered, either in isolated places, or successively all over with spots of a moderately vivid redness, which very speedily become raised throughout their whole extent and filled with a transparent fluid, so that little by little the whole crowd of these spots seems transformed into vesicles surrounded with a copper-colored areola which is in all respects like the areola of the original macula. These vesicles are circular, globular, prominent, and of different sizes, from that of a pin's-head to the size of a pea, and even much larger. The spreading of this varicella takes place very slowly, not only with respect to the general spreading of the eruption, which is very gradual, but likewise with respect to the development of each single vesicle. Such a vesicle may sometimes remain unchanged for a whole week, on which account the eruption, after a certain period, may acquire a very peculiar appearance. We may see, for instance, on the one hand, fresh, well-rounded, elastic, transparent, perceptibly raised vesicles, surrounded by not very dark, but perceptibly copper-colored areolæ; whereas on the other hand, older vesicles are seen by the side of the former, that have already become depressed, are rather broad than projecting, and only contain a small portion of the re-absorbed fluid; others again, though flattened, are thick and hard to the feel, and contain a turbid fluid; whereas another set has become converted into thick, blackish crusts. All of them, however, exhibit in all their stages the specific color which marks all syphilitic products, although this color runs into a variety of tints, all of which, however, betray by their characteristic appearance the original color from which they spring. When first arising, for instance, the vesicles occupy the whole of the original spot, whose redness disappears entirely, but soon reappears again in the shape of a red areola by which the vesicle is surrounded. At first this areola has a coppery color, which vanishes away in the dirty, yellowish-brown, gray tint left behind by the vesicle, after its disappearance, so that these dirty-gray spots are much broader than the original vesicles. If this syphiloid is carefully examined and contrasted with the eruption which, according to some authors, constituted the first manifestation of syphilis, in the shape of a general protopathic cutaneous disease described as *Variola venerea*, it would seem as though the form of varicella, which we have just now delineated, might be the first and true, though very badly degenerated type of the whole disease. This syphiloid is frequently seen accompanied by angina syphilitica, or even by exostoses and bone-pains.

Sec. 98.—Pemphigus Syphiliticus, Rhypia.

This occurs in two distinctive forms; a) as syphilitic pemphigus, and b) as rhypia or rupia. The former of these forms, which is described in our books as pemphigus of new-born infants, has so far been only met with among this class, without the syphilitic nature of this disease having ever been suspected, until Professor Dubois of Paris demonstrated it by the most incontrovertible testimony. This pemphigus always shows itself in the form of several blisters in the palms of the hands, or on the soles of the feet, of the size of a hazelnut, and generally broad, flat, not very extensive, regularly rounded, filled with a sero-purulent fluid, and surrounded by a copper or violet-colored areola. Sometimes, though rarely, this fluid dries up, forming a blackish-brown crust; in the majority of instances the bulla bursts, the fluid runs out, and the bulla ulcerates, which never happens with the non-syphilitic pemphigus. The syphilitic pemphigus is generally present already when the infant is born, or develops itself at any rate shortly after birth. It seems remarkable that this syphiloid should never be accompanied by any of the ordinary phenomena of secondary syphilis, as happens to so many other syphiloids; nor that the skin of these new-born infants should never exhibit the dryness and shrivelled appearance which authors consider as a diagnostic sign of congenital syphilis and which imparts to these infants the well-known appearance of old age. Wherever this form has been seen, the mother was either still affected with syphilis, or had had the disease at some former period. Up to the present time, as has already been stated, this pemphigus has only been noticed among infants, where it is not by any means a very rare occurrence.

The other form, known as syphilitic rupia, is somewhat less frequent. It consists of broad, flattened, not very full bullæ, surrounded by areolæ of a deep copper-color, and containing a blackish fluid which speedily dries up and becomes converted into a blackish crust whose centre is thicker than the circumference, forming, by this means, a cone which is considerably raised above the epidermis. The surrounding areola deepens in proportion as the crust is older; not unfrequently an ulcer forms, which dips down to the subjacent textures sufficiently to be designated as a true *ulcus consecutivum*, round the crust, by which means the elevation of the crust over the skin becomes still more prominent; this is more particularly the case when the ulcer is somewhat advanced in age. The number of these bullæ varies; at all events it is larger than in pemphigus, though even in the form rupia they do not exceed fifteen to twenty in number. If with the larger bullæ smaller ones are associated, these may become renewed several times, whereas the larger ones remain; these it is that may be changed to ulcers. If these bullæ cover the whole body, as is sometimes, though rarely, the case, they are generally of the same size, and the eruption might easily be mistaken for ecthyma, from which it is almost only distinguished by its broader, more superficial bullæ, by their coniform crusts, and by the fact that the bullæ continue to appear in successive numbers even while the process of ulceration is still going on in other localities. The course of rhypia is always very slow; if the ulcers disappear, they always leave, without an exception, round scars which still retain for a long time their characteristic peculiarities

Sec. 99.—Syphilitic Pustules.

All syphilitic pustules have this in common, that they may break out in all parts of the body, and that they are frequently accompanied by the worst secondary phenomena, such as secondary chancres, exostoses, bone-pains, etc., or that they have become evolved with other syphilidæ as a final consummation. According to Cazenave, they may break out as a truly protopathic product immediately after infection has taken place. But the case upon which he bases his opinion was an infection, not contracted by sexual connection, but by inoculation. The victim was a physician with a sore finger, who assisted a woman who had a chancre, in confinement. Two or three months after infection, red spots broke out, followed by numerous pustules on the lower and upper extremities, shoulders, and head, which were at first mistaken for varioloid, but afterwards revealed their syphilitic character by *chancrous ulcers*, whose aspect reminded one of the descriptions of syphilis from the times when syphilis was an epidemic disease. Be this as it may, in our day these pustules, if we except inoculation by the skin, do no longer occur as protopathic products of impure connection. Upon examining such cases as Cazenave's more closely, we shall see that, where inoculation results in the formation of pustules, the ulcers arising from them, in which the original characteristics of chancre are found slightly altered in form, not in essence, nevertheless exhibit essential differences from the syphilitic pustules, notwithstanding all their apparent similarity with this syphiloid. He who, after the fashion of Willan, deems the anatomical form equivalent to the essence of the eruption, and from analogous forms infers an identity of pathological essence, may readily be induced to conclude that protopathic chancres, if occurring in different forms, may not only be represented by protopathically appearing pustules as products in all respects identical with chancre, but likewise by any form of syphiloid ulcers. Admitting that the ulcers in Cazenave's case were not a pustulous syphiloid, but true chancres, we shall insist upon our proposition, that all pustulous, ulcerated eruptions, which have been observed hitherto, never have been protopathic products, but can never have been any thing else than *secondary* eruptions. In the following paragraphs, we shall see, from a description of each particular form of these syphilitic pustules, in how far they are essentially distinguished from chancres by their course, and even by their frequently spontaneous disappearance, after having run through all their different stages, not to mention other distinctive signs, which every attentive reader can readily discover for himself. The best description of these eruptions has been given by Cazenave. But it is not only by this description that he has facilitated the diagnosis of this syphiloid, and its distinction from other similar non-syphilitic eruptions, but by rigidly arranging this syphiloid in accordance with its external forms, which had hitherto been imperfectly and obscurely described by authors under the common name of syphilitic pustules, under three distinct heads: *a*) *Acne syphilitica; b*) *Impetigo syphilitica;* and *c*) *Ecthyma syphiliticum.* Let us adopt this arrangement in considering each of these forms.

Sec. 100.—Acne Syphilitica.

This is the most frequent of all the pustulous forms of syphilis, and is more frequently overlooked than any other. It always occurs in the shape of isolated, scattered pimples of the size of a small lentil, that are irregularly scattered over various portions of the surface of the body, not very prominent, but of characteristic color, suppurating more or less imperfectly, and finally changing to crusts that are smaller than the original pimples. This acne may affect every part of the body, the face, back, chest, and extremities, but assumes a somewhat different form, according as it breaks out in one place or another. In the face, on the chest and back, it resembles most generally the common non-syphilitic acne; the pimples are rather large, prominent, and rounded, one half of a pimple being in a state of suppuration; they are usually covered with a small, more or less thick scurf, which, after it falls off, leaves a rather broad and depressed scar, often resting for a long time upon a tubercular base. On the limbs, these pimples are flat, especially at their base, which is broader, and not so round, and surrounded by a rather deep copper redness. The pimples themselves first have the shape of not very much elevated and sometimes painful spots of the size of small split peas; afterwards their centre becomes raised, after which a small collection of pus is perceived at its point, which disappears in two or three days, either in consequence of being absorbed, or the point being accidentally lacerated; or else it may become converted into a small, not very firmly adhering scurf. In this condition, the pimple forms a small papulous, copper-red elevation, offering but a slight resistance to the pressure of the finger, and showing a small depressed cicatrix at its point; sometimes the centre is perforated and surrounded for some time by remnants of epidermis. The longer this eruption lasts, the more it loses its pustulous form, and approximates the form of papules, for which it might easily be mistaken. Here, too, as in most other syphilitic eruptions, successive crops of new pimples make their appearance while the old ones are still running their course, so that these different and simultaneously-occurring formations offer great facilities for studying the whole course of the eruption ; though, after all, in spite of the great importance which Cazenave seems to attach to it, it matters very little whether this form is considered as of the pustulous or papulous variety, provided we are sure that it is a *syphilitic* disease. In this respect, it frequently happens that this acne is confounded with eruptions of an entirely different kind, even with the itch, more particularly if the pimples are scattered in great numbers over the extremities. I have met with a case where the flexor-surfaces of both arms were covered with these pimples, and where the nocturnal itching of which the patient, a very unclean woman, complained, and which was caused by vermin, made me doubt for a while the true nature of this disease, until I administered a dose of *Mercurius*, 12, after which the pimples rapidly disappeared, leaving only spots of the characteristic, unmistakable syphilitic color. This acne always runs a chronic course ; its pimples, which are always isolated, never terminate in ulceration ; their base almost always becomes indurated, until gradually the whole disappears, leaving only a small scar, which remains forever.

Sec. 101.—Impetigo Syphilitica.

This syphiloid may present itself in two different forms, according as the pustules either remain isolated or become confluent. In the former variety, the tolerably large pustules remain isolated, or, if they become confluent, it is mostly by accident, and never more than two or three at a time. When first appearing, they look like copper-colored spots of a tolerably vivid redness, the epidermis on which becomes raised in its whole extent, without showing a hardened base. When perfectly formed, they are small, soft, rather closely congregated pimples, filled with a purulent fluid, and surrounded by a red border ; as to the characteristic copper-color, however, it is confined to the portions of skin between the pimples, rather than to a definitely circumscribed areola around each pustule, the color of which areola at first even is very faint, but becomes more distinct in proportion as the pustules are more completely formed. The first appearance of this impetigo is very frequently preceded by a general feeling of malaise and of weariness and lameness in the limbs; the eruption may, moreover, spread over a more or less extensive surface. It is most usually seen on the abdomen, nates, and on the inner surface of the thighs, less frequently on the upper extremities, and still less frequently on the face. If once fully formed, these pustules, unless they are accidentally lacerated, may remain for several days at the same point of development; in every case, however, the purulent fluid which they contain coagulates, resulting in the formation of a small, brownish scurf, which is broader than the original pustule, and, in the majority of cases, dries up more and more, until it falls off and leaves only a cicatrix behind. In some cases, the pustules increase in size, the purulent fluid becomes more copious, and raises the epidermis in a larger circumference, in which case, several of these pustules approximate and run together under one crust, beneath which an ulcer may form which, although not very deep, may leave a cicatrix, that is larger and more depressed than the cicatrix formed by an isolated pustule.

The second or confluent form of this impetigo, which, in reality, is nothing more than a pustulous eruption setting in at the very commencement with an increased pathological activity, is, in every respect, more virulent. The confluent pustules, by their union, cause a suppuration which, although superficial, results in the formation of broad and more or less scattered cicatrices. This form is not often seen on the lower limbs, but more especially on the chest, neck, and, which is much worse, in the face and on the forehead. This form, likewise, is preceded by a general feeling of malaise, attended with more or less marked febrile motions; after which, the eruption itself is ushered in with a more or less vivid redness and swelling of the parts, upon which small pustules soon break out, and run into each other the more rapidly the more inflamed they are at their base, soon after forming broad scurfs, surrounded by copper-colored areolæ, whose crusts are unequal, raised, greenish, soft to the feel, and arched at their centre, deeply adhering to the surrounding skin, and betraying, by their very sight, the existence of a subjacent ulcerated surface, which, after the scurfs have fallen off, is found transformed into more or less disfigured cicatrices. This syphiloid may break out in several localities at once; if once formed, it does not spread any further, like serpiginous tubercles, for instance, but remains located where the original redness had first made its appearance.

Sec. 102.—Ecthyma Syphiliticum.

This syphiloid is distinguished from the former by the larger size of its pustules, not unlike the pustules of the common non-syphilitic eczema. The eruption is formed by a rising of the epidermis, underneath which pus is secreted; at their base, the pimples are more or less hardened, and very soon are transformed into thick crusts, which, when falling off, leave depressed cicatrices. According as these ulcers are either superficial, or more deeply penetrating to the subjacent tissues, we distinguish a *superficial* and a deep-seated eczema. Each of these varieties again admits of different forms.

In the former of these two varieties, the superficial ecthyma, the pustules, though more voluminous than those of impetigo, are never larger than a dime; they are perfectly round, run to a point like a cone; are filled with a thick, yellow fluid, and surrounded by copper-colored areolæ, without, however, any induration of their base. Offering but little resistance to the pressure of the finger, they generally break very easily, and very soon change to brown, round, not very firmly-adhering scurfs, with raised edges and a uniform thickness throughout, and always resting upon a very superficial ulcerated surface. These superficial pustules are generally scattered over large portions of the surface of the body, although they occur most frequently on the hairy scalp, yet they likewise show themselves in other localities, and even in several places at one and the same time. In most cases, they come out isolatedly, but they may likewise form clusters, in which case, the crusts arising from them are larger, thicker, not unlike the scurfs of the above-mentioned impetigo, from which they differ in this, that the scurfs of ecthyma are always perfectly round, not raised in the centre like a cone, but depressed and raised at the edges, not very firmly adhering to the skin, and never exceeding a common dime in size.

In the second form, the deeply-penetrating ecthyma, we have larger pustules of an oval form, which, when first breaking out, look like violet-red spots, soon become filled with a *bloody* pus and surrounded by bluish areolæ, around which the skin has a copper-colored appearance. Where the epidermis ceases to be tense, a swelling is perceived which causes these pustules to appear somewhat flattened. If these pustules tear and gradually pour out their contents, this bloody matter finally forms a scurf that increases in size during the first days of its existence, but finally dries up more and more, and almost resembles the scurf of a burn. This crust, which has the form of the original pustule, is thicker in its centre than that of the superficial ecthyma, and sometimes is even arched. If the crust is removed before it becomes detached of itself, a deep ulcer is seen with grayish, small granulations at the bottom, abruptly circumscribed edges, close to which a whitish border is raised above it, composed of remnants of the epidermis. If the crust runs its course unimpeded, it dries up more and more, becomes pitted at the centre, shrinks, and, after falling off, leaves, like all other syphiloids, a round and more or less depressed scar behind, which retains for a long time the characteristic color. The pustules, in this form of the ecthyma, are rather scanty, five or six, scattered at large intervals from each other, and most frequently seen on the arms and legs.

Sec. 103.—Lichen Syphiliticus, Venereal Itch.

Syphilitic papules are hard, firm, full, little blotches, and solid to the feel; containing neither pus nor any other serous fluid, irregularly scattered over large surfaces, and, in their totality, exhibiting the characteristic syphilitic color. They may break out on almost every part of the body, but are most generally observed on the extensor-surface of the extremities; likewise on the back, shoulders, and nape of the neck, where they usually have the appearance of thin, small, coniform, numerously-scattered pimples, which may likewise occur in groups, but may likewise appear less numerous and of larger size, even of the size of a small split pea. Hence we distinguish two kinds: a) the *syphilitic rash*, and b) the *syphilitic papules.*

The former, more especially known under the name of *lichen syphiliticus*, or venereal itch, has very small, sometimes innumerable, pimples that almost run into each other, and show a sort of lustre, which, in addition to the copper color, imparts to them a very peculiar appearance. This form, especially when it breaks out in the second stage of the primary, during the presence of protopathic phenomena, may be attended with all the symptoms that generally precede common, non-syphilitic exanthems; such as headache, weariness and lameless of the limbs, and more or less fever. In this case the eruption is generally all over; not only on the back and extensor surface of the extremities, but likewise, and more particularly, in the face and on the neck. If very acute, this form of the eruption does not last longer than a fortnight; in a few days the pimples begin to decay, break up in fragments and disappear, leaving only short-lasting spots, but never any scars. Sometimes their breaking is followed by slight desquamation. This eruption does not always appear in an acute form, but, after the complete disappearance of all protopathic products, may likewise break out as a true *secondary* syphiloid, of indefinite more really *chronic* duration. It is only this chronic form that I have had an opportunity of witnessing.

The other *papulous* form of this eruption has larger and broader pimples which, mostly arising from small spots of a dirty-yellow color, are rounded, never appear in groups, but always singly, scattered over large surfaces, which they invade gradually, not all at once. Hence this eruption may be observed, in all its stages, on persons afflicted with it, at one and the same period; in one locality we may observe firm, raised, copper-colored papules, whereas in another locality they appear shrunk, soft, and less red; and in other places we only see yellowish-red spots on the point of changing to papules; and still in other parts, spots of a grayish color, and more depressed, being remnants of former papules; the skin between all these different appearances exhibits a livid color. These larger papules are generally located on the extremities, shoulders, nape of the neck, especially on the forehead, where they form the so-called *corona veneris*. They always run a chronic course; like the former, they never change to ulcers, crusts, or scales, but frequently appear intermingled with other syphiloids, and not unfrequently simultaneously with ulcers in the throat, exostoses, etc.

Sec. 104.—Tubercular Eruptions.

This syphiloid generally assumes the form of small, firm, dense, raised blotches, resisting the pressing of the finger, and, like the papules, containing neither pus nor any serous fluid. These tubercles are somewhat raised above the skin, sometimes scattered, and sometimes less numerous and limited to small blotches; sometimes combined in more or less regular groups, and in other cases scattered over a large portion of the surface of the body. The same diversified appearances exist in regard to their form, size, and general course. Some have scarcely the size of a pea, are round, shining, copper-colored; others are broad, flattened, globular, round, or oval, and as if seated within the layers of the integuments; whereas in other cases they are raised a few lines above the skin, as if placed upon it. Some of them are smooth and even, scaly, and even ulcerated and covered with scurfs; in some patients the disappearance of the tubercles is followed by nothing but light grayish spots that gradually disappear, whereas in other cases they cause inextinguishable, uneven cicatrices. Some, finally, achieve their whole course, together with all the disorganizations of which such tubercles are capable, without extending beyond the boundaries of their original site; whereas in other cases they spread far beyond their original limits, destroying the integuments in their course. Moreover, they may attack every part of the body; their favorite localities, however, are the face, nose, ears, eyebrows, and hairy scalp; though they have been known to spread over the whole surface of the body. The same differences are perceived in regard to the course they pursue, as in regard to their form. At times appearing slowly and by degrees; at times suddenly and unexpectedly; they frequently announce their advent by a general sensation of malaise, or supervene in company with syphilitic affections of the mucous membranes and bones; and, in almost every case, their appearance is superinduced by some accidental circumstance, such as an emotion, fever, etc. Sometimes they are accompanied by a considerable swelling and painfulness of the affected parts; very frequently they remain perfectly indolent, without affecting the surrounding parts. In other respects they may remain unchanged for months; but, starting from a given point, be it dispersion or ulceration, they may either disappear in an incredibly short space of time, or they may cause the most terrible disorganizations. In accordance with these different characteristics, Cazenave has enumerated the following five kinds of tubercular syphiloid eruptions: a) grouping; b) scattered; c) perforating; d) serpiginous, and e) flattened. We will examine them more closely in their order.

Sec. 105.—Simple Grouping and Scattered Tubercles.

In spite of apparent differences of form, these two kinds have so many points in common that they may be very properly ranged in one class.

a) Grouping Tubercles.—These tubercles are generally of inconsiderable size; they do not seem very much inclined to ulcerate, and the characteristic copper-color is not very marked, although it may show itself in two different ways. In most cases these groups are regular, perfectly rounded, and composed of more or less tubercles of the size of a large pea, in such a manner that each adjoining group forms, as it were, a ring with an elevated border, which is interrupted again by every subsequent tubercle, leaving an intermediate copper-colored space. According as the tubercles which form this ring are more or less in number, the length of its diameter varies. These tubercles, which are often covered with small, hard, grayish scales, never ulcerate, run a slow course, and generally disperse without leaving the least scar. They break out most frequently on the arms, sometimes on the forehead and neck. On the other hand, *irregular* groups of tubercles appear on the cheeks and lips; they are ranged close to each other without order, generally shining, but small and resembling papules, occupying, however, a much broader base than these latter. They are of a genuine copper-color which often extends beyond the locality where the tubercles are seated, especially in the face; moreover, the tubercles are hard, projecting, and resisting the pressure of the finger, like large-sized pin's heads. Although they never become moist, nor easily ulcerate, yet, after having stood a long while, they may become inflamed, run into each other, and cause a swelling of the part, which may break out in more or less deep ulcers; in the majority of cases, however, they pass away by dispersion after a certain period, decreasing at the same time in size as well as in color, and finally disappearing without leaving a trace behind. Whenever these grouping tubercles appear, they always constitute a symptom of fully developed secondary syphilis.

b) Scattered Tubercles.—These tubercles pretty generally break out at considerable distances from each other; the intermediate skin looks wilted and dingy; they are more prominent, more raised, and have a broader and more hardened base than the former variety; they are more irregular, imperfectly rounded, oval; they are of a bright copper-redness; the epidermis that covers them is tense and shining. Being perfectly indolent, they appear to be the result of a slowly progressing inflammation; they never become either scaly or ulcerated, but remain shining, without ever secreting a moisture. Sometimes, though rarely, the appearance of the eruption is preceded by headache and nocturnal bone-pains; they appear principally in the face and on the limbs, but may show themselves on almost any other part of the body, and even appear in company with grouping tubercles, although in different localities. They run a slow course; after they have gradually grown to the size of an olive, they may remain stationary for a long time, until, in consequence of some accidental cause, they become inflamed and afterwards ulcerate, which, however, is a rare occurrence; at the end of two or three weeks they generally disperse without scarcely ever leaving a spot behind, the color of which never continues longer than a month after the eruption has disappeared. A small scar is sometimes seen on their original site.

Sec. 106.—Perforating Tubercles.

This form, so named from the destructions which these tubercles may cause by ulceration, is distinguished by the production of large papules or deep-seated indurations in the integuments that at first are inconsiderable, but soon increase in size. They are not usually very numerous, and break out in the face, especially on the lips, alæ nasi, and in front of the ear near the meatus; even if they appear in other localities, they are always present in the face. In most cases they are broad and semi-globular; their base looks as if it were grown together with the integuments, and penetrated deeply into the cellular tissue which they show a great tendency to perforate by ulceration. Very often they remain stationary for a long period, even for a whole year; after this period they begin to look red and, for some time, change their color; sometimes they appear of a coppery-red, sometimes gray, and then again of a simple red color, until the suppurating process begins at the outermost point of the tubercle. As soon as suppuration has set in, the ulterior course of the tubercle may take two different directions. Most frequently the course is slow and almost painless; the tubercle gradually softens at one or more circumscribed points which sometimes coalesce, and, either after or even before the complete discharge of the pus, change to a thick, not very humid, and lightly adhering crust which, after falling off, forms again until the tubercle is completely destroyed, cicatrization not taking place until the last remnant of the indurated tubercle has passed away by suppuration. If cicatrization should take place at an earlier period, the process of suppuration will again recommence sooner or later until the whole tubercle is gone. Not always, however, the softening takes such a slow course. Very often the tubercles at once become tense, painful, and are surrounded by an inflamed, red areola, after which the ulcerative process, beginning at the terminal point, rapidly penetrates through the whole thickness of the induration, and a black, dry, thick crust forms, that soon falls off and reveals a cup-shaped ulcer having all the characteristic signs of a syphilitic sore. New crusts keep forming, with new destructions, until the whole tubercular mass is removed and a final cicatrix has formed. In every case this cicatrix is pitted, of a violet color, with abrupt edges, and always retains the indestructible traces of a former tubercle. If these tubercles break out on the lips, nose, and on other parts, it frequently happens that these organs are irremediably lost. Even if the destruction should not be complete after a first ulceration, it will certainly result in the entire loss of the parts after a second or third renewal of the ulcerative process, and we can never be sure of having achieved a perfect cure until a long period elapses after the last cicatrization without any new outbreak taking place. This syphiloid is most frequently seen already towards the end of the second stage of the primary period of syphilis, it being a not very remote sequela of protopathic products. This syphiloid is most likely the most hideous of all, which, if occurring in the face or on the nose, might easily be confounded with lupus, carcinoma, or even with elephantiasis, where this disease prevails, if it were not that here, too, the previous history of the case, and the characteristic signs which are peculiar to all syphiloid eruptions, render the diagnosis all but certain.

Sec. 107.—Serpiginous and Flat Tubercles.

The first of these two forms, the so-called serpiginous or creeping tubercles, are distinguished from the former by this, that, in their case, the suppurative process does not spread downward to the subjacent textures, but onwards over the adjoining surface. At its appearance, this form is known by large, red, round, hard papules, breaking out irregularly, here and there; they are not very numerous at first, do not exceed the size of a hazelnut, and sometimes are no bigger than a pea. Though they can occasionally be seen on other parts of the body, yet they break out most frequently on the back, chest, and in the face, whence they afterwards spread over the whole body, except the palms of the hands and soles of the feet; their favorite locality, however, is the forehead, hairy scalp, nape of the neck and shoulders, and no less the hairy parts of the body, or the parts adjoining the hair, such as the temples, eyebrows, inguinal regions, and sexual parts. The tubercles themselves are smooth, shining, of a copper-red, and never covered with scales; very frequently they remain indolent for a long time, without changing; suddenly, however, after a longer or shorter period, they commence to inflame, and to suppurate at their terminal point, after which the tubercles are rapidly destroyed, and become converted into thick, hard, coniform, sometimes black, at times gray, and always firmly-adhering crusts. If these crusts are removed before they become spontaneously detached, a rather superficial ulcer becomes visible, which soon covers itself with a new crust, which is neither as black nor as thick as its predecessor, but continues to be thicker at the centre than at the edges. As soon as this ulceration commences, new tubercles form by the side of the former, or on the borders of the cicatrices of former tubercles. By coalescing into one, these new tubercles form extensive sores, or else a number of smaller ulcers may arise in succession, at short intervals from each other. The destruction of neighboring parts, arising from this continued formation of new tubercles, may extend over a large surface of a few inches in diameter, or may give rise to several ulcers of a rounded shape, and separated from each other by free intervals. It seems as though the process of ulceration would have a spontaneous termination, if it were not fed by new tubercles starting up in proportion as their predecessors are removed by ulceration. Hence it is that they may cicatrice at one end, after the fashion of the serpiginous chancre, while the ulcerative process continues at the other end, where it is fed by the formation of successive crops of new tubercles, whose cicatrices continue for a long time to betray their origin by their form and peculiar distribution. Moreover, we may observe on every patient the different stages which this syphiloid runs through, at one and the same time. In this way, we may see at one place more or less numerous, prominent, copper-colored, irregularly-scattered tubercles, more particularly within the limits of the affected parts; whereas, at some other places, we see more or less thick and broad, hard, centrally-raised, and somewhat dry crusts, the intermediate space between which is occupied by gray ulcers, with raised, abrupt edges, some of these ulcers being round, others irregularly-shaped, or spirally contorted, beside which, we witness the most diversified cicatrices, the older of which appear white and fibrous, whereas the more recently formed are violet-red, etc. This syphiloid runs a very slow course; it generally does not make its appearance until a long time after the primary syphilitic phenomena have disappeared.

Concerning the *flat tubercles*, which Cazenave likewise ranges among his syphiloids, but which are, for the most part, primary phenomena, see *mucous tubercles*, §§ 68–72.

Sec. 108.—Lepra Syphilitica, seu nigricans.

(*Syphilitic Leprosy.*)

Several authors have not been willing to regard this eruption as an independent form, but maintain that the formation of scales is a termination peculiar to all syphiloids. This is indeed true, in most cases; but, inasmuch as there are some forms where the formation of scales plays an important part, and even constitutes the whole phenomena exclusively, as it were, a correct and easy diagnosis of syphilitic cutaneous eruptions would seem to render a more particular consideration of these scaly syphiloid eruptions indispensable. Cazenave, who is the most correct observer of all syphilitic forms, classes lepra under three different categories: 1) *lepra nigricans*, or syphilitic lepra; 2) *psoriasis*, or *scaly tetter;* and 3) *psoriasis cornuta*, or *horny scales.*

The first of these three kinds, *lepra syphilitica*, consists of an eruption of circular, violet-red spots, of different sizes, somewhat raised at the edges, and rather depressed in the centre. These spots, which never attain to the large size of common, non-syphilitic lepra spots, generally are of the size of a dime, sometimes even much smaller. When first breaking out, the spots are like little papules, raised above the skin, and looking like points of a coppery color, which spread and become pitted in the centre, or rather raised at their edges, while gradually the spots assume a dark, dingy, violet-red color, with a somewhat blackish tint, and become covered at their borders with gray, hard, dry scales. The eruption may continue in this condition for a long time, except that the scales fall off and become renewed again, or else do not return at all, in which case, these spots retrograde in the same manner as they had gradually developed themselves, leaving only dark vestiges, which continue to mark, for a long time after, the rounded form of the affected parts, and are darker at their edges than at the centre, which first loses its characteristic color. These spots can show themselves at every point of the surface of the body, but the extremities seem to constitute their favorite site; Cazenave has seen them scattered over the whole body. I have seen them, in the case of a rather careless woman, and whose face alone had remained free, covering the limbs, abdomen, chest, and back, at the same time as they were associated with other syphilitic cutaneous forms in other parts of the same body. Their first appearance is sometimes preceded for some days by a general feeling of malaise, headache, sadness, even bone-pains, all of which symptoms generally disappear in proportion as the eruption breaks out upon the skin. In the case of my woman, the patient had had a chancre two years previous, which had become cicatrized a long time ago; and the different syphilidæ, which generally selected the skin for their locality, had already been out over a year, attended with a sort of sadness or joylessness, from the very moment when the eruptions first made their appearance, and which did not cease until they had been completely removed.

Sec. 109.—Psoriasis Syphilitica (Diffusa, Guttata et Cornuta).

That form of psoriasis which approximates most nearly the common, non-syphilitic psoriasis, is psoriasis diffusa; and more particularly the variety designated as psoriasis guttata. Psoriasis *diffusa* consists of rather large, round or irregular, yellowish, pale-red, or copper-colored spots, that become covered with hard, brittle, faint-white scales, the centre of which frequently ulcerates and forms a blackish scurf; the scaly spot frequently shows slight cracks, from which a clear serum oozes out, which may be succeeded by ulcerations and condylomatous growths. This form is most frequently seen in the face, though it may likewise break out on the hands and around the ankles, and, according to some, even around the anus and on the scrotum.

Psoriasis guttata, which occurs much more frequently, is not, as some assert, confined exclusively to the hairy scalp; on the contrary, it may spread over the whole surface of the body. On the body it is seen in the shape of small, prominent spots, of the size of a three-cent piece, generally round or oval, not pitted in the centre, generally isolated and scattered in tolerably large numbers. These small spots, which are of a marked copper red, and retain this color for a long time before it changes to gray, soon become covered with a gray, rather firmly-adhering scale, which, after it once drops off, is not apt to form again, and leaves a small, red, somewhat raised spot, surrounded by a narrow white border. These spots often remain a long time before they flatten down and grow paler; even after they have sunk to a level with the skin, the redness often perseveres for a long time, and imparts to the spots an appearance of being elevated above the skin. After a time, their color changes to brown and then gray, and the eruption disappears without leaving a trace behind.

Psoriasis cornuta, also designated as *palmaris* and *plantaris*, because it breaks out almost exclusively in the palms of the hands and on the soles of the feet, may break out in two different forms. In one form it may assume the shape of small risings, of the size of a pea, somewhat wart-shaped, and seated upon a red, not always distinctly perceptible base, with a hard, white, horny centre, that sometimes can be picked off with the nails, but in other cases seems to be sunk into the integuments, like a wedge. This horny elevation is generally surrounded by a ring, of one or two lines in width, having the characteristic color but not always distinctly visible, if the hands are not clean, and becoming more prominent after the hands have been washed with *cold* water. I have seen this form break out, sometimes even after the lapse of a fortnight, in individuals in whom a chancre had been suppressed by external means, without the use of Mercury; whereas the second variety has only been seen by me on persons who had taken a good deal of Mercury for chancre, and even after chronic mercurial poisoning, in cases where no syphilitic taint was present. This variety consists of a more or less broad, scaly spot, or of several of them, on which the epidermis seems to become detached in large scarlet flaps, whose scales are sometimes so thick that it seems as though several layers might be torn away. These scales sometimes crack, forming painful rhagades having a very *clean* appearance, and being entirely devoid of any of the signs of similar rhagades at the anus, or between the toes. These scales are very often surrounded by a tolerably broad border of an unmistakably syphilitic color; in such cases a so-called mercurial syphilis, or a coalescing of syphilis and mercurial disease most likely prevails.

Sec. 110. Syphilitic Affections of the Nails and Hair.

In order to facilitate their diagnosis, we will consider these affections more particularly.

1. *Affections of the Nails.*—In treating of the consecutive, and sometimes likewise protopathic ulcers of the primary period of syphilis, we have already made mention of *syphilitic ulcerations of the nails* (*onychiæ syphiliticæ*), which often break out around the nails as irregular rhagades, with fungoid borders, and betray their syphilitic origin by their gray, bluish color, and by their secretion of a fetid ichor. Beside these ulcerations, in consequence of which the nails often drop off, these may likewise undergo important structural alterations, without any ulcerous disorganization, simply by the syphilitic virus diffused through the organism. In consequence of such alterations, they may likewise drop off the same as when they are destroyed by ulceration, although such structural alterations almost always involve the matrices of the nails. In most cases of this kind, the internal border of the nail secretes a sort of purulent fluid, sometimes in considerable, and, at other times, in scarcely perceptible quantities, the color of the skin remaining unchanged all the time. Very frequently the nail is more or less painful, the pain being, if not always, at least very often felt when pressing upon the ball of the finger or toe, and sometimes preventing the use of these parts. The affection is very often associated with other syphiloid eruptions.

2. *Falling off of the Hair.*—This symptom is one of the most frequent accompaniments of secondary syphilis. I do not know of

a single case of this disease, where the above-mentioned symptom did not occur. Three of my female patients, so far, not only lost their head-hair, but likewise their eyebrows, eyelashes, the hair of the private parts, so completely that no trace of it could be seen; although it grew again after a time, and the face became again invested with its noblest ornament. Older authors have attributed this sad result to the abuse of Mercury, which *may indeed produce similar results;* but in the cases where I witnessed this spoliation, not a grain of Mercury had ever been taken. The pityriasis described by other authors as an affection of the hairy scalp that is said to precede the falling off of the hair, is likewise no permanent symptom; in many cases the loss of hair may indeed be caused by syphilitic affections of the hairy scalp; but in many, and indeed in most cases, this loss takes place without the least sign of a syphilitic affection of the scalp being perceptible. On the other hand, the hair may fall off in consequence of secondary, and even primary syphilis; sometimes even during the fungoid stage of protopathic chancres. The older the disease, and the more remotely from the period of protopathic chancre the falling off of the hair takes place, the more unfavorable the prognosis. Among older patients the prognosis is likewise more unfavorable than among young people. Among young people, if the hair fell off shortly after the appearance of protopathic phenomena, and the disease was otherwise *rationally* treated, and cured with appropriate means, the hair grows again as thickly and as rapidly as if it never had been lost. It is only in places where the roots of the hair had been completely destroyed by ulceration, that the most celebrated pomatum, as well as any other remedy, will prove inefficient to restore it.

III. AILMENTS ACCOMPANYING SYPHILOID ERUPTIONS.

Sec. 111.—General Observation.

The phenomena which we intend to mention in the following paragraphs under this designation, are described by most writers on syphilis as "complications of syphiloid eruptions;" this term, however, conveys a wrong idea of what would have been said, if the matter had been examined from the right point of view. Complications are, generally speaking, extraordinary and embarrassing phenomena, supervening during the course of a malady, in addition to its main symptoms; phenomena that would not have appeared, if the malady had run a simple and natural course, and which are caused either by the violence of the malady itself, or by other accessory circumstances outside of its proper range. This is not the case in regard to the syphilitic phenomena coexisting with the syphilidæ, for the reason that the main disease is not the existing syphiloid, but the *syphilitic disease itself;* so that the syphilitic phenomena appearing simultaneously with the syphiloid, which itself is only a symptom, cannot be considered as *complications* of the latter. The case is indeed different, if it is not the disease, but the symptomatic syphiloid that is viewed as the main object of cure; in such a case we may indeed talk of complications that impede, or embarrass the plan of treatment; but such complications would only be therapeutical, not pathological complications, since they all constitute integral parts of the malady, as the false membrane is an integral part of croup, and the stitch in the side an integral part of pleurisy. Inasmuch as it is our aim never to convey to our readers a wrong idea, on any page of this work, of what we mean by the object of cure, and inasmuch as the term "*complications of syphiloids*" does convey a wrong idea, we have preferred the expression "Simultaneous, or accompanying complaints," by which we mean, complaints that may break out in other localities simultaneously with a syphiloid, or other complaints, simultaneously with which the syphiloid may co-exist; since in many of these cases the main phenomena are not to be found on the skin, but on the primarily affected parts. A proper knowledge of these accompanying complaints is equally important for a homœopathic physician, as for an allopath; though not in the same manner for the former, as for the latter. It facilitates the diagnosis of syphiloid eruptions, as such; and aids us in discovering the proper remedy in the case. We will, therefore, consider this subject further: 1) by pointing out the *primary* symptoms, during the presence of which syphiloid eruptions may supervene; 2) the *secondary* symptoms, by which syphiloids may be accompanied; and 3), the non-syphilitic cutaneous diseases, during which syphiloid eruptions may break out as a complication of the former.

Sec. 112.—Primary Symptoms simultaneously with which Syphiloids may occur.

In a former paragraph (§ 84), we have already stated that secondary phenomena may not only arise after the disappearance of primary symptoms, but likewise even during their presence. This is more particularly true with reference to syphiloids, some of which initiate, and, as it were, announce the advent of the secondary period in the character of premonitory symptoms. In this respect, however, not all syphiloids hold the same rank. While some of them almost always justify the suspicion that syphilitic phenomena are still perceptible on the sexual organs, such as old chancres during the period of reproduction, older or more recent buboes, incipient or older mucous tubercles, figwarts, with or without gonorrhœa, etc., there are other syphiloids, on the contrary, that do not reveal any thing of the kind, and where every trace of the primary symptoms has disappeared. Primary phenomena are still most frequently to be found coexisting with syphilitic measles (roseolæ syphiliticæ), sometimes with syphilitic eczema, the venereal itch, and, in general, all forms which, like those just mentioned, set in with general symptoms of malaise and fever. Less frequently will primary symptoms be found with syphilitic herpes, rhypia, syphilitic acne, impetigo, ecthyma, and tubercles; in their case secondary affections, such as ulcers in the throat, affections of the mouth, bone-pains, etc., will shed light on the true nature of these eruptions; although a closer inspection may reveal even here, if not open chancres, at least suspicious-looking cicatrices somewhat raised above the sound skin, and having a more or less copper-colored appearance. In the case of women, these eruptions are often accompanied by a suspicious discharge from the vagina, which is not a genuine gonorrhœa, although the French class all these discharges under the same general name of *blennorrhœa* or *blennorhagia.* This suspicious discharge corresponds to the balanorrhœa of males, which is likewise very apt to supervene during the presence of the secondary symptoms, and may enlighten us concerning the true nature of the existing syphiloid, which, in its turn, may shed light on the real character of the blennorrhœa. In general, these eruptions have no fixed rule, either as regards time or pathological relations; after the *primary* stage is past, they may break out at any time, when and how they choose, without its being possible to explain why, in one case, they act differently from another; in one patient, for instance, the same syphiloid may make its appearance while the primary symptoms are still in full bloom, whereas in another patient it may not manifest itself until the primary symptoms have all disappeared.

Sec. 113.—Accompanying Secondary Complaints of a Different Kind.

We have already directed the reader's attention to the fact that a syphiloid, especially in constitutional syphilis of long standing, scarcely ever appears alone, but always in company with other eruptions, such as syphilitic papules with pustules, scaly eruptions, or tubercles; or eczema, impetigo, pemphigus, etc., with macûlæ, and so on, presenting an exceedingly checkered combination. Beside this, these syphiloids may be accompanied by secondary and (falsely-named) tertiary phenomena of various kinds. Hence nothing is more erroneous than the proposition, that used to be taught as a dogma in our schools, "The course of syphilis is divided in four periods: 1) chancre and buboes, and after they disappear; 2) chancre in the throat and cutaneous eruptions, and *after their disappearance;* 3) affections of the bones, gummata and other phenomena; 4) general syphilis and—death!" More correct recent observations have shown that this is not exactly the course of things. As soon as the secondary period has commenced, all the syphilitic phenomena occurring subsequently to the primary invasion, may manifest themselves successively or simultaneously, without any definite order as to time. Hence, syphiloids may coexist with other syphilitic phenomena, if not with all of them, at least several at once, though, in severe cases, the whole series may manifest themselves at the same time: secondary chancres, mucous affections of the throat, mouth, and nose, exostoses, bone-pains, caries. There is scarcely a syphiloid of some extent and importance, where, even if all primary symptoms had disappeared years ago, the diagnosis is not facilitated by coexisting affections of the throat and mouth, or by bone-pains, gummata, exostoses, etc. During the presence of these syphiloids, it likewise happens that simple wounds of the skin become disproportionately severe, suppurate and change to ulcers that have all the characteristic signs of chancre, by which means a flood of light may likewise be shed on the character of the existing eruption. In a syphiloid eruption where the constitutional affection has already lasted a long while, a remarkably characteristic symptom, which may supervene independently of the specific color of the syphiloid, is a peculiar *affection of the pigment of the skin*, especially in the face and on the forehead, sometimes on the chest, neck, and lower limbs, consisting of spots that almost represent *liver-spots*, continuing unchanged for years, of a brownish hue, irregularly rounded, and remaining visible after or during the appearance of the most varied syphiloids, without passing off in the least until the whole of the syphilitic disease is extirpated. Another, much more dangerous condition, may become associated with the syphiloids, which is nothing less than a general *cachexia;* this, however, only sets in when several other syphilitic affections in other tissues accompany the syphiloid eruptions. In consequence of this cachexia, the poor patients may become covered with wounds, sores, and cicatrices of every description, and, deprived of one or more of their senses, especially of the senses of vision and hearing, may wander about as disgusting and emaciated cadavers, with a wilted, lax, dry, sallow and livid skin, reminding one of the cachexia of cancer. Fortunately, a condition thus aggravated is exceedingly rare, and indeed occurs only in cases where all care had been neglected, and the patients had been of feeble health previous to the infection; although it may likewise be occasioned, as is not unfrequently the case, by bad management with mercury, at least to a certain extent.

Sec. 114.—Non-syphilitic Eruptions accompanying the Syphiloids.

Another point, which cannot be sufficiently attended to in a case of syphiloid eruption, is the fact that not only several of them may appear together, mixed up indiscriminately one with the other, but that they likewise manifest themselves associated with other *non-syphilitic* exanthems, on which account the diagnosis of the existing combination may become very difficult, and the physician may find it a hard task to make up his mind regarding the true nature of the case before him. For this reason, it is important and useful to know what eruptions may possibly appear together; this knowledge may enable us to see light even in obscure and dubious cases. In respect to these combinations, which may really be regarded as true complications, we have to distinguish two possibilities: *a*) a syphiloid may supervene while some other cutaneous disease is already present; or, *b*) this disease may break out while the syphiloid is already developed. The former of these two cases, where the syphiloid supervenes during the presence of an already existing exanthem, can only properly refer to *chronic* cutaneous diseases, since all acute diseases temporarily suspend the course of syphilis, which, even if actually and fully developed in the organism, would not break out until the acute disease had run its course. As regards *chronic* exanthems, the syphiloids may indeed become associated with them, either by coalescing with them, and imparting to the former a syphilitic appearance; or else both exanthems may coexist independently of each other, in which case, syphilitic and *non*-syphilitic scales, scabs, tetters, lichen, eczemata, etc., may be observed and contrasted on one and the same patient with considerable interest and advantage. Such cases, however, are not very frequent; whereas other cases, where syphilitic pustules, for instance, are seated on old, large liver-spots, occur much more frequently. As regards the other case, where a *new* exanthem becomes associated with an existing syphiloid, this *new* exanthem must always be one of an acute form, such as measles, smallpox, scarlatina, etc., inasmuch as the organism being saturated with the chronic syphilitic miasma, the existing diathesis does not leave room for the development of another chronic eruption; though I have seen more than one patient who, even while affected with a chronic syphilitic exanthem, was, at the same time, attacked with the itch. If *acute* exanthems supervene during the presence of syphiloid eruptions, the former may assume a very malignant form, especially if the syphiloid had already shown symptoms of malignancy, and had become deeply rooted in the tissues. On the other hand, if the syphiloid and the other symptoms of secondary syphilis were but slight, I have seen every syphilitic sign become suspended, and utterly disappear, in consequence of the supervention of an acute exanthem, and not reappear again until this exanthem had run its course without the least untoward result. As to the assertion, that the syphilitic diathesis may be completely extirpated by the supervention of typhus, smallpox, etc., I am unable to confirm it. I have seen two such cases; in both of them the syphilitic symptoms were indeed suspended during the course of the acute disease; in both of them, however, though the disease ran a very favorable course, the final convalescence was attended with malignant syphilitic ulcerations, as a last sequela.

IV. DIAGNOSIS OF SYPHILITIC EXANTHEMS.

Sec. 115.—General Observation.

One who has carefully perused our description of the different syphiloids, but has not observed them in practice, might be led to imagine that nothing is easier than to recognize their true character at first sight whenever they occur. This is indeed true in many cases, especially if other primary or secondary symptoms of syphilis are present at the same time. Even in cases where these accessory symptoms are wanting, the characteristic color; the rounded form of single pimples, or whole groups of them, which always approximate to the circle; the successive crops in which these eruptions appear; in one word the whole look of such a syphiloid, and above all, its contrast with a similar, *non*-syphilitic exanthem, together with a knowledge of the previous history of the case, will lead the physician, if not to the positive conviction, at least to the supposition that he is dealing with a syphiloid in the present case. A mere supposition is of course no certainty; and if it is necessary in any disease to have certainty, it is in syphilis; not only on account of the danger involved in a misapprehension of its true nature, the danger of increase and aggravation of the symptoms, but likewise on account of the inconvenience to which a physician might be exposed, if in a case of obscure and chronic exanthem, but perfectly free from all syphilitic taint, he should allow himself to express the suspicion that the exanthem might possibly betray the presence of some hidden syphilitic infection. But how is the physician to acquire certainty in the absence of all other syphilitic signs, or if the patient out of modesty or in consequence of other important considerations, should insist upon never having been affected with syphilis; or if he should even have remained ignorant of the fact in consequence of drying up an incipient chancre-vesicle with lead-water, or suppressing it with some cauterizing agent, and if the rapid disappearance of this primary sign of the syphilitic infection should have led him to overlook the danger and to mistake this first manifestation of the disease for something unimportant and perhaps a mere accident? But supposing we discover symptoms of a former syphilitic infection, would this justify us to pronounce the existing exanthem of a syphilitic character, even if the absence of all positive signs of syphilis should be calculated to excite a doubt in our minds? We have already stated (§ 85), that in cases where syphiloids break out years after the primary phenomena have disappeared, we shall discover a continued series of syphilitic phenomena from the first moment of manifestation of the syphilitic infection down to the appearance of the present exanthem. It is to this circumstance that we desire to direct the special attention of practitioners in cases where a careful inquiry into the previous history and origin of the case neither reveals a present infection, nor any other, unless perhaps one that had been forgotten for years. If we can find out that the patient, who pretends never to have been infected with syphilis, has had several exanthems, (*the nature, form, color, and course of which the physician* cannot investigate with too much care,) and if the character or the nature of these exanthems corresponds to that of analogous syphilitic exanthems, we may almost rest assured that the present eruption, if some of its leading appearances resemble the symptoms of one of the former series, is of a syphiloid character. And vice versa, if a patient who had not been exposed to any new infection for the last three years, and had been treated *rationally* for the former infections, applies for treatment, and the eruption, according to all appearances, is decidedly of a dubious character, no other secondary symptoms being present, and the patient having been perfectly exempt, during this period of three years, from all suspicious eruptions, from all equivocal spots upon the chest, face, or hands, we may as safely conclude that the existing exanthem is *non-syphilitic*, as it was fair to conclude in the former case that it was of an opposite nature.

Sec. 116.—Certain local Diagnostic Signs.

As has already been stated, these are: 1) the peculiar *color;* 2) the disposition inherent in the isolated spots, pustules, or pimples, or in whole groups of these eruptions to assume a *circular* form; and above all, 3) the succession of crops, which is never seen as significantly in any other dermoid disease, and which gives us an opportunity of observing a syphiloid eruption in all its different stages at one and the same time. This sign is of the utmost significance. It alone, if fully present, together with the other characteristic symptoms, is sufficient to decide the diagnosis even when no other syphilitic phenomena are present. These exanthems, however, are not always seen at this period; very frequently they present themselves during the first stage of their existence, when no succession of crops has as yet taken place, and the *color* and *form* of the eruptions have to be the sole guide of the physician. In relation to these two characteristics, we shall therefore offer a few suggestions. As regards *color*, we have already stated a number of times that the characteristic color of syphilitic eruptions is the color of *copper;* but we have likewise seen that this red, during the course of these eruptions, passes from the simple *red* through a bluish brown or yellow to the dark reddish-gray color of venison, and to a dingy gray-yellow, through so many shades, that it requires a well-practised eye to recognize, amidst so many different shades, the *peculiar* syphilitic color, which, nevertheless, can never remain unrecognized by any one who has once had a chance to observe it. Inasmuch as not every practitioner has seen all these different shades, and the general definition of *coppery-red* might easily lead to wrong conclusions, the question will be, under what general appellation these different shades should be comprehended so that they may be recognized even by a physician who has never seen them. The solution of this problem has been vainly attempted by most of the older as well as modern writers on syphilis; fortunately, however, this question admits of a ready answer at the period when the characteristic succession of crops has not yet taken place, and when the *color* of the eruption is to decide its syphilitic character. For it is during this period, when the exanthems first make their appearance, that the copper color is most deeply marked, and only vanishes at the time when the period of the succession of crops sets in, when with every new crop the deep copper-red will again appear: so that the peculiar copper-red, whether of the whole exanthem or only of parts of it, is and always will be the characteristic *diagnostic sign* which, in addition to the tendency to the *circular form*, will almost always be sufficient to determine the syphilitic nature of the eruption. At all events, this color is a safer diagnostic sign than the mere form, although this will likewise prove a valuable indication provided we do not look at the eruption in a one-sided manner; but view it as a *whole*, as we see it simultaneously on the face, chest, back, limbs, etc.; if seated on the fingers, for instance, we tell the patient to place them close together, so that we may have a chance of observing the full shape of the exanthem, whether pustules, spots, or pimples. The difficulty, in this respect, is not, however, limited to a recognition of these circular forms; for, as we shall see in the subsequent paragraph, there are other, non-syphilitic eruptions that assume a round form, such as herpes circinnatus (ring-worm), etc.

V. COMMON DERMOID DISEASES, WITH WHICH SYPHILOIDS MAY BE CONFOUNDED.

Sec. 117.—Rubeola, Varicella, Smallpox.

What we have said at the conclusion of the preceding paragraph, of the circular form as being common to some non-syphilitic eruptions, applies equally to some other symptoms which both *syphilitic* and *non-syphilitic* exanthems have in common. In order, therefore, to furnish all the means which may assist in establishing a correct and discriminating diagnosis, we deem it indispensable to present a list of the non-syphilitic cutaneous affections with which the syphiloids are most easily confounded. These are, in general: 1) some *exanthematic* and *epidemic* eruptions; 2) certain *dermoid affections of the face;* 3) various *herpetic eruptions;* and 4) some forms of mercurial syphiloid eruptions, all of which we will consider more particularly in the following article.

1. *Exanthematic* and *Epidemic forms.* Under this head, *rubeola, varicella* and *varioloid* deserve our first attention. As regards rubeola (roseola communis), with which, in case the patient should deny the existence of any previous syphilitic infection, syphilitic spots (roseola syphilitica) might be confounded, we have to observe in the first place that the febrile motions with which the breaking out of this last-named exanthem may be attended, are never as violent as the fever accompanying acute exanthems. Moreover, the redness of the common roseola-spots pales off in proportion as the eruption runs its course, and disappears under the pressure of the finger; their final disappearance leaves nothing but a slight desquamation; whereas the spots of the syphilitic roseola are of a coppery-red, deepening and finally changing to a grayish color as the spots run their course; moreover, they progress

slowly, disappear but imperfectly under the pressure of the finger, and, long after their disappearance, leave brown, or dirty yellowish-brown tints which, though not very distinct, become more prominent in the cold or after washing in cold water. As regards *varicella* and *variola*, with which some syphiloids are likewise apt to be confounded, the fever accompanying these non-syphilitic eruptions at their first appearance, is likewise much more intense than the febrile motions attending analogous syphiloids; in addition to which, the syphilitic vesicles are always surrounded by a copper-colored areola, which is wanting in simple varicella, whose vesicles moreover rapidly incline to suppurate, whereas the syphilitic vesicles remain for a long time in the same condition, and finally become converted into blackish crusts which fall off, leaving dingy-gray spots behind. The absence of *acute* fever during the prodromic stage of the *syphilitic ecthyma*, where the febrile motions, as in the case of all other syphilitic eruptions, are much less marked than the fever accompanying the breaking out of an acute exanthem, may be sufficient to distinguish that ecthyma from common variola, though the syphilitic pustles may lead a superficial observer into error, as they indeed have done in many cases, for a few days at least. But even here all uncertainty will undoubtedly disappear after the lapse of a few days, were it only if we consider the slow course and the more circumscribed spreading of syphilitic pustules, not to speak of the different cicatrices and marks which these pustules leave behind.

Sec. 118.—Continuation of the former Subject.

Facial Eruptions.—The different eruptions in the face, more particularly *acne*, *mentagra*, *lupus vorax*, and even *carcinoma*, are much more readily confounded with syphilitic products than the ordinary exanthems, or any other febrile eruptive diseases. Errors of this kind having frequently taken place, we will give a full description of the diagnostic signs, a knowledge of which may prevent all misapprehensions.

As regards *acne*, and more particularly the *indurated acne*, *acne indurata*, nothing is easier than to mistake it for a pustulous syphiloid, or to mistake the latter for simple acne; a mistake that may occur so much more readily as the distribution of the pustules is about the same in either disease. What sheds light on the diagnosis is the fact that in syphilitic acne, beside the copper-colored areola which surrounds the tubercular indurated pimples, instead of a simple erythematous blush, the number of these pustules is much less, and the cicatrices they leave behind are round and pitted, whereas the cicatrices of simple acne are oblong, elevated, and lax, if folded upon themselves; a diagnostic sign which is the more important, since both forms break out more particularly in the face and on the forehead, and, on the shoulders, appear sometimes simultaneously. Beside these eruptions we have a kind of *syphilitic tubercles* on the nose and cheeks, that might likewise be confounded with the common acne indurata, if the former were not distinguished from the latter by their greater hardness, their coppery-red color and generally oval form, as well as by their larger size, their more deep-seated base in the integuments, and their disposition to ulceration and the formation of crusts, without mentioning the peculiar cicatrices they leave behind.

It is these last-mentioned signs that constitute the main difference between the so-called mentagra and syphilitic tubercles; in addition to which, mentagra is accompanied by a sort of hypertrophy of the whole of the subjacent cellular tissue, which is never perceived in the case of syphilitic products.

Lupus likewise, especially when seated on the nose, has been falsely mistaken for a syphilitic product; or, which is more frequently the case, syphilitic products have been mistaken for lupus, which, considering that the diagnosis is not very easy, is indeed not a very difficult matter. While in their tubercular condition, they can be distinguished from each other by this, that the tubercles of lupus are flatter, softer, more yellowish, and never shining at their surface, but always having a shrivelled appearance, with œdema of the subjacent cellular tissue, and pale lead-color of the skin; whereas syphilitic tubercles are always hard, copper-colored, shining and semi-globular, and moreover surrounded by a copper-colored areola. In addition to this, the ulcers of lupus are always superficial, soft, spongy, and resting upon a soft, œdematous base, whereas the syphilitic ulcers are deep-seated, having a lardaceous base and abrupt edges.

Almost the same *diagnostic signs* distinguish *carcinoma of the face and lips* from *syphilitic tubercles;* the former never has the characteristic hardness, nor the peculiar copper-color of syphilitic tubercles, not to mention the fact that cancer always arises from a scarcely ever salient induration (scirrhus) in the interior of the tissues.

Sec. 119.—Continuation of the former Subject.

Herpetic Eruptions.—More frequently than with any of the preceding forms have syphilitic eruptions been confounded with *herpes circinnatus*, *ecthyma simplex*, *impetigo*, *lichen*, *psoriasis*, and *pityriasis*, and likewise with various spots on the skin. Let us, therefore, discriminate them with great care.

1) *Herpes Circinnatus* has undoubtedly its annular shape in common with the analogous syphiloid, from which, however, it is distinguished by its fainter blush, whereas the color of the syphiloid is of a *deep copper tint*, and covers the whole spot, whereas in the simple herpes circinnatus the skin inside the ring preserves its natural whiteness.

2) *Ecthyma simplex* is distinguished from the syphilitic ecthyma by the fact that the former only occurs among old people, has no *succession of crops*, only causes superficial ulcerations, the skin between the pustules being neither wilted nor dingy-looking; their cicatrices never are as round, pitted or deep as those of the syphilitic eczema.

3) *Impetigo simplex* is readily confounded with the syphilitic impetigo, and vice versa. In the non-syphilitic impetigo the scurfs are never as green, as little raised, firmly adhering, and are never surrounded by as broad, copper-colored areolæ as in the syphilitic form, nor is there any suppuration going on beneath the scurfs.

4) *Lichen simplex* has a great deal in common with the syphilitic lichen; the vesicles of the non-syphilitic form are less elevated and more confluent, the skin preserving its natural somewhat rosy hue; the eruption is likewise attended with more or less *itching;* whereas the vesicles of the syphilitic lichen are of a copper color, raised, less confluent, of a peculiar lustre; they never ulcerate, as is sometimes the case with *lichen agrius*.

5) *Psoriasis*, when appearing on the palms of the hands and

soles of the feet, is almost always of a syphilitic kind, more particularly if the spots are surrounded by a more or less copper-colored border.

6) *Pityriasis* might mislead one by its more or less rounded, desquamating spots, especially if they have a reddish tint; nevertheless, with a little attention, the syphilitic form is easily distinguished by the absence of all *pruritus*, and by its brown copper-color, its more definitely rounded form, and the wilted, sallow appearance of the surrounding skin, from the well-known spots of the common pityriasis, which have mostly a yellow or vividly red color, and only show a very slight, scarcely perceptible, mealy desquamation.

7) Among the various cutaneous spots, it is particularly the *liver-spots* (ephelides hepaticæ), and the *spots in the faces of pregnant females*, that may give rise to mistakes, and may induce a careless observer to diagnose a syphilitic affection, more especially since syphilitic and non-syphilitic spots frequently appear mixed up together. In these cases, in order to avoid mistakes, it may perhaps be sufficient to remember that all syphilitic spots, in this affection more perhaps than in any other syphilitic forms, are distinguished by their well-known *copper* or *brown-gray* color, and their sharply-circumscribed, round shape.

Sec. 120.—Continuation of the preceding Subject.

A few other Chronic Cutaneous Affections.—Besides the *non*-cutaneous affections mentioned in the preceding paragraphs, we still have: 1) *Eczema* (eczema rubrum); 2) *Scabies* (itch); 3) *Mercurial* eruptions; 4) *Lepra;* and 5) the *Elephantiasis* of the Greeks; these eruptive diseases likewise deserve a more particular consideration, in order that they may not be confounded with analogous syphiloid exanthemata.

1) *Eczema*, which a superficial inspection might lead one to diagnose as a simple eruption, where, on the contrary, we have a syphilitic exanthem before us, is distinguished from the latter by its much smaller, more numerous, and more confluent vesicles, by the pruritus with which it is always attended, and by its very fre-

quently fiery-red color; whereas the syphilitic eczema shows larger, less numerous, less frequently confluent and never-itching vesicles, which are, moreover, surrounded by copper-colored areolæ. As regards the eczema impetiginosum, the syphilitic form which corresponds to it always exhibits, besides its peculiar black crusts, ulcers and cicatrices, such as they never appear in the non-syphilitic variety.

2) *Scabies*, with which a syphilitic affection has very frequently been confounded, is easily recognized, even if no acorns should be found by the microscope, by the nocturnal itching which no syphiloid eruption has in the same degree; if the itch is mingled with syphiloids, the latter readily distinguish themselves from the itch-pustules as heterogeneous phenomena.

3) *Mercurial* eruptions, which may not only take the form of vesicles, papules, and small tubercles, but upon the hairy scalp may break out in tolerably large ulcers, and form a sort of dark-brown crusts, resembling in color very nearly the syphilitic crusts, are distinguished from the latter both at their origin as well as during the period of desiccatiou, by the almost voluptuous *itching* by which they are always accompanied, and which invites the patient to scratch them open; and likewise by the fact, that they always appear singly, and never leave the characteristic cicatrices of syphiloid exanthems behind them. The surface of these mercurial ulcers, which are never very deep, looks as if it had been corroded by insects, or like a honey-comb, full of fine perforations.

4) *Lepra* is distinguished from its analogous syphiloid, for which it is often mistaken, by its border, which is not, as in the analogous syphiloid form, formed by a ring of tubercles, with occasional interruptions, but by a uninterrupted circle, having a blackish rather than a copper-colored hue, and always detaching numerous scales, sometimes in such large quantities that a whole handful may be picked up in the patient's bed, whereas in syphilitic lepra these scales are not very numerous, and frequently scarcely perceptible.

The *elephantiasis of the Greeks* (lepra ulcerosa), has likewise been confounded with syphiloid exanthems, although its tubercles never show the hardness of syphiloid tubercles, but consist of small, livid, soft, doughy and unequal swellings, which are frequently accompanied by a characteristic insensibility of the skin, and a horrid-looking hypertrophy of the affected limb; its ulcers resemble lupus rather than ulcerous syphiloid exanthems. Only at the commencement of the disease, when, as is well known, elephantiasis commences with the breaking out of *spots*, it may be possible to confound it with syphilitic spots, but scarcely even then, provided we remember that the skin, in the spots of elephantiasis, is *perfectly insensible.*

VI. PROGNOSIS AND TREATMENT OF SYPHILIDÆ.

Sec. 121.—Prognosis.

Rigorously speaking, the prognosis of these exanthems is the same as that of syphilis itself; where this is cured, the syphilidæ will likewise disappear; where syphilis is not cured, the prognosis of the syphilidæ is neither more nor less favorable than that of chancre, bubo, mucous tubercles, and figwarts, with or without gonorrhœa. Respecting syphilidæ, the prognosis is in so far more dubious, as the existence of these exanthems implies a more or less general infection of the constitution with the syphilitic disease, and hence an increased difficulty of removing the eruption. So far as their dangerous character is concerned, not all syphiloids are of the same importance, since some of them seem to be more transitory in their course, and almost disappear without leaving a vestige behind, whereas others prove exceedingly inveterate, and cause the most horrid disorganizations of the face and other parts. Viewed in this light, the *exanthematic*, and perhaps also the *papulous* form, are the mildest exanthems, since they not only cause no pain, but do not leave a trace behind them. The *squamous* syphiloids, likewise, are not very dangerous in themselves. Notwithstanding they may sometimes spread over a large extent, and notwithstanding the occasional hardness of their scales, they never cause any destructions in the integuments, and never leave cicatrices, but always terminate in spots that never leave a vestige of disease behind. More or less dangerous are *pemphigus* and *rhypia*, not only because they always leave deep, disfiguring, and indestructible cicatrices, but likewise because they always show that the syphilitic poison has already begun to taint the very foundations of the constitution. Under certain circumstances, the vesicular form, and more especially the syphilitic impetigo, may become dangerous disorders, not only on account of their obstinate character, but likewise on account of the bone-pains with which they are attended, and on account of the irregular, disfiguring cicatrices which they leave behind. Among the *pustulous* exanthems, the syphilitic acne and the non-confluent eczema are not very dangerous, leaving only inconsiderable cicatrices; whereas the confluent eczema and the ecthyma constitute some of the worst forms of syphiloid exanthems, the former occasioning very extensive disfiguring cicatrices, more particularly in the face, in which respect it is in no degree behind the ecthyma, although, as a rule, it is less obstinate than the latter. The worst forms of any are, without contradiction, the *tubercular*, not only because their presence always implies a thorough poisoning of the organic tissues by the syphilitic virus, but likewise on account of the enormous destructions which their termination in ulceration, especially in the face, that seems to be their favorite site, may cause, leaving the most horrible cicatrices and disfigurements, which, in spite of a perfect eradication of the poison, remain unchanged during the whole life-time of the patient. However, it is not so much by the individual conduct of each single syphiloid, but, above all, by the inclination of all syphiloids to break out afresh, and by the number, form, and locality of the accompanying ailments, that the amount of danger to the patient is to be determined, who may sink from misery into misery, until finally death releases him from his sufferings. Death, however, is never the direct consequence of syphiloid exanthems, but is always superinduced by the destructive workings of cachexia depending upon the action of the syphilitic poison in the tissues of the organism. Viewing the matter from this point, the general prognosis of syphiloids will be found to depend: 1) upon the number of the existing syphiloids, and upon the frequency of their return; 2) upon the number, form, and locality of the simultaneously-occurring ulterior, secondary symptoms; 3) upon the more or less rational method of treatment of the original primary symptoms; and, 4) upon the constitutional condition of the patient generally.

Sec. 122.—Treatment of Syphilidæ.

It seems scarcely necessary to premise that this treatment should coincide perfectly with that of syphilis generally; all, therefore, that may be required at our hands, is to indicate the remedial agents that seem best adapted to these forms of the syphilitic disease. In this respect we have to observe, in the first place, that so far as the selection of a remedy is concerned, it makes very little difference to what dermatological form the syphiloid before us belongs; whether exanthematic, papulous or vesicular, pustulous, squamous or tubercular; the question will be more particularly under what circumstances and conditions the syphiloid has become developed. In this direction, we have to consider three leading points that should guide us in the selection of a remedy: 1) the manner in which the patient had been treated heretofore, whether with or without mercurial preparations; 2) the accessory, primary, or secondary ailments accompanying the syphiloid; and 3) the character of the prognosis as determined by the nature of the syphiloid itself; whether the exanthem is transitory, and may finally disappear without a vestige remaining, or whether it is inveterate and destructive.

If the patient has not yet been treated with Mercury, I always commence the treatment, irrespective of accessory symptoms or the particular nature of the syphiloid, with *Merc. sol.* or *Præcipit. ruber*, and do not discontinue its use (including perhaps a change to *Sublim. corr.*, *Mercur. nitros.*, or *Cinnabaris*), unless no improvement follows in ten days or a fortnight, or the improvement that had been obtained, ceases to continue. I pursue the same course, if the patient has been treated with Mercury and the primary products have been cauterized at the same time; it is only where the treatment has been exclusively conducted with Mercury, that I at once employ some other remedy, according as one or another remedy may be indicated by the accessory symptoms and the nature of the exanthem.

In regard to the accessory symptoms, every thing depends whether they are primary or secondary. If primary (chancre in the second stage, buboes, mucous tubercles, figwarts), I pay no attention to the exanthem, as if it did not exist, and content myself with treating the primary symptoms, according to circumstances, either with *Merc. sol.*, or, if the nature of the symptoms should require it, with *Cinnabaris*, *Nitri ac.*, or *Thuja;* by pursuing this course, the syphiloid disappears in the same degree as the cure of the primary products progresses favorably. If, instead of the primary symptoms, other secondary symptoms are present (chancres in the throat, bone-pains, etc.), I select my remedy agreeably to the whole series, the nature of the secondary phenomena, as well as that of the exanthem.

In regard to the indications furnished by the nature of the syphiloid itself, I distinguish two kinds of exanthems: *a*) exanthems of a transitory character, disappearing of themselves; and *b*) inveterate exanthems, terminating in destruction by ulceration. If the former are accompanied by secondary phenomena, I pay no attention to the exanthem, and treat the other phenomena according to the method indicated for affections of the mucous membranes, in the following chapter (§§ 131, 138, and further). If, on the contrary, the syphiloid is one of the ulcerous and destructive kind, I direct my attention exclusively to the syphiloid, without noticing the secondary phenomena, and, if no Mercury has been used by the allopathic attendant, and the syphilitic products have been treated exclusively with cauterizing agents, derive the most distinguished results from the various mercurial preparations, such as *Merc. sol.*, *Merc. præc. ruber*, etc., which I do no longer administer, as when treating primary chancre, in two daily doses, of half a grain of the first centesimal trituration each, but give only one dose of the second or third trituration every other day (see also § 131).

Sec. 123.—The leading Remedies for Syphilidæ.

For the various syphiloids, we scarcely require any other remedies than those which are used for primary products (chancre, buboes, mucous tubercles, and figwarts); such as *mercurial preparations*, *Cinnabaris*, *Nitri ac.*, *Thuja;* to which, in case secondary symptoms are to be considered, we may add: *Aurum*, *Lycopodium*, *Staphysagria*, *Kali iodatum*, *Lachesis*, and in some cases, *Sulphur*, *Hepar sulphuris*, and *Sarsaparilla*. There are cases where the syphilitic exanthem stands all alone, without any primary or secondary symptoms. From my own experience, I am prepared to assert that these cases are not very rare, but that the exanthems, in such cases, are trivial and not very dangerous. Nevertheless, if continuing too long, they may become very troublesome to the patient (such as neglected roseolæ, scales in the palms of the hands and soles of the feet, papulous scabies, etc.), and, at the same time, evidence the presence of uneradicated remnants of the syphilitic disease. In these forms, which have occurred to me only where the chancre or bubo had indeed been satisfactorily treated with Mercury; but where the treatment had only commenced in the second or fungoid period of this product, *Mercurius* will scarcely ever do much good, and I have cured most of these syphiloids with *Phosphorus*, *Nitri ac.*, *Sarsaparilla*, and *Lycopodium*, in the 18th to the 30th attenuation, pellets, much more effectually than with Mercurius. Nor have I seen any good effects from *Kali iodatum*, although I have administered it in comparatively large doses—four grains, to one ounce of water. Otherwise it is very strange, that, considering the large number of chancre, gonorrhœa, and figwarts cures, with which our homœopathic literature abounds, we only meet with general recommendations of certain remedies, like *Kali jodatum*, for syphilitic cutaneous affections, and scarcely a single report of a cure. In general, we find recommended:

1) By Lobethal (All. hom. Zeit., vol. 30), following the recommendations of allopathic physicians, in large doses: The *Hydriodate of potash* for, so-called, tertiary and quarternary multifariously-shaped, cutaneous affections; for large cutaneous ulcers, of a sickly color; tubercular and papulous eruptions in the face, etc. The doctor, however, neglects to inform us, what particular forms of syphiloid exanthems (which are, however, always of a secondary character) he understands by "tertiary" and "quaternary" forms.

2) By Clotar Müller (All. h. Zeit., vol. 34): *Mercurius bijodatus* for syphilidæ. This excellent practitioner at the same time remarks, that in many cases of syphilitic exanthems, the mercurial preparations are altogether inappropriate. This is undoubtedly correct; but I cannot agree with him in opinion that, where the mercurial preparations are altogether indicated, Merc. sol. and Merc. præc. ruber are less efficient than *Merc. bijodatus*. This last-named preparation has seemed to me very unreliable, and I do not make much use of it.

3) By Trinks (All. h. Zeit., vol. 15): *Præc. ruber* as preferable to *solubilis* in syphilitic exanthems; generally speaking, this ob-

servation is correct; but, if presented in too sweeping a manner, may lead to grave errors.

4) By Rummel (All. h. Zeit., vol. 18): *Nitri. ac.* for broad, red spots resembling psoriasis, subsequent to the treatment of primary ulcers with large doses of Mercury. According to my experience, this observation is correct.

5) By Fielitz (Prak. Beit., vol. 2); *Nitri. ac.* for isolated, burning, ulcerated surfaces on the hairy scalp, accompanied by ecthymatous pustules in the face, forming crusts, and surrounded by broad, red areolæ.

6) By Hofrichter in Prague (All. h. Zeit., vol. 35): for brown spots on the glans, of the size of lentils, and vanishing after their membranes become detached, together with brown tubercles near the seam of the scrotum, and on the perineum as far as the anus; these tubercles are of the size of peas, and terminate in ulceration.

(Füllgraf, in the sixth vol. of North Amer. Journal, relates a case of *syphilitic* pustules, which was cured in twelve days by three galvanic baths of forty-five minutes each, administered at intervals of two or three days.—H.)

THIRD CHAPTER.

INTERMEDIATE FORMS OF SECONDARY SYPHILIS.

I. DEFINITION AND ENUMERATION OF THESE FORMS.

Sec. 124.—Definition of the Intermediate Forms.

If we consider that the living human, or, more generally speaking, the animal body is an organism, whose constant endeavor it seems to be, in a circle of living action, on the one hand, to receive substances that come in contact with the surface of the body (skin or mucous membrane), and, in a spiral course, as it were, to conduct them onward through the different tissues by a process of assimilation to the very centre of life; and, on the other hand, by a similar course to reconduct all heterogeneous, non-assimilable matters to the periphery, and to excrete, by the skin, all those things which the other excretory organs had failed to remove from the tissues: we shall find that the primary chancre and the syphilidæ, of which we have treated in the preceding chapters, are the limits within which the syphilitic disease runs its course, from the moment of its first appearance to the time when the virus would, perhaps, be forever eliminated through cutaneous eruptions, if such an elimination were always possible with perfect completeness. As the chancre is, as it were, the initial point of the syphilitic disease, so the syphilitic exanthems should be the termination of all syphilitic phenomena, and perhaps would be, if the excretory process were not in any way disturbed in its course towards completion. This elimination not taking place as completely as it should, it follows that between the above-mentioned two extremes, there must be other points, in greater or less proximity to the periphery of the vital functions, where the organism endeavors to perfect this elimination, but where, if the eliminating process should fail, it sees itself, contrary to its endeavors, assaulted in tissues that are not capable of conducting this process any further. Hence we have, between these two terminal points, the chancre and the syphilidæ, a whole series of intermediate phenomena, which we have designated as "intermediate forms of secondary syphilis." The mucous membranes, being the internal continuation of the external integumentary periphery of the organism, constitute the locality where these intermediate phenomena first manifest themselves. These may, however, if the excretory process should either fail to take place on these membranes, or should only take place imperfectly, become localized in other tissues, such as the bones, as symptoms of an imperfect or unsuccessful elimination. According to this view, syphilitic affections of the bones may, therefore, manifest themselves prior to, or simultaneously with, or subsequent to the affections of the mucous membranes, although the former, in their capacity of pathological retro-formative manifestations of a morbid process that originally tended to find an outlet on the mucous surfaces, are necessarily much less frequent than the diseases of the latter organ. What the affections of the mucous membranes are to the syphilidæ, this the affections of the bones, as far as their frequency is concerned, are to those of the mucous membranes. It is not because the different secondary phenomena occur in a certain chronological order, but because some of them occur more frequently than others, that we place the affections of the osseous system after those of the mucous membranes. We do not regard the former as a new *tertiary* manifestation, but simply as a purely passive phenomenon, occurring subsequently to the ordinary secondary phenomenon, which tertiary manifestations may take place from the moment when, after the termination of the protopathic morbid process in the first stage of chancre, the organism makes more or less *ineffectual* attempts to transmit the syphilitic affection to the external skin, and, in case of failure, to the mucous membranes.

Sec. 125.—Tissues where the Intermediate Forms are located.

These intermediate forms may not only occur on the mucous membranes or in the bones, but likewise in other tissues. Hahnemann already mentions, as a consequence of suppression of sycosic, and hence syphilitic gonorrhœa, "*a contraction of the flexor surfaces;*" and several recent authors not only speak of "*bone-pains,*" but likewise of "*muscular pains,*" or even of "*muscular swellings,*" which are said to take place together with other secondary phenomena, and which may be located in the *tendons* and *aponeuroses.* The so-called *gummata* or *gummatose* swellings, which, as some would have it, do not occur in the osseous system, but in the cellular tissue, are as well known at the present time as exostoses or tophi, with which the former, more especially if they happened to be seated in the neighborhood of the bones, were apt to be confounded. The lymphatic vessels are less frequently affected, although a species of secondary buboes may occur, but not often. Whether, as some assert, the syphilitic disease may show itself in other tissues, causing, for example, organic affections of the bowels, stomach, lungs, liver, spleen, etc., and affecting even the heart, and, lastly, the brain and spinal cord, is another question, that may, perhaps, never be decided with certainty, and may be doubted so much more, as there are authors who, without any further examination, attribute every morbid symptom of internal organs that may happen to manifest itself during the presence of syphilitic phenomena, to the action of the syphilitic virus; not to mention those who, if individnals had a gonorrhœa or chancre once in their lifetime, trace even cancer of the stomach, pulmonary tubercles, softening of the brain, indurations of the liver, and other similar affections, even if they should only occur twenty or thirty years subsequently to the syphilitic infection, to the action of this virus; yea, even scrofulosis, tuberculosis, in fine, all the derangements that Hahnemann sets down to the account of psora, are charged to syphilis as their fountain-head. There is no doubt that, beside the already known syphilidæ, affections of the mucous membranes, osseous system, etc., there may be many other syphilitic products that are overlooked, and have remained unknown up to the present time. Pathological forms, such as rhagades or secondary ulcers, which are as yet distinguished from syphilidæ by their isolated appearance, may, perhaps, hereafter be recognized as intermediate forms of secondary syphilis. Be this as it may, we can never do too much for the perfect investigation and complete knowledge of syphilitic phenomena, and it is for this reason that we mention in the subsequent articles of this chapter not only the known intermediate forms, but likewise those regarding which opinions still differ. We shall class the affections to be described in the following four categories: 1) *syphilitic rhagades* and *secondary ulcers;* 2) the *phenomena occurring on the mucous membranes;* 3) the affections of the *osseous system;* and, 4) phenomena in other tissues.

II. SECONDARY ULCERS AND SYPHILITIC RHAGADES.

Sec. 126.—Symptomatic description of the same.

These phenomena, among which we do not number the ulcers occurring on the mucous membranes, show themselves on the skin in the shape of *ulcerated sores*, which are distinguished from the syphiloids proper, or from syphilitic exanthems, by this, that they are not eruptions, properly speaking, but *true sores*, not developing themselves out of previous syphilidæ, but breaking out at once in their original specific form, and likewise by this other feature, that they do not, after the fashion of syphilidæ, spread over large surfaces, but, like primary chancre, are confined to definite localities. In most cases they appear several weeks after the cicatrization of the protopathic primary ulcer, but may not break out until several years after, in which latter case they are preceded during this whole period by secondary phenomena. They break out most frequently around the arms and on the sexual organs; but they may likewise show themselves on the mammæ, even on the umbilicus, eyelids and ears, and not unfrequently between the toes. With few exceptions, these ulcers, as a general rule, resemble primary chancres, and, like these, may remain stationary, whereas, in other cases, they become painful, inflamed, dipping down to the subjacent textures, and even assuming a phagedænic character. In common with primary chancres, they first appear in the shape of a red spot which soon becomes sore, ulcerates, dips down like a cup, and assumes all the signs of a syphilitic ulcer. In some rare cases they are preceded by a painless induration and swelling of the subjacent tissue, which, as in the case of primary chancres, may continue long after cicatrization has taken place, provided the ulcers were closed by purely external means, without the internal use of suitable specific antidotes. On the body of the penis, scrotum, mammæ, and on other similar parts, they first begin with a red, hard, round, isolated pimple, which rapidly bursts, discharging an acrid serum, and forming a hard and thick crust, whose thickness and size increase in proportion as the ulcer continues to spread. If breaking out in some fold of the skin, or on parts that are in constant motion, for instance around the arms or between the toes, they almost always form open ulcers, and, instead of the round chancre-form, they may assume an oblong shape, which, however, will always become rounded, if the fold where they are located is drawn out into a level. Hence, wherever, they may appear, they are readily recognized, and, by their chancre-resembling properties, can be easily distinguished from non-syphilitic ulcers, even if no other syphilitic phenomena should be present, either on the skin or mucous membranes, although in such a case, which is indeed not very rare, a certain degree of uncertainty must necessarily exist. We will therefore subjoin a few remarks on such ulcers, when they break out on the *sexual organs*, and likewise when they show themselves at the *anus* and *rectum*, or in other localities.

Sec. 127.—Secondary Ulcers on the Sexual Organs generally.

Among the different forms which writers on syphilis describe under this name, and of which some authors declare that they show themselves as frequently, if not more so, on the inner surface of the prepuce, behind or upon the glans and on both sides of the frænulum, as upon the outer skin of the prepuce or penis, there are undoubtedly many that have nothing further in common with syphilis than that the name of syphilitic ulcers is falsely attributed to them, on which account it is absolutely necessary to establish their diagnosis upon a firm basis. In the first place, *herpes præputialis* may be mistaken for a secondary ulcer in persons that had been afflicted with chancre at some previous period. Herpes, however, always announces itself by the breaking out of several closely-crowded vesicles upon an inflamed, but not circularly circumscribed spot of the inner or outer side of the prepuce, forming very superficial ulcers, whose surface has a bright red appearance, and never exhibits the lardaceous base of the chancre. Besides this præputial herpes, we have another most likely mercurial symptom that has to be carefully distinguished from syphilitic chancres. These are perfectly *red* and exceedingly superficial *erosions*, mostly on the prepuce, and lined with a yellowish-white mucus, which superficial practitioners, more particularly among the French, class, under the name of fugitive chancres or *chancres volants*, among secondary syphilitic products, and which break out again every three or six months, especially if the patient has already undergone a mercurial treatment. Of an entirely different nature are the true *secondary* chancres, which, when breaking out on the glans, always denote the prevalence of a very old constitutional syphilis. These secondary chancres have more or less shaggy borders, a red-brown and granular base, or, if they had become phagedænic, are covered with a dirty-gray scurf, and, like many other secondary symptoms of syphilis, break out in most cases after a very hard and painful swelling of that portion of the glans where they threaten to become located. Very frequently the phagedænic destruction spreads to the meatus urinarius, which, unless the accident is prevented by the timely introduction of a bougie, may remain permanently and irremediably constricted, even after cicatrization has taken place. When appearing on the prepuce, they easily give rise to a malignant phimosis or paraphimosis, which, after a time, and unless precautionary measures are taken in season, may lead to gangrene, and, in case the body of the penis becomes involved, cause the most violent hæmorrhage, and compel the amputation of the diseased organ. The prepuce is not unfrequently perforated by these secondary ulcers, even as the frænulum is often destroyed by the primary chancre. If located on the body of the penis, they frequently destroy the spongy portion, and by this means may, like those located on the glans, cause very violent and dangerous hæmorrhages. Otherwise these chancres are probably *consecutive* phenomena belonging to the transition period, rather than *secondary;* in many cases they may not be any thing else than old and neglected primary ulcers; in my practice they have occurred to me so often, that I had almost doubted the existence of *secondary* chancres, and, to judge by the descriptions which I had read of them, had fancied that they had been confounded with *old, neglected primary chancres,* until quite recently I observed two cases, one after the other, one on the glans, the other on the body of the penis, where these new chancres, after the primary chancres had been removed by cauterization, had broken out simultaneously with pustulous eruptions; in a third case, where a horrid-looking pustulous exanthem of the face had been considerably improved by *Merc. sol. Hahn.* 2, a dose every other day, two chancres broke out anew on the outer border of the labia majora, in places where the cicatrices of two former chancres could be seen; they were not mercurial but *syphilitic* ulcers, and were readily healed with *Nitri. ac.*

Sec. 128.—Secondary Ulcers on the Female parts.

Most of these ulcers which present themselves for treatment are, most likely, consecutive symptoms of the transition stage from the primary into the secondary period, although I have met them in company with unmistakably secondary phenomena. They are most frequently seen near the inferior commissure, at the entrance of the vagina, and on the perineum. The pratings of old-school physicians concerning the difficulty of curing ulcers located near the inferior commissure must, however, not be referred to the nature of these ulcers, but should be understood of the peculiar manner in which these gentlemen treat such ulcers, exclusively by external means, and thus securing their cicatrization. If treated with appropriate specific remedies internally, they yield to such treatment neither sooner nor later than any other ulcers of the same class, no matter where located; only those which are seated at the entrance of the vagina (if of a phagedænic character, and after having lasted a long time, may perforate the walls of the vagina, and may penetrate into the rectum; and those that are seated anteriorly, may find a passage into the urethra, and give rise to incurable fistulæ of this canal. Even on the neck of the womb, these secondary chancres have made their appearance; and it is here that—on account of the accompanying stinging pains; of the badly-colored ichorous discharge from the vagina, and of a peculiar feeling of weight in the rectum; as well as on account of the swelling, of the increased warmth, and of the ulcerations of the neck of the womb, which are readily discovered by exploring the parts with the finger—these ulcerations have frequently been mistaken for cancer, until their true nature was ascertained. But even in such cases, where the physician should never lose sight of the possibility of confounding syphilitic with cancerous ulcerations, the previous history, and the initial symptoms of the case, in addition to other syphilitic symptoms that may likewise be present, may excite suspicion, which an examination with the speculum may soon clear up. It is true that such an examination is not always easy, for there are cases where the physician—even if he should suspect a syphilitic infection—cannot, and dare not give utterance to such a thought. If we consider how many pure-minded, virtuous, and sensitively-modest women, whose husbands fancied themselves cured, and radically freed from all syphilitic taint, have been infected by them with this horrid disease, without the poor patients having the least suspicion regarding the true nature of their ailments, it is not difficult to understand that so many syphilitic ulcerations have been mistaken for cancerous disease, and have been treated accordingly. I have had women come to me, who had been treated by allopathic physicians for cancerous ulcerations, and who, being unwilling to submit to another examination, were treated by me, for a long time, without any abatement of the pains or the discharge (although with our present means relief can be afforded, even if patients are suffering with cancer), until, suspecting a syphilitic taint, I finally had recourse to *Merc. sol.* and *Nitri ac.*, by which means I not only effected a rapid improvement, but a complete cure; in no case did the treatment last beyond three months.

Sec. 129.—Syphilitic Rhagades at the Anus and entrance of the Vagina.

These rhagades consist of narrow, elongated ulcers, or cracks in the folds of the anus. They are more or less numerous, scarcely ever show themselves except in cases of unmistakable constitutional syphilis, and may be confounded by inexperienced persons with rhagades, or lacerations caused by the passage of hard excrements, by the introduction of a foreign body, or even by hæmorrhoids. These last-mentioned rhagades, however, are easily distinguished from syphilitic ones, by the fact that they are seldom very numerous, and always exhibit a red (more or less bleeding) surface, and not very elevated borders; whereas, syphilitic rhagades are numerous, rest for the most part upon a rather hard and swollen surface, and have a rather hard and lardaceous base, with red, hard, raised edges. According to some authors, these rhagades are, in some cases, quite superficial, not very painful, with soft and smooth edges, and secretion of a whitish pus, in which case it would undoubtedly be very difficult to decide whether they are of a syphilitic nature, or not. If I may trust my own experience, I am disposed to assert that rhagades of this description are *never* syphilitic; I have met with such rhagades when all primary or secondary syphilitic symptoms were entirely wanting, but a disposition to hæmorrhoids or common tetter existed, or where the patient suffered with nothing else than mercurial symptoms. The authors who have stated such anomalous doctrines, in their rage to discover everywhere symptoms of masked syphilis, go so far as to regard the common *pruritus of the anus and scrotum* as ordinary signs of the syphilitic disease, in all cases. The case is different where these rhagades are deep and painful, with hard and raised edges, and secretion of a bloody, acrid serum, which corrodes the neighboring parts. In such a case, their syphilitic nature can almost always be taken for granted; and a further examination will almost invariably reveal the existence of other secondary symptoms, either upon the skin or on the uneven surfaces.

Beside these *rhagades*, true chancres often are seen on the border of the anus as well as in the rectum, close above the sphincter. These chancres are never *secondary*, but always *primary*, caused by direct infection, in consequence of a criminal attempt at sexual connection, and in all cases one of the most terrible products of the syphilitic virus. If these primary chancres occur at the anus, they frequently occupy the same folds where the rhagades are located, but are not as numerous as these; very frequently they constitute a single ulcer, are less in circumference, and distinguished in nothing from primary chancres, either as regards appearance or edges, except by their oblong form, which is owing to the shape of the fold where they have become located. When seated at the entrance of the rectum, they are located higher up than the rhagades, always *above* the sphincter of the anus, so that externally not the least trace of them can be discovered, except by the oozing, which, however, is not always perceptible, and generally passes off with the excrements.

Sec. 130.—Secondary Ulcers on other portions of the external skin.

Among these we mention, as first in rank, the syphilitic *rhagades between the toes*, which are almost always overlooked, although they are scarcely ever unaccompanied by other secondary syphilitic phenomena, principally affections of the throat. Always in a state of ulceration, they resemble pretty accurately the rhagades at the anus; they are somewhat raised, oblong, deep, and of a violet-red; at the same time they incline to spread towards the balls of the feet, and may render walking very troublesome and painful. They may likewise show themselves in the shape of cracks around the rounded borders of the nails, where they secrete, like the former rhagades, a purulent, ichorous, very fetid serum.

On the mammæ, on the contrary, truly secondary ulcers are very rare; most of these ulcers, which are principally seen on the mammæ of nursing women in the shape of *mucous tubercles*, are undoubtedly caused by infection communicated by syphilitic infants; they do, however, exist on the mammæ of other women, in which case they are always accompanied by syphilitic phenomena on the skin, or mucous membranes.

Such chancres have likewise been perceived on the *umbilicus*, where they generally commence with a more or less vivid redness, deep in the tissues of the umbilicus. This redness is succeeded by an ulceration that very soon assumes all the characteristic appearances of chancre. In most cases, these ulcers are likewise attended with other symptoms of constitutional syphilis.

Ulcers breaking out on the eyelids (where figwarts may likewise become located) are sometimes perhaps of a primary nature, and are caused by contact with the fingers, to which some of the syphilitic matter was adhering; nevertheless, they are more frequently *secondary* than primary ulcers. If secondary, they generally break out on the free margin of the eyelids, very soon spreading over their outer or inner surface, if not over both at one and the same time; they are most generally accompanied by violent inflammation, in which the conjunctiva becomes involved. After healing, they generally leave irregular cicatrices behind, resembling those after burns; and not unfrequently they cause a falling out of the eyelashes, which, in such a case, never grow again.

Such ulcers may likewise break out *on the ears*, where they usually become seated on the posterior or anterior surface of the concha, or even in the outer meatus auditorius. If seated between the ear and the mastoid process, they generally resemble oblong rhagades; whereas, if located on other parts, they look more like slimy tubercles and herpetic excoriations, but are always of difficult recognition, unless other syphilitic signs are simultaneously present. Some of these ulcers likewise assume the form of deep phagedænic ulcers, with abrupt edges, a lardaceous and uneven base, occasionally exhibiting red and bleeding spots, or covering themselves with a scurf. If phagedænic, they may penetrate deep into the internal meatus, destroy the ossicula, and, in this manner, cause an incurable deafness. In most cases of such deeply-penetrating ulcers, nothing, fortunately, remains but a buzzing in the ears, which will, however, bid defiance to all the remedial agents that are employed against it.

Sec. 131.—Treatment of these Ulcers.

Regarding the diagnosis and prognosis of these ulcers and rhagades, we have nothing to add to what has already been said on the same subject in previous chapters, when speaking of other forms of secondary disease. The complaints of old-school physicians, regarding the desperate obstinacy with which these ulcers and rhagades resist all treatment, only refer to the foolish use of cauterizing agents with which these appearances are sought to be managed, especially in hospitals. Under homœopathic treatment, with truly rational, and rationally used, remedies, the management of these ulcers becomes comparatively easy, and the cure certain and complete. Among these remedies, *Mercurius* occupies the first rank; for this reason, that such secondary ulcers almost always break out as ultimate sequelæ, where the primary symptom had either been treated without Mercury, or with cauterizing agents and external mercurial applications. I always accomplish a cure with *Merc. sol.* 2, giving half a grain at a dose every other day; nor have I ever been obliged to resort either to another remedy, or to another mercurial preparation, except in two cases, where these secondary chancres came to me out of the hands of beginning colleagues, who, by deluging the patient with Mercury, had aggravated his case; and where, in one case, I derived benefit from *Lachesis*, and in the other case from *Sulphur* and *Nitri ac.*, and where, in both cases, the rest of the disease was radically and permanently removed by means of two doses of *Merc. sol.* 3, giving one dose every four days. If, in treating secondary affections, I give *Mercurius* in smaller and less frequently repeated doses than when treating primary phenomena, I do this for the simple reason that, be the organism "*saturated*" ever so thoroughly with Mercury, the cure of secondary affections will not be hastened by such a course, were it only because these affections naturally run a slower course than primary products of the syphilitic disease. Owing to this more inveterate duration of secondary ulcers, Mercurius will have to be continued in all such cases for a longer period. If it is given *as often* as in primary ulcers, double and treble the quantity that may be required for the cure of a primary chancre, may have already been used before the treatment of the secondary ulcer is half accomplished; if, at this stage, the use of Mercury is continued, it frequently happens not only that the cure of the ulcer remains stationary, but that the symptoms of the case become terribly aggravated. Such aggravations are exclusively due to an excess of mercurial action. Such aggravations have occurred in my own practice, when, dazzled by the hue and cry of anti-Hahnemannians against triturations and attenuations, I was induced to try the use of massive doses in syphilis. I, too, undertook to *saturate* my patients with Mercury, until, taught and made wiser by experience, I returned to my former employment of Mercury, giving one dose every other day, since when I cure my patients not only more rapidly, but without exposing them to the pernicious effects of Mercury. For chancres on the *penis* and *scrotum* that were most likely of a secondary character, Clotar Müller (All. h. Zeit., vol. 37) has employed, with great benefit, the *Muriate of Gold.* Others have employed *Præc. ruber*, *Cinnabaris*, *Merc. sol.* (and Biniodide of Mercury. H.)

III. SECONDARY AFFECTIONS OF THE MUCOUS MEMBRANES.

Sec. 132.—General view of these Affections.

Secondary affections of the mucous membranes are really nothing else than secondary chancres and syphilidæ of every variety, transferred from the external skin to the mucous surfaces. It may be asserted, without fear of contradiction, that they occur most frequently in the form of ulcers, which may be classed in four more or less distinct categories: 1) *superficial* ulcers that may break out in any part of the mouth and throat, and which form a sort of whitish-gray, obscurely-circumscribed tetter or cyst, with a dark-red border, and showing but indistinct traces of ulceration. By French pathologists these appearances are attributed to their so-called *blennorrhagia*, and by the Germans to gonorrhœa pure and simple. 2) *Deeper ulcers*, resembling simple chancre, which, though not very deep, penetrate the whole thickness of the mucous membrane, are distinguished by their lardaceous and granular base, as well as by their shaggy, somewhat everted edges, and their slightly reddened areola, and are mostly located in the throat, and very frequently in the region of the wisdom-teeth, where they are easily confounded with the little ulcers which sometimes break out about the time when the wisdom-teeth are about to protrude; 3) the so-called *chancres of the throat*, which appear more particularly npon the tonsils, and resemble the *Hunterian chancre;* without any previous swelling of the subjacent tissue, they cause a cup-shaped perforation of the affected part, have a yellow base with a dark-red border, and not only penetrate to the subjacent tissues, but likewise spread on the surface; and, 4) *phagedænic* ulcers, which betray the analogous chancre at the very outset, and, if they break out in the throat, may not only destroy the uvula, the velum and pharynx, but the palate-bones themselves.

In regard to *syphiloid affections* of the mucous membranes, we have: 1) the *exanthematic* form, consisting in the breaking out of more or less irregular, not always very red, spots, sometimes white in the centre, occurring at every point of the fauces, and on the inside of the cheeks, and frequently disappearing of themselves after a short period; 2) the *papulous* form, appearing in the shape of small, rough, oblong granules, of the size of a pin's head, and most generally seated on the edges and at the tip of the tongue; this eruption often disappears again spontaneously; 3) the *tubercular*, coming out in the shape of flattened, so-called *mucous tubercles*, in the corners of the mouth, on the inside of the cheeks and lips, on the velum palati and root of the tongue; it is, in fact, nothing else than the *mucous tubercles* that have been transferred from the sexual organs to other mucous surfaces; and, 4) an eruption of circular patches, resembling *syphilitic psoriasis*, which may break out anywhere in the mouth and throat, and is one of the most obstinate of these different forms.

All these ulcerous and non-ulcerous forms, which, it is true, occur most frequently in the mouth and throat, may yet break out on other portions of the mucous membranes, more particularly on the sexual organs, and likewise in the nasal cavity, in the larynx, meatus auditorius, eye, etc., in which case they show a variety of modifications that deserve a more particular notice.

Sec. 133.—Syphilitic Affections of the Mouth and Throat.

Rigorously speaking, we might omit these parts, inasmuch as every thing that we have stated in the preceding paragraph applies more particularly to these organs; nevertheless, inasmuch as these different forms do not manifest themselves with equal frequency, a few additional remarks, having reference thereto, may not be out of place.

1) The most distinctly-marked form of syphilitic ulcers of the throat, which resembles most closely the Hunterian chancre, breaks out on the tonsils, where, first along, so little pain and swelling are experienced, that the patients do not heed the symptoms until the ulcer has become distinctly recognizable. This has a yellowish or brownish scurf, which dips down into the interior of the tonsil without the surrounding parts being either much swollen or red, and without any other pain being felt except a stinging sensation, more particularly during the act of deglutition, which, however, is not near as much interfered with as the extent and appearance of the ulcer might lead one to suppose. It is only if the ulcer continues to spread that deglutition becomes more difficult, the voice acquires a peculiar husky sound, and the sense of hearing becomes impaired.

2) *Phagedænic chancres* in the throat set in with *putrid ulceration* that soon changes to a wide-spread *gangrenous destruction*. These ulcers not only break out on the tonsils, but likewise on the velum palati, and in the pharynx, but break out most frequently on the superior and posterior wall of the pharynx, and behind the pillars of the palate, where they sometimes, unless the parts are examined by turning them up with the spatula, have made considerable progress before they are discovered. In most cases, they are accompanied by great pain, inflammation, and some swelling of the parts; the least attempt at deglutition causes the most violent

pain; there is considerable ptyalism, and a good deal of cough, so that one might suspect a tolerably far advanced laryngeal phthisis, which suspicion may be heightened by the fact, that with the purulent expectoration a general emaciation and an accelerated pulse are apt to supervene. In regard to the destructions which these ulcers may cause, they are not inconsiderable; at the posterior nares, the bones are sometimes denuded of all their coverings, the nose destroyed, and even the cervical vertebræ invaded and attacked with fatal caries. Even if these phagedænic ulcers do not terminate in gangrene, and present a less formidable appearance, their destructive progress is ever onward; beginning at the velum with a small yellow scurf, which is surrounded by a crimson areola, they often spread with incredible rapidity, and frequently succeed in destroying a large portion of that organ before their disorganizing action is checked in the least. In most cases, these ulcers are accompanied by a cutaneous exanthem resembling rhypia.

3) Beside these two kinds of chancre of the throat, some authors range in this class the *annular herpetic ulcer*, of which mention has been made in the former paragraph. It is distinguished by its *faintish-white circular* patches, on the surface of the tonsils, velum palati, columns of the palate, tongue, and even cheeks and lips, and is always accompanied by a scaly eruption on the skin, of which it may be regarded as a continuation. Many pathologists deny its syphilitic nature, and only view it as a mercurial affection; this opinion, however, may be erroneous; at any rate, it is not substantiated.

4) Among other affections of the mouth and throat, the balance of which have already been described in the last paragraph, we only mention *mucous tubercles* and *figwarts*, which, though rarely, yet sometimes show themselves at the root of the tongue, where they are sometimes mistaken for cancer of the tongue, on the velum palati and in the neighborhood of the posterior molares.

Sec. 134.—Continuation of the preceding subject.

Distinctive diagnosis of syphilitic and non-syphilitic affections of the mouth and throat.—We have shown that the secondary syphilitic products on the mucous membrane of the throat and mouth may appear: 1) as superficial, whitish, *tettery ulcerations;* 2) as *simple chancres of the tonsils;* 3) *as phagedænic chancres of the fauces;* 4) as spots or papules that soon disappear again; 5) as *mucous tubercles,* and 6) as circular *herpetic ulcers* accompanied by a squamous exanthem on the skin; and that these ulcers may not only be attended with condylomatous growths, but may likewise cause the most fearful destructions; may eat away the palatine and nasal bones, and may result in caries of the cervical vertebræ. Usually, at least very frequently, these phenomena set in with a simple redness and puffiness of the mucous membrane, which is nowhere ulcerated, but very frequently streaked with varicose vessels, and sometimes here and there covered with a layer of tenacious mucus; this condition, which is known under the name of *angina syphilitica,* may continue for a long time without showing any signs of ulceration.

As a general rule, these ulcers of the mouth and throat are readily distinguished from *non*-syphilitic ulcers, although it may happen in a few rare cases that the former are mistaken for *mercurial, scorbutic* and even *simple* ulcers. To enable the reader to avoid such mistakes, we will subjoin the following remarks:

1) *Mercurial ulcers* are generally seated on the inside of the cheeks, near the gums and on the borders of the tongue, do not, like syphilitic ulcers, spread from behind forwards, but from before backwards, and usually spread more rapidly than syphilitic ulcers; they have no grayish or lardaceous, but a milky-white base, are never surrounded by an erysipelatous redness, and may in some cases occasion very dangerous rhagades.

2) *Scorbutic* ulcers always exhibit a dark-red, bluish and blackish base, with similarly-looking edges, are of a relaxed consistence, of fungoid appearance, have an irregular form, bleed readily, and are generally seen on the gums and around the roots of the teeth.

3) *Simple* ulcers, especially when arising after an ordinary inflammation of the throat, always have a simple, distinctly inflammatory character, run a proportionately rapid course, and are generally consequent upon small abscesses in the tonsils.

4) Simple *aphthæ,* which some might possibly mistake for

syphilitic ulcers, break out, especially in children and when attended with fever, in greater number than syhilitic ulcers; they are of a milky-white or yellowish color; it is only in the case of full-grown persons, when they break out in consequence of using heating food or beverages, at most one or two at a time, on the inside of the lips or cheeks, that they may readily be confounded with syphilitic ulcers, so much more easily since these so-called gastric aphthæ have sometimes a whitish, lardaceous, mother-of-pearl base, are always surrounded by a more or less inflamed areola, and not unfrequently are more or less deep and painful. However, they disappear in all cases of themselves in five days, or, at the latest, in a fortnight.

5) With carcinomatous ulcers they might possibly be confounded in cases where fungoid chancres or numerous fungoid condylomata have broken out on the tongue; in such a case, however, the balance of the symptoms will soon shed light on the true nature of the case.

Sec. 135.—Secondary phenomena in the Larynx and Nose.

Although in most cases the symptoms in these organs are caused by the spreading of the disease from the fauces, yet they may likewise be attacked by themselves, and, inasmuch as in such cases the true nature of the malady may easily be overlooked, it seems indispensable that these forms should be considered more in detail.

1) *Syphilitic affections of the Larynx.*—Syphilitic ulceration of the larynx, if occurring by itself, generally sets in a long time after the disappearance of the primary symptoms, in which case it is accompanied by all the symptoms of ordinary affections of the larynx, such as: a certain uneasy feeling and a seated painfulness in the region of the larynx, alteration or even loss of voice, difficulty of breathing, short cough, with a desire to hawk up the stuff which obstructs the larynx, and expectoration of a purulent substance streaked with blood. If the affection progresses, fever may supervene, with night-sweats and all the other signs of laryngeal phthisis. Sometimes the cartilages of the vocal organs become involved. In such a case the prognosis becomes much more unfa-

vorable, since, even after the ulcers are completely healed, aphonia, or at least an incurable hoarseness, may remain behind. I have seen this disease develop itself in the case of a young, vigorous German, who had been treated for laryngeal phthisis by the greatest physicians in Paris, and whose affection I likewise mistook for this disease until syphilitic pustules broke out on the forehead, when he placed himself in the hands of some other homœopathic physician, of the Specific School, under whose treatment he died in six months.

2) *Syphilitic affection of the Schneiderian membrane* (*ozœna syphilitica*).—Like laryngeal affections, these may likewise break out by themselves, without any previous ulceration of the fauces; they manifest themselves sooner or later, subsequent to the disappearance of the primary symptoms, in the form of a dry coryza; indeed, the patient fancies he has taken cold. Soon, however, he commences to blow out of his nose a thick, yellowish, purulent matter, which is often mixed with thin, blackish crusts; at the same time he becomes aware of a diminution of the sense of smell; after which a more careful examination of the nasal cavity reveals a fungoid swelling of the Schneiderian membrane, extending in both nostrils as far as the eye can reach. At the same time, or soon after, on the inner walls of the alæ nasi, or higher up, ulcerations break out which, like those in the throat, are phagedænic, and may affect the nasal bones. If these become destroyed by the ulcerative process, the patient, when blowing his nose, generally blows out pieces of these bones, until the nose caves in, without the outer skin having become injured. This is the ozœna syphilitica of older authors, during which condylomatous growths in the nostrils may supervene which have often been confounded with polypi. In other respects this affection is one of those that may break out sooner than any other after the disappearance of the primary phenomena, but which at the commencement is heeded no more than so many other apparently trifling syphilitic symptoms, which may continue unnoticed for years, until the disorder suddenly becomes more manifest, five, six or seven years after the chancre had been healed, and is then regarded as a recent affection.

Sec. 136.—Affections of the Ears and Eyes.

Conjunctivitis and Iritis.—Although not very frequent, yet both these affections are not so very rare either, provided we choose to heed them.

Beside the secondary ulcers that here break out, syphilitic affections of the ears consist in a syphilitic derangement of the mucous membrane of the meatus auditorius, characterized by a yellowish-green, viscid, thin, and more or less copious discharge from the ears, which, like all other constitutional syphilitic discharges, are generally painless, and attended with more or less difficulty of hearing. Sometimes we notice, at the same time, syphilitic ulcerations of the outer ear, or at the entrance of the meatus; if located more interiorly, they can be discovered by means of the speculum. Soft, cauliflower excrescences and other *figwarts*, as well as *mucous tubercles*, have been seen in the meatus.

Syphilitic Affections of the Eyes.—Here we distinguish two kinds of affections: 1, *Conjunctivitis Syphilitica*, which is a disease of the mucous membrane; and 2, *Iritis Syphilitica*, which has nothing to do with the mucous membrane, and is entirely confined to the iris.

(*a.*) Syphilitic conjunctivitis is recognized by a peculiar, brick-red, sharply circumscribed wreath of vessels in the conjunctiva and sclerotica surrounding the latter organ, where it unites with the cornea, with a wall about a line in width. This inflammation is always very painful, and attended with great photophobia.

(*b.*) *Iritis Syphilitica* is characterized by contraction or distortion of the pupils, with immobility of the iris, which projects beyond the cornea like a pad; there is profuse lachrymation, violent pains in the orbits, and discoloration of the iris. Syphilitic iritis is distinguished from simple *traumatic* iritis by its less rapid course, which is always chronic, and by the pains setting in more particularly *at night*, and being felt not only in the orbit and eye, but invading the whole of the affected side of the face and head. If left to itself, syphilitic iritis often causes, after a short period, the most extensive destructions of all the tissues of the eye, commencing with the iris. At the commencement of the disease, it is not always easy to distinguish it from rheumatic iritis, so that it often becomes necessary, in case of a dubious diagnosis, to examine the throat of the patient, and the whole surface of the skin, with a view of ascertaining the existence of other secondary signs of syphilis in these localities; for this inflammation seldom makes its appearance during the primary period of chancre, but is almost always accompanied by simultaneously existing affections of the skin and throat; nor can the ring-shaped redness, nor the distortion of the pupil, or the discoloration of the iris and the effusion of lymph, be regarded as diagnostic signs, since all these changes occur in every case of iritis. *Condylomata* or *tubercles*, however, growing out of any portion of the iris, are diagnostic signs. At first, they are brown-red; afterwards, yellowish; project beyond the level of the iris, and sometimes increasing in size, so as to press the iris back. In other respects, in no disease are relapses so frequent as in iritis; even if the disease terminates favorably, the eye remains for a long time sensitive to cold and damp weather, dreads the light, and discharges a more or less copious quantity of tears.

Sec. 137.—Prognosis of the previously named Diseases.

In most respects, the prognosis is the same as that of syphilis generally. Some of the above-mentioned forms, however, involve more or less danger, both on account of the organs affected, as well as on account of the nature of the phenomena characterizing the invasion of the poison in each special case. For this reason, it seems desirable that a few remarks should be offered on this subject. The most dangerous of all are, undoubtedly, the *phagedænic ulcers;* and among this class, more especially those that are seated in the throat and eyes. For all that, the prognosis of *chancres in the throat*, as long as the bones and cartilages have not yet been destroyed, is not so very unfavorable, particularly if no other secondary phenomena are present, and relapses have not yet taken place. Ulcers on the velum are likewise much worse than those that are seated on the palate, and in the pharynx, for the reason that the former, after being healed, may leave the velum lacerated by irremediable perforations. Of course, the prognosis is somewhat dependent upon the existence of syphilidæ that may happen to coexist with the ulcers in the throat. If the syphilidæ are but slight, and of a transitory nature, there is not so much danger of seeing the disease of the throat converted into speedily-destroying ulcers. On the contrary, if the accompanying syphilidæ are of a malignant and destructive nature, the affection of the throat may assume a similar character, unless the disease is speedily arrested in its course.

This remark concerning the accompanying syphilidæ, likewise applies to affections of the nose, larynx, ears, and eyes. The danger, or absence of danger in these affections, is proportionate to the more or less dangerous character of the accompanying accessory phenomena. If these are malignant, syphilitic ozœna, even if cured, may result in permanent loss of smell, and in an irreparable caving in of the nose. Laryngeal ulcers, where they do not terminate fatally, by the supervention of phthisis, may entail an incurable aphonia. Syphilitic otorrhœa may leave a permanent buzzing in the ears, or an incurable deafness, behind; and syphilitic iritis may not only cause loss of sight, in the affected eye, but likewise the most hideous destruction and disfigurement of the tissues.

As regards prognosis, syphilitic iritis is the very worst disorder of any that can arise, after badly-managed or neglected primary ulcers. Not only is there great danger of a complete destruction of the eye, but, even if the disease is healed, the eye remains much smaller; or, if the treatment had been badly managed, horrid fungoid growths may shoot up from the body of the organ, so that, unless they can be cured by internal treatment, it would have, after all, been more desirable to lose the eye than to carry such horrid malformations about through life.

In a great measure, the prognosis is, fortunately, determined by the treatment instituted for all these different affections. If conducted with powerful escharotics or mercurial frictions, we cannot expect to accomplish much good; on the contrary, if these affections are treated internally, with appropriate specific agents, and the treatment is begun in season, we may, even in the worst cases, promise a reasonably satisfactory cure.

Sec. 138.—Treatment of Syphilitic Affections of the Mucous Membranes.

For the same reasons as those that have already been detailed (Sec. 131), I use *Mercury* in all *chancrous ulcerations;* if resembling the *simple* or *Hunterian* chancre, I employ *Merc. sol.;* in the *phagedænic* form I prefer *Merc. corr.*, until an improvement sets in, after which, I continue the treatment with *Merc. solubilis.* If *condylomatous growths* have started up, I give Nitri. ac., or Cinnabaris, less frequently *Thuja*, from which I have never derived any benefit in deep-seated phagedænic chancres, but a good deal in ulcerated erosions of the throat. Regarding the dose: I never give, in urgent cases, lower than the second trituration of Mercury, in one-half-grain doses, morning and night, giving only one dose every morning on the third and fourth day, and after this period, one dose every other day. Until now, I have had every reason to be satisfied with this proceeding, even in a case of phagedænic chancre of the throat, attended with incipient iritis, where *Corr. subl.*, followed by *Mercurius*, first induced an improvement, and afterwards achieved a perfect cure of both the chancre and the affection of the eye. I have never yet had a chance to treat a full case of syphilitic iritis, with the characteristic tubercles or condylomata, but should not hesitate to give *Cinnabaris* first, and if this should not speedily improve the case, should change to *Nitri ac.* In the above-mentioned case of ulceration of the larynx, I had produced some little improvement with *Lachesis*, even before being acquainted with the syphilitic nature of the case, until it was distinctly revealed by the corona veneris on the forehead. For syphilitic crusts and ulcers in the nose, which I have never had occasion to treat, except in cases where a good deal of Mercury had already been used, I have always used *Aurum* 3, with the best success.

Whereas mercurial preparations have always helped me out in secondary chancres on the different mucous surfaces, on the contrary, I have never derived much benefit from them in *exanthematic*, *herpetic*, but slightly ulcerated erosions of the throat or other mucous surfaces. All such cases are benefited by Lachesis, more especially by Lycopodium, and no less by Nitri ac., Thuja, Cinnabaris, or even. sulphur. I explain this by the circumstance that all these higher forms, according to my observations, only break out in cases where the primary ulcers had already been treated with Mercury; but where the treatment had only commenced towards the termination of the transition stage, or where the internal use of Mercury during the primary stage had been associated with cauterization of the ulcer, in both of which cases Mercury had, indeed, abated the intensity of the malady, but, on the other hand, had allowed it time to coalesce with other morbific principles in the body. Be this as it may, the physician can never investigate with too much care the history of any syphiloid that presents itself for treatment; more particularly, he should endeavor to find out *how soon after the first appearance of the primary symptoms* their treatment had commenced, and in what manner it was conducted.

Sec. 139.—Therapeutic Observations of other Physicians regarding the above-mentioned Forms.

In comparison with the cures of primary ulcers, with which our literature abounds, we have but few cases of secondary affections of the mucous membranes, and, in fact only general remarks, the most important of which we will here recapitulate, accompanied by our own additions.

1) Clotar Müller (All. h. Zeit., vol. 37), recommends very properly *Corr. subl.* for chancres in the throat. This may, however, apply more particularly to phagedænic chancres, where *Corr. subl.* is undoubtedly preferable to any other mercurial preparation.

2) Hartmann (Therapeutics, vol. 2), prefers *Acidum phosph.* to *Nitri. ac.* in cases of sore, ulcerated velum palati (syphilitic ulcerated tetter in the throat). I cannot share this opinion. Phosphori ac., in my hands, has never seemed as effectual as *Nitri. acidum.* This author's remarks concerning the curative virtues of *Lycopodium*, in herpetic affections of the mouth and pharynx, are abundantly confirmed by the results of my own experience.

3) Trinks (All. hom. Zeit., vol. 15), denies the curative virtues of *Merc. sol.*, as utterly insufficient in *secondary* affections, whereas he recommends this very agent for recent affections of the soft parts of the mouth and fauces, and even for syphilitic iritis, without in-

forming us whether, by "recent affections," he means chancrous or herpetic phenomena; for in the former, *Merc. sol.* would help as surely as it would be absolutely inappropriate in the latter. It is true that, in destructive ulcers of the fauces, *Merc. præc.* is more efficient than Merc. solubilis; *Merc. subl.* is superior to either as a curative agent in these affections. *Nitri ac.*, recommended by Trinks, is most likely superior to *Merc. sol.*, only if Mercury had already been used, or where fungoid growths have already made their appearance.

4) Wolf, in Dresden (Archiv., vol. 11, number 1), considers *Thuja* as adapted to syphilitic ulcers of the throat after abuse of Mercury. This is undoubtedly correct in some cases, especially where condylomata are present.

Moreover, the following remedies have been used by myself and others with advantage:

a) for *herpetic eruptions* in the mouth and throat: Lycopodium, Nitri. ac., Phosphori. ac., Zincum.
b) for *excoriations, erosions:* Merc. sol., Nitri. ac., Phosphori ac., Lachesis.
c) for *ulcers on the tongue:* Merc. præc., Nitri acidum.
d) for *ulcers in the throat:* Merc. sol., Præc. ruber, Sublimat. corr., Lachesis, Aurum, Lycopodium, Iodium, Kali jod.
e) for *angina syphilitica:* Lycopodium, Lachesis, Aurum, Nitri ac., Merc. sol., Argentum, Mezereum.
f) for *affections of the nose:* Merc. sol., Aurum, Lachesis, Kali Iodatum.
g) for *iritis syphilitica:* Sublim. corr., Nitri. ac., Thuja.

Where mercurial preparations were indicated, they were generally employed in the first and second or third trituration, all other remedies in an attenuated form, even globules of the thirtieth attenuation. After a practice of forty years, during which I have tried every imaginable size of dose, I have come to the conclusion that this mode of exhibiting the drug is about the most efficient and successful.

IV. SYPHILITIC AFFECTIONS OF BONES.

Sec. 140.—General Review of these Affections.

Without overlooking the anatomical difference existing between bone and periosteum, we range the affections of both in one category, not only because the periosteum is part of the osseous system as well as the bone itself, but likewise because in syphilitic affections both are generally involved, and, though the organs are different, yet the disease with which we have to deal is one and the same. However, if we wish to distinguish the affections of the bony system with reference to their anatomical locality, we may distinguish three essentially distinct varieties; a distinction that may be of no avail whatever as far as treatment and diagnosis are concerned, but may be somewhat useful with regard to our prognosis, which it may enable us to determine more satisfactorily to ourselves, and perhaps to the patient.

1) If the *periosteum* alone is diseased, we ascertain this fact by a thickening of this membrane, attended with a keen painfulness to pressure; the disease generally terminates in a deposition of bony matter under the periosteum, in consequence of which the bone at the affected part becomes hypertrophied. Such a hypertrophy is termed *syphilitic node*, or *syphilitic exostosis*, and is generally seated on the tibia. If the periosteum should become ulcerated (which is a rare occurrence), it may happen that a portion of the subjacent bone becomes *necrotic*, and exfoliates, which, however, does not constitute caries, but simply a *syphilitic necrosis*.

2) If the bone itself is affected, caries begins independently of the periosteum, in the retiform tissue of the bone, gradually perforating the outer layer of bone, in which case the disease does not result in the formation of a hard swelling, like exostosis, but in that of a *soft* swelling, which can be seen and felt externally, and which, when opened, discharges a slimy fluid; the periosteum, at this place, is somewhat thickened and detached from the bone. In the centre of this denuded portion of bone, a small perforation is seen passing through the cortical layer of bone, until it reaches its inner substance. These carious swellings occur most frequently on the skull-bones, but are likewise seen on the lower jaw and the

radius. They constitute the worst of all syphilitic affections of the osseous system, and frequently invade a large surface of the skull.

3) Beside these swellings, there occurs another phenomenon, although less frequently than the former, likewise more particularly on the skull-bones. At first, it seems to have been a simple inflammation of the bone, in consequence of which the bone has become hypertrophied, and its tissue has become thickened and heavier. The periosteum may remain sound for a long time, but may likewise, in the course of the malady, become inflamed at some points, and may become raised in the shape of small *periostoses* or *tophi*. These tophi frequently disappear of themselves, sometimes in the space of ten days or a fortnight, but are generally replaced by others in a short time, which likewise disappear again in order to give place to new ones; if suppuration sets in, carious ulcers form, which soon, however, likewise become cicatrized.

These three anatomical changes may occur with or without bone-pains; the last-mentioned, when the bone alone is affected, may take place without any alteration of substance, so that, if we desire to acquire a perfect knowledge of syphilitic affections of the bony system, we have to consider the following four points, each by itself: 1) *bone-pains*; 2) *inflammation of bones*; 3) *exostoses*; and, 4) *caries*.

Sec. 141.—Syphilitic Bone-pains.

These pains may make their appearance either long or shortly after the primary symptoms have been got rid of. They generally manifest themselves by keen tearing, *deep-seated* pains, accompanied by a disagreeable sensation of pressure, boring, stinging, and other similar pains following the direction of the long bones, sternum, clavicles, or over the bones of the skull. At night these pains generally exacerbate, when they almost become intolerable. Unattended by any change in the pulse, or by a swelling of the affected parts, and neither aggravated by contact nor pressure upon the parts, they neither resemble *neuralgic* pains following the course of a nerve, nor *rheumatic* pains, which are disposed to wander about, decrease rather than increase in the warmth of the bed, and are felt in localities that can be definitely pointed out;

whereas the patient is unable to indicate the precise spot where the syphilitic bone-pains are seated. When affecting the skull, these pains are severer than in other parts, and may lead to very dangerous symptoms; whatever bone, however, they may attack, they always hinder the night's rest, raging, in most cases, from nine o'clock in the evening until two or three o'clock in the morning, interfering with the proper preservation of the body, undermining the patient's strength, and often causing considerable emaciation. In many cases these pains remain seated in one bone without producing the least material change in its tissues; but very often they are the precursors of subsequent exostosis, necrosis or caries; at all events, however, they do not constitute an independent disease *per se*, but must always be considered, wherever they appear, as the first stage of all the other syphilitic affections of bones. The disease may, indeed, remain stationary in this first period, but, in most cases, these pains are preliminary to the structural alterations of the bones.

These pains are generally associated with other simultaneously-appearing phenomena of secondary syphilis, such as syphilidæ, affections of the mucous membranes, etc., in which case it is not difficult to determine their true pathological nature; whereas, in cases where these symptoms are wanting, the diagnosis of syphilitic bone-pains is not always as easy as some people imagine. What we have said above of the noctural appearance of these pains as a diagnostic mark by means of which they can be distinguished from rheumatic pains, is not true as a rule without exception, since rheumatic pains, although usually abating in the warmth of the bed, very frequently exacerbate *at night;* on the other hand, there are syphilitic bone-pains that are felt only during the day, but leave the patient perfectly easy at night, as I have seen in more than one case. In such cases, however, the seat of these pains, together with their nocturnal appearance and the difficulty of fixing their exact locality in the affected bone, may render the diagnosis certain beyond all doubt. This difficulty is principally owing to the fact, that the true seat of these pains is not, as in rheumatic pains, in the coverings, nor at the surface of the bones, but most generally in the *medullary membrane;* although it may likewise be located in the periosteum, in which case it increases on pressure, and its precise locality can be definitely ascertained; so that this definiteness regarding the precise seat of the pain, becomes just as sure a diagnostic sign, as its indefiniteness in the former case. Nevertheless, however excruciating these pains may be, their prognosis is not, by any means, the worst in the different forms of syphilis; since they yield more easily than many other syphilitic phenomena, to a truly rational treatment.

Sec. 142.—Inflammation of the Bones and Periosteum.

Although bone-pains very frequently exist without any material changes in the periosteum or bone, yet, as Ricord has satisfactorily demonstrated, they are frequently attended with inflammation, not so much of the periosteum, as of the substance of the bone itself.

Inflammation of the periosteum, if it does at all exist, most likely never occurs independently of the bone. That which has been more recently described, under the names of periostosis and exŏstosis, as terminations of inflammation—we mean the exudations that take place beneath the detached periosteum, and form hard swellings—most probably arises from a superficial inflammation of the bone itself, rather than from inflammation of the periosteum. If the periosteum should be inflamed, more or less circumscribed swellings may arise, more particularly on bones covered with simple integument, which swellings afterwards form the true *periostoses*, and are seen, for instance, on the tibia, clavicle, radius, ulna, skull-bones, and metacarpal and metatarsal bones. These swellings are sometimes without any sensation; if there is no distinct fluctuation, they at least have a doughy feel, and the integument over them may remain for a long time movable and without any perceptible alteration. Capable of dispersion in certain cases, these swellings may, under other circumstances, terminate in suppuration, forming true abscesses, which, when opened, may show the bone simply denuded of its periosteum, or a portion of it attacked with caries or necrosis, down to a certain depth, and, in fortunate cases, provided already with new granulations.

Otherwise, the more deep-seated inflammation of bones from syphilitic infection is like any other form of ostitis. It may affect the very same parts which we have described a little while ago, as the seat of periostitis. Very often it only attacks the surface of the bones; not unfrequently, however, it penetrates the whole of the bony tissue. Generally they run a chronic course, although, exceptionally, they may likewise assume a sub-inflammatory form. But for the known bone-pains, it might exist for a long time without betraying itself by any perceptible swelling of the bone; however, should it continue for a long time, it results in the formation of *exostoses;* in either case, it generally terminates in dispersion, and but very seldom in caries or necrosis. Like simple bone-pains, ostitis has been regarded by many physicians as a *mercurial* affection, which it undoubtedly is in many cases. In many cases, however, it may occur in patients who have never made any use of this metal, and where a syphilitic taint is evidenced by the simultaneous manifestation of other syphilitic phenomena upon the skin, or in the throat. If these phenomena are wanting, and the patient has been drugged with Mercury, the diagnosis remains undoubtedly doubtful, inasmuch as not only Hahnemann, but other physicians likewise, have found that Mercury will not only cause inflammation, but a variety of other affections of the bones; any one who doubts this fact, may become convinced of its truth by examining, in the University of Bonn on the Rhine, the half-corroded skull of a man who had died of what is called *syphilis of the bones*, where he can distinctly perceive the mercurial globules shining in the bony tissue, showing that this metal, in spite of all assertions to the contrary, is capable of causing such frightful disorganizations of the bones.

Sec. 143.—Exostoses and Periostoses

Among the swellings occurring on the bones, we distinguish two kinds with reference to prognosis: 1) slight swellings, which often disappear of themselves, and are occasioned by morbid depositions of the inflamed periosteum, and hence are designated as *periostoses;* and 2) much more serious swellings, where the substance of the bone itself is inflamed, and furnishes these depositions; these swellings are termed *exostoses.* Let us endeavor to give a discriminating description of both forms.

1) *Periostoses*, which some German authors, among whom Hartmann, falsely describe as gummata (see § 147), are small, roundish, imperfectly circumscribed, mostly soft, doughy swellings, known as *syphilitic nodes*, or tophi, arising, as has already been stated, from a previous inflammation of the periosteum, and

are principally located on the tibia, clavicle, ulna, radius, skull-bones, and sternum. Although consisting of a swelling of the inflamed periosteum and the subjacent cellular tissue, these swellings frequently show, without any doubt, whether the inflammation is confined to the periosteum, or whether it does not rather emanate from the outer bony laminæ. In this latter case, it may occasion the effusion of an albuminous fluid between the bone and the periosteum, in consequence of which the former becomes more or less thickened, forming a painless, indolent swelling, which may terminate in dispersion. In other cases, on the contrary, the inflammation of the periosteum may progress and terminate in suppuration, in which case the bone, after the abscess is opened, is found denuded of its periosteum; after which the bone, according to circumstances, either exfoliates or becomes necrosed, or else may become attacked with a progressive caries. This last-mentioned termination occurs more frequently with the broad bones, skull-bones, sternum, etc.; whereas the long bones, tibia, bones of the arm, etc., are more frequently attacked with necrosis. The periosteum may, however, remain inflamed without the substance of the bones becoming involved, and, amid an abatement of the pains, may terminate in chronic thickening and hypertrophy, which, however, does not preclude the possibility of final dispersion.

2) *Exostoses* always depend upon inflammation of the bone itself, and, according as the superficial laminæ or the whole parenchyma of the bone are inflamed, may assume different forms. If the inflammation is merely superficial, the periosteum is always involved, in which case, if nothing but albuminous exudations take place, the disease may be confined to the above-mentioned periostoses; on the contrary, if suppuration of the bone or deposition of inorganic substances takes place, the exudations or simultaneous suppurations of the periosteum are accompanied by semi-globular, conical, flattened or oblong *exostoses*, which may continue for years in the shape of hard, more or less circumscribed swellings, without dispersing, and which, if occurring on the internal surface of the skull-bones or sternum, may materially interfere with the functions of these organs. If the whole parenchyma of the bone is attacked, the bony swelling is uniformly developed in all directions, as may be noticed on the tibia, humerus and femur; such an exostosis or

rather hypertrophy of the bone is distinguished with great difficulty from an analogous scrofulous disorganization. Nor is it always easy at the commencement of such swellings to distinguish periostoses, exostoses and hypertrophies from each other; if more advanced, the first-named can always be recognized by their increased *softness*, the second by their *hardness* and *semi-globular shape*, and the last-named by the uniform extension of the hard swelling.

Sec. 144.—Necrosis and Caries of the Skull, Nose and Palate.

These disorganizations, which, after all, are nothing else than the not very rare termination of a syphilitic inflammation of the bones or their periosteum (*ostitis* and *periostitis*), do not exhibit any symptomatic peculiarities that are not likewise seen in non-syphilitic affections of the same kind. In regard to their site they show, however, some peculiar features deserving of a more especial notice.

1) Syphilitic affections of the skull-bones very frequently announce themselves in the shape of simple bone-pains, which, after having lasted for a longer or shorter period of time, give rise to swelling of the bone and sensitiveness of this part to pressure; if the cerebral surface of the skull-bones is the seat of the affection, it manifests itself at most by more or less impairing the cerebral functions; in such a case we have no means of ascertaining whether there is necrosis, caries or a simple exostosis, or whether the dura mater is attacked or not. If seated on the outer skull, these affections, like similar affections in other cases, are characterized by tumors or open ulcers; they have been known to cause terrible disorganizations, to corrode the whole outer layer of the skull-bones, and even to penetrate to the inner layer and expose a large portion of the cerebrum.

2) Equally dangerous are these affections if the bones of the *orbits* and of the *ear* are the seat of the disorganizing process. By exercising a pressure upon the optic nerve they may not only cause a considerable diminution of the optic nerve, but likewise complete blindness; or they may cause deafness by attacking the ossicula of the ear. As long as the pains remain internal, and the destruction of the bones is not yet revealed by any external dis-

charge, the diagnosis of these affections remains very obscure, and, even if other syphilitic phenomena should be present, can only be cleared up within the limits of probability.

3) The affections of the nasal bones are of more easy recognition. If caries or necrosis should set in, we soon perceive painfulness and swelling on one side of the nose, the swelling having a doughy feel, without the color of the skin being in the least altered. Soon, however, the skin assumes a red color, the bones show less resistance to the pressure of the finger; pressure is even attended with a peculiar creaking or crackling sensation; at the same time the patient begins to discharge a purulent matter from his nose, which afterwards is mixed up with small bony splinters; in other cases, which are, however, less frequent, these splinters may find a passage through the outer integuments, in which case a small abscess forms, that opens spontaneously. After the dead pieces of bone have been removed, the nose caves in at that spot, so that, if both sides of the nose have thus become affected, and if the septum and other cartilages and bones of this organ have been destroyed, the most hideous disfigurement may be the consequence. In case caries of the nasal bones should be associated with syphilitic tubercles, the skin itself may become destroyed, and the whole organ be lost, so that nothing remains but the posterior nares lying open, like horrid chasms, on a level with the cheeks. It is scarcely necessary to remark that speech and voice soon become impaired in the presence of these disgusting disorganizations.

4) Destruction of the palatine bones likewise commences with a seated pain in the arch of the palate, soon after which the mucous membrane of the affected part assumes a violet-red color, and becomes swollen and spongy. Soon after, from a small opening in the swelling, an ichorous pus is secreted, and afterwards bony splinters; at the same time the patient's breath becomes very offensive. In consequence of this destruction of the palatine bones, an outlet is effected from the posterior nares, which, if the loss of substance is not too considerable, may close again; but, if too considerable, may leave an open, oval or irregularly-shaped opening, which can only be partially remedied and covered up by means of an artificial palate.

Sec. 145.—Necrosis and Caries of other parts.

Less frequent are syphilitic affections of the jaw-bones, pharyngeal and laryngeal bones, vertebræ and articulations ; nevertheless they occur likewise, and not unfrequently are overlooked, as we shall see presently.

1) The jaw-bones are generally attacked only with syphilitic necrosis, not caries ; the upper maxillary bone is more frequently attacked than the lower.

2) Carious destructions of the larynx are generally the sequelæ of previous syphilitic affections of the mucous membrane, which, by destroying the cartilages, may lead to laryngeal phthisis. These destructions are almost always preceded by syphilitic ulcers at the root of the tongue, the epiglottis, or on the walls of the pharynx, at the same time that the balance of the symptoms do not differ in any thing from those of a true laryngeal phthisis, so that the diagnosis can only be cleared up by the previous history of the case, in connection with other simultaneously-existing affections.

3) In the region of the pharynx likewise, carious destructions of the anterior portion of some of the vertebræ have been observed, which, associated with grave symptoms of syphilitic action in the soft parts of the pharynx, or, rather, spreading from these to the vertebræ, have resulted fatally to the patient.

4) It is doubtful whether truly syphilitic destructions can occur down the vertebral column, although some authors assert that they have seen the lumbar vertebræ destroyed by syphilis, or congestive abscesses caused in consequence of the lateral portions or the spinous processes of the vertebræ being invaded by the disease, or spinal curvatures result from the anterior portions of the vertebræ being affected and destroyed by the poison. There is no doubt that the lumbar and dorsal vertebræ can be attacked by caries; but, in order that we may be certain whether caries is not of a scrofulous but syphilitic nature, the knowledge that this individual had been affected with gonorrhœa or chancre once in his life-time is not sufficient. If we desire to be perfectly sure of our diagnosis, other syphilitic phenomena have to be present beside the caries;

although even the presence of these phenomena does not furnish indubitable evidence in the case of a scrofulous individual that had been affected with diseases of the bones at a previous period.

5) The same remark applies to caries of the joints, where, according to some authors, syphilis may likewise erect its throne, causing the so-called "*white swellings,*" where a nocturnal exacerbation of the pain is supposed to constitute a diagnostic sign. Syphilis may possibly cause such disorganizations; but it is equally true that a good deal that owes its origin to other causes, has been set down to the account of syphilis. If so much has been said against Hahnemann's *psora,* what shall we say of those who behold in every abnormal structural change a result of syphilitic or even gonorrhœal poisoning, dating perhaps back to the third or fourth generation!

6) We need hardly state that necrosis or caries may befall all those parts where periostoses or exostoses may develop themselves, such as the tibia, sternum, clavicle, etc.

Sec. 146.—Diagnosis, Prognosis and Treatment of Syphilitic Affections of the Bones.

As regards diagnosis, it is evident that, if there is any difficulty, it can only be to determine whether the disease is of a scrofulous or mercurial nature, excepting, however, the bone-pains, the diagnosis of which has been indicated, § 141. In such cases, a most careful investigation of the previous circumstances sometimes affords all the light that can be obtained. If neither scrofulous complaints nor abuse of Mercury, but a whole list of syphilitic phenomena had preceded, the syphilitic nature of the case is all but certain, more particularly if the existing symptoms had been preceded by nocturnal bone-pains. In the absence of all syphilitic signs, however, all suspicion of a syphilitic taint must be abandoned, and, if signs of scrofulosis and mercurial abuse are present, the diagnosis can only turn upon the difference between these two orders of symptoms. The case is different if scrofulous and mercurial symptoms exist, mixed up with old symptoms of constitutional syphilis. In most of these cases, a correct and satisfactory diagnosis is all but impossible; and all we can accomplish is to obtain, by means of a careful and discreet investigation of the previous history of the case, a certain degree of probable knowledge concerning that one of these three different diatheses which the phenomena that happen to be the most prominent, for the time being, may lead us to regard as their exciting cause.

In regard to *prognosis*, what has been said in treating of the other syphilitic affections is likewise applicable in these cases. So far as particular affections are concerned, we may state that, of all syphilitic affections of the bones, the periostoses are the lightest, and the least dangerous. These periostoses often disappear of themselves, whereas the exostoses sometimes bid obstinate defiance to all treatment. In *caries* and *necrosis*, as well as in *simple inflammation* (ostitis, periostitis, and bone-pains), the prognosis is almost exclusively dependent on the treatment instituted against these conditions; a complete cure can always be promised, provided the treatment is conducted in a rational manner, with appropriate specific remedies.

As regards the treatment of these syphilitic affections of the bones, I ought to state that, except ulcerous destructions of the nasal and palatine bones, arising from syphilitic affections of the mucous membranes (for which I always use *Merc. sol.*, and *Aurum*, with the best effect), I have never yet met with syphilitic affections of the skull-bones, tibia, clavicles, sternum, etc., where the patients had not already been drugged with Mercury, and where *Aurum* proved the most efficient remedial agent. Only in two cases of caries of the tibia, associated with chancres in the throat, and where no Mercury had been previously used, this agent cured both the caries and the chancrous ulcerations. Beside this remedy, I have used, with the utmost advantage:

For *bone-pains*, *ostitis*, and *periostitis:* Mezereum, Phosphorus, Staphysagria, Phosphori acidum, Nitri acidum, Aurum, Guaiacum.

For *swelling of bones*, *periostoses*, and *exostoses:* Aurum, Fluoris acidum, Phosphorus, Staphysagria, Mezereum (Calcarea), Silicea, Sulphur, Phosphori acidum.

For *caries* and *necrosis:* Aurum, Nitri acidum, Fluoris acidum, Silicea.

I have likewise used *Kali Iodatum* in affections of the bones, even in large doses, as recommended by allopathic physicians, and I have seen excellent effects from its use in such quantities; but they were never as lasting as the good effects obtained by means of small doses of other remedies. Usually, the symptoms yielded to Kali Iodatum in a very short time, but returned again (perhaps in the shape of excessive effects of the drug?), in six or twelve months, which never occurred in cases that had been cured with the eighteenth or thirtieth attenuations of other drugs. This has induced me to adhere to the latter, without ever using Kali Iodatum. As regards *Aurum*, I give it in the third trituration, one half of a grain every four days.

V.—SYPHILITIC AFFECTIONS OF OTHER TISSUES.

Sec. 147. Syphilis of the Cellular Tissue, Gummatose Swellings (gummata.)

Ranging the secondary syphilitic affections that may occur in other tissues beside the mucous membranes and bones, according to the frequency of their occurrence, we shall have to assign the first rank to the affections of the *cellular tissue*, where the so-called gummata are located, which, even now, are considered by many physicians who value their diagnosis quite highly, as identical with periostoses, from which they are, however, as far apart as bones are from cellular tissue. A periostosis is seated on the bone; a gummatose swelling, between the integuments and muscles, and is seen in all the different layers, and in every portion of the cellular tissue, on the thighs, calves, arms, and neck, even on the head, where, as in any other portion of bone without much fleshy covering, the swelling may develop itself close to the bone, which may even become involved in the swelling, and affected with caries, provided the gumma penetrates to a sufficient depth. Nevertheless, the true seat of these tubercular swellings is in the *cellular tissue*, where they commence in the shape of a lump, which, without any sign of inflammation, and only accompanied by dull pains and some tension, continues to grow very gradually for months, and even a whole year, until it has reached its full development, after which it terminates in suppuration. The cutaneous covering remains intact for a long time; after a time, however, it begins to turn red, and to coalesce with the swelling, until it tears, and several small foramina arise, that soon unite in one large ulcer with hard, everted edges, and a grayish base. If such a tubercle is opened before it passes into a state of suppuration, it is found to contain a cellular substance filled with a yellow, honey-like fluid; the suppuration never spreads over the whole swelling, which always secretes only a small quantity of a thin, ichorous pus, and continues to suppurate until the outer shell, in which this tubercular swelling seems to rest, is gone, after which the loss of substance begins to be repaired, leaving a cicatrix like those that are caused by burns. If these gummata break out on the head, they may be associated with caries of the skull-bones, of which they seem to constitute the proximate cause. These gummata seldom break out at once at every point; in most cases, they succeed each other in different parts, for months, and even years; very often, several of them are found congregated in the same locality. Although their true locality is beneath the integuments of the extremities, yet they are likewise met with beneath the mucous membrane of the mouth, palate, and fauces, even in the parenchyma of the tongue, which feels as if stuffed with hazle-nuts, that may lead one to suspect schirrous indurations, and even carcinoma, after suppuration has set in; indeed, such a pathological condition bears some resemblance to carcinoma of the tongue. Most authors are of opinion that such gummatose swellings always denote a deeply-rooted constitutional syphilis, and that syphilitic phenomena of the worst sort will invariably follow in its train, even if they should not yet have made their appearance at the first outbreak of the gummatose disorganizations. This apprehension is undoubtedly well founded, in some cases; on the other hand, other authors have seen such gummata run their whole course without giving rise to any signs of constitutional syphilis. I have only seen two cases of gummata—one case being a woman, and the other a Russian traveller. Both patients had had a chancre six and eight years ago, had been affected with several secondary symptoms, and for the last three years had been affected with these gummata, being the remaining isolated symptoms of the syphilitic disease.

Sec. 148.—Syphilitic Affections of the Muscles, Tendons, and Aponeuroses.

We have already stated, at the beginning of this chapter, that, among the sequelæ of suppressed sycosic gonorrhœa,

Hahnemann mentions a *contraction of the flexor tendons of the extremities* as one of them. In corroboration of Hahnemann's testimony, it may be said that even the greatest skeptics among the allopaths, Lagneau, Bell, Ricord, and others, regard this symptom of contraction of tendons as one that not unfrequently occurs simultaneously with other syphilitic phenomena.

Another morbid manifestation in the tendons and aponeuroses consists of a sort of *aponeurotic swellings* and *tendinous tophi* that sometimes grow to a considerable size, and are seated in the fibrous tissue of the tendons and aponeuroses. Most usually the swellings are of firm consistence, and seem to consist in a circumscribed hypertrophy of the fibrous tissue of the tendons, with effusion of plastic lymph in the interstices. They are generally the seat of a greater or less degree of painfulness, which is increased by moving the affected part. Not unfrequently they appear simultaneously with exostoses of the neighboring bones. If lasting for a long period without suppurating, they may become ossified, and this ossification may involve the whole tendon, or may be limited to a small portion thereof, and may form a sort of *sesamoid bone.* Most frequently they occur on the surface of the tendons, in which case the swelling is more perceptible, and forms a sort of abrupt prominence in the course of the tendon, not unlike a ganglion. If seated within the substance of the tendon, the swelling has either an oval or spindle-shaped form.

Beside the above-mentioned, there are, according to the observations of Benison, of Strasburg, still other tubercles in the *flesh of the muscles.* These tubercles commence like a local, circumscribed, *soft* swelling, of a somewhat firmer consistence than that of œdema, and, on being cut through, are seen filled with a plastic, grayish-looking substance, which, as it slowly progresses, softens into a glutinous, ropy fluid, not unlike a solution of gum. If, from some cause or other, the course of such a tubercle becomes acute, *pus* forms in the interior of the muscle; the softened fibres are destroyed, and far-spread disorganizations may be the consequences of such softening; it is not by any means impossible that the psoas- and lumbar-abscesses in the pelvic region should originate in a syphilitic taint, on which account practitioners *cannot be sufficiently mindful of such a possibility.* In other cases, these swellings terminate in *indurations*, first assuming the consistence of cartilage, and afterwards of bone; the remarkable masses of bone that have been discovered in the muscles of the thighs, in the glutei muscles, etc., of some cadavers, are probably derived from syphilitic tubercles in the interior tissue of muscles. In other respects, these swellings may occur in all muscles; yea, certain organs whose parenchyma is like that of muscles, or where muscular tissue predominates, such as the *lips* and *tongue*, seem to be more particularly liable to such a disorganizing process. If located in the tongue, these swellings may appear on the edges, at the tip or root of this organ, in which case they almost always interfere with speech, and must not be confounded with the condylomatous growths on the mucous surfaces, from which they are, moreover, distinguished by their structural differences. On the lips, they might be more easily confounded with carcinoma; here, however, they occupy most generally the central portion, whereas carcinoma manifests itself on the free border of the lips in the shape of a wart-shaped tubercle, with stinging pains. These swellings may finally develop themselves in the muscles of the velum palati, as well as in those of the larynx, where they may run through all the above-mentioned stages, from simple, soft or suppurating swellings to cartilaginous or ossified indurations.

Sec. 149.—Syphilitic Affections of Internal Organs.

Authors entertain very different opinions on this subject. Whereas, some of them assert that the syphilitic virus does not exert the least influence on any other organs than the external skin, the mucous membranes, and the bones; others, on the contrary, pretend to have seen the liver, kidneys, and stomach, even the lungs and heart, the brain and the spinal cord affected by syphilitic phenomena. There is no doubt that in caries of the skull-bones or vertebræ, the membranes of the brain and spinal cord can become involved in the ulcerative process; the statement, however, that syphilitic affections can originally develop themselves in these organs will have to be substantiated by more reliable testimony.

As regards the abdominal viscera, the celebrated Doctor Cazenave, of Paris, indeed, relates a case where the syphilitic character of the intestinal phenomena is almost demonstrated. A man of thirty-five years, whose body was covered with syphilitic ulcers, was at the same time attacked with a violent purulent dysenteric diarrhœa. The patient had upwards of sixty discharges a day. This condition justified the conclusion that the same ulcerative process that was going on on the skin, had likewise developed itself in the bowels; a conclusion that was the more justifiable, since the diarrhœa, which had almost destroyed the patient's life, improved in the same ratio as the tubercular ulcerations on the skin began to heal under appropriate treatment. The same author quotes other cases where the autopsy of individuals who had died of syphilitic cachexia, revealed syphilitic ulcers in the bowels, more especially at the termination of the ileum, and in the whole tract of the cæcum, some of which resembled the elevated, some the Hunterian chancre, with everted, abrupt edges, the destructive process not being arrested till it reached the serous covering. All such patients had been suffering during the latter part of their sickness with colic and diarrhœa.

We have already made mention of the syphilitic phenomena on the mucous lining of the larynx, and in the cartilages of this organ (§§ 135 and 145); whether these phenomena can spread from those points to the bronchial mucous lining, or even to the lungs and heart, is another question. At any rate, we shall have to look for further evidence as regards the lungs and liver, whose tissues have not the least affinity either with the mucous membrane or the muscles or bones, any more than with the epidermis. The heart, being a muscular organ, might, under certain extraordinary circumstances, be attacked with the muscular swellings described in § 148, no less than the tongue, lips, and velum palati; in this respect, similar swellings might even become developed in the substance of the stomach. The only case of which we know, that bears upon this point, is a case related by Dr. Baumès, of Lyons, in his treatise on the venereal diseases, where a girl of fifteen years, who had become syphilitic a year previous, and who, not knowing what a chancre and mucous tubercles were, had not paid the least attention to these symptoms, and had employed no other means of treatment than washing with cold water, was attacked a few months after with palpitation of the heart, difficulty of breathing, and an obstinate cough, with which, at a later period, violent headache, severe attacks of cardialgia and hysteric complaints became associated. All these symptoms disappeared suddenly, as if by magic, when, all at once, syphilitic pustules broke out on the legs, which had repeatedly shown symptoms of œdema, since the commencement of her malady. The evidence of her transgression having been laid bare in this undeniable manner, she related the whole history of her case. That the heart, lungs, and stomach were affected in this case is evident beyond a doubt; but whether this was owing to the syphilitic virus is not quite so certain.

[NOTE. In connection with this subject, we wish to direct the reader's attention to a work of Professor Arnold Beer, of Tübingen, published by H. Laupp, Tübingen, 1867, and entitled "*Eingeweide-syphilis*," syphilis of internal viscera; in this work, the Professor, by means of extensive pathological inquiries and microscopical examinations of the tissue, furnishes satisfactory evidence of syphilitic disorganizations of the ileum, rectum, liver, spleen, kidneys, meningeal membranes, lungs, valves of the heart, endocardium, and other organs. The student of morbid anatomy is furnished in this work with a multitude of valuable and interesting contributions to a more extensive and accurate knowledge of the destructive effects of secondary syphilis.

Of the few cases which this work contains, we will relate two, one of them showing the adequateness, and the other the inadequateness, of the allopathic treatment of syphilis.

One was the case of a robust man of thirty years, whose legs were swollen, which he supposed to have been owing to a cold. The albuminous deposit in the urine was of moderate quantity, but remained unchanged for a long time; the specific weight of the clear urine varied between 10.11 and 10.15. At first the œdema continued to increase, so that the thigh became somewhat involved; it now remained stationary for several weeks, in spite of all the diuretics and sudorifics that were used against it. The patient then informed me that he had had an ulcer on the penis for some time that would not heal. It had the characteristic form of chancre, and the edges were slightly indurated. The patient was directed to take the Iodide of Potassium, under whose use the diuresis increased considerably, whereas the albuminous deposit and the œdema decreased, until, after using the drug for three weeks, the patient was completely restored.

According to the Professor's observation, œdema of the lower extremities and albuminous urine, together with shrinking of the liver, are characteristic of incipient syphilitic degeneration of the kidneys, provided there is otherwise positive evidence of the existence of syphilis.

In the other case, the patient, a young man, complained of

diffuse rheumatalgia in various parts of his body. His complexion had had a peculiarly sallow appearance, somewhat yellowish, although not icteric, properly speaking; this color was particularly marked on the hands. His liver was shrunk considerably. There was no œdema, but the urine was slightly albuminous, and remained so for a long time. This patient had had a chancre some time previous. Although no other syphilitic signs were present, yet I diagnosed incipient syphilitic disorganization of the kidneys, and gave the patient Iodide of Potassium. Very soon he was attacked with the most violent iodism. I diminished the dose, but the iodism continued as violent as ever. The remedy had to be discontinued, and the patient remained uncured.

In this case, if the Iodide was the proper remedy, a much smaller dose than the one given would undoubtedly have been sufficient.—HEMPEL.]

Sec. 150.—Diagnosis of the previously-mentioned Diseases.

We have already stated, in speaking of each of these diseases in particular, in what respect gummata, tendinous tophi, and tubercles of the muscles are distinguished from analogous non-syphilitic products; nevertheless, the diagnosis of these affections, as the reader may have already inferred from our statements, is not very easy, since even practitioners of considerable experience, through inadvertence and deficient investigations concerning the previous history and circumstances of the case, have mistaken gummatose swellings and tubercles of the muscular tissue for carcinomatous affections, and tendinous tophi for simple ganglia. On the other hand, true carcinomatous ulcers, purely inflammatory abscesses in the muscles or cellular tissue, and harmless ganglia, might be mistaken for constitutional syphilis. For this reason, whenever physicians are called upon to treat swellings and abscesses in the above-mentioned parts, or even simple inflammations or contractions of tendons, and circumstances justify the suspicion of a syphilitic taint, we advise such physicians never to neglect the most minute investigation of the anamnestic circumstances of the case; and even to examine the condition of the skin and of the mucous lining of the mouth, throat, and nose. By pursuing this course, I have often succeeded in discovering the syphilitic character of such products, and, tracing them back through a whole series of successive crops of syphilitic phenomena, in being led to the primary chancre as the fountain-head of the existing disorganizations. I may remind the reader of the case of a married woman, mentioned in § 147, where tubercles had formed under the integuments of the thighs and legs, that evidently were located in the cellular tissue, and, at first sight, would at once have been taken for gummata, if this opinion had not been somewhat shaken by the fact, that these swellings were totally scattered by suppuration; and likewise by the shape of the subsequent ulcers, which, without having the lardaceous base of the gummata, resembled the holes that are seen immediately after the cellular tissue of a boil becomes detached; and finally, by the long-continued suppuration of these swellings, and by their size, which, in some of them, increased to the size of half a dollar. That all these symptoms must emanate from a syphilitic origin, was made evident to me by the fact, that during the suppuration of the tubercle, the ulcer became surrounded by a brown-red areola; and likewise by this other fact, that previous to the last cicatrization, new tubercles continued to make their appearance, and that the disease, which was said to have been cured several times, had broken out again, after the lapse of six or nine months. There were no other syphilitic symptoms perceptible; after questioning this woman's husband, he finally admitted, that more than six years ago, he had a chancre, which he had cauterized immediately; shortly after which, however, his wife had become attacked with a suspicious-looking discharge from the vagina, on account of which he had sent her, under cover of some plausible pretext, to her relatives in the country, and had placed her under the care of a physician of his acquaintance. Subsequently to this period his wife, who had remained in perfect ignorance of her true condition, had been attacked with pains in the throat, rhagades between the toes, and other eruptions, until, with the appearance of the tubercles, all these symptoms vanished. Since that time, the husband himself had never been free from suspicious eruptions, and was even to the present time affected with a slight syphilitic angina.

Sec. 151.—Prognosis and Treatment.

Beside the prognosis common to all syphilitic affections, the prognosis in the case of all these disorganizations is unfavorable, in so far as all these swellings constitute some of the most obstinate phenomena in the whole domain of syphilis. What, in all such cases, renders the prognosis still more dubious, is the succession of such attacks which authors very improperly designate as "relapses." True relapses, rigorously speaking, only occur under allopathic treatment, or under homœopathic treatment with overwhelming allopathic doses; if the disease is once arrested by the specially appropriate remedy, a true relapse can no longer take place. Most previous writers on syphilis having been allopathic practitioners, who were in the habit of treating syphilis with the most massive doses, they must necessarily have regarded as relapses what was really a mere recurrence of the syphilitic phenomena, which must continue to take place until the disease itself is eradicated from the organism. Inasmuch as a period of six or twelve months may elapse before the syphilitic symptoms break out again, the physician, even under homœopathic treatment, cannot be sure whether his remedy acted merely as a palliative or as a curative agent, until a whole year, at least, has gone by; more particularly if the patient had been previously drugged with large quantities of the hydriodate of Potash. Such recurrences scarcely ever, or perhaps never, take place if the syphilitic phenomena are removed by means of small, or even the smallest homœopathic doses; he, after all, is a true master of the healing art, who knows how to cure a disease with the smallest possible dose; not he who prides himself in prescribing massive doses for mere names of diseases, such as *tertiary* or *quaternary* syphilis.

As regards treatment, I, unfortunately, have not much to say. These forms of the syphilitic disease are very rare, and, in my own practice, I have only seen two cases. In the case of the Russian traveller, mentioned § 147, *Silicea*, after many other uselessly employed drugs, finally effected such a permanent cure, that five years after, when I had an opportunity of seeing the patient again, no new symptoms had made their appearance. In the case of the woman mentioned in the same paragraph, and afterwards more in detail § 150, whose symptoms had been palliated by the hydriodate of Potash, the most striking improvement was effected by means of *Arsenicum*, which I prescribed more particularly for the putrid appearance and the burning pains of the ulcers. For two years past, I have used this agent with changeable success for dubious affections of the skin, having a syphilitic appearance about them. However, all I can say in favor of this agent is, that it seems to me more worthy of commendation than the hydriodate of Potash. It is undoubtedly true, that the hydriodate of Potash renders excellent service in more than one form of secondary syphilis, especially after the complete disappearance of the primary symptoms; but whenever this agent is capable of effecting a cure, it never need be given in larger quantities than at the rate of four grains to four hundred grains of water. The cures which I have so far effected with this drug, have so far proved lasting cures. If I tried to hasten the cure, by giving larger doses of this drug, I have seen the syphilitic phenomena break out again, six or nine months after the supposed cure, taking it for granted that these new symptoms did not indicate an excess of hydriodate-of-potash action. If this agent does not effect a speedy improvement in doses of one-hundredth of a grain, I at once have recourse to some other drug. Further remarks on this subject will be offered in the next two following divisions; and more particularly at the termination of the fourth.

THIRD DIVISION.

GENERAL PATHOLOGICAL OBSERVATIONS

ON

SYPHILIS AND ITS COURSE GENERALLY.

FIRST CHAPTER.

PATHOLOGICAL NATURE AND ORIGIN OF SYPHILIS.

I. PATHOLOGICAL NATURE OF SYPHILIS.

Sec. 152.—Pathological Unity of the Syphilitic Phenomena.

ALTHOUGH, in treating of the secondary phenomena of syphilis, we have taken the existence of this disease for granted, and have deemed it unnecessary to adduce corroborative evidence in its favor as an idiopathic pathological condition, yet, on the other hand, we must not forget that more than one reputable author not only denies the venereal origin of the syphilitic phenomena, but rejects even their idiopathic nature, and their derivation from one and the same pathological unity, even as a great many of Hahnemann's disciples deny even to this day his doctrine, that psora is the fountain-head of most chronic diseases. In order not to omit any thing in our argument concerning syphilis, we will therefore state what seems to us the irrefutable truth in this respect. Casting only a superficial glance at both the primary and secondary symptoms of syphilis, we see at once that, owing to the peculiar pathognomonic character of each of the primary symptoms, it is just as impossible to bring these different primary symptoms under one generalization, as it is not only possible, but becomes absolutely necessary to establish such a generalization with regard to the secondary phenomena. Whereas the primary phenomena do not seem to have a single feature in common: among the secondary phenomena, on the contrary, there is not one that does not show the characteristic signs of the whole series, so that, even if we should be unable to prove the venereal origin of each member of the class, yet we shall have to consider them as symptoms of one and the same unitary disease. In further examining the form which the different secondary phenomena have in common, we meet with the copper color of the cutaneous exanthems, with the circular shape of the single pustules, tetters and tubercles, as well as of whole groups of these eruptions, and with the cup-shaped depressed form of the ulcers, with their callous and everted edges, in a manner so striking, and even so uniform, even to the destructions of the cellular tissue, muscles and bones, together with all the characteristic signs of chancre, that we feel tempted to regard this disease, without any further evidence, as an universalized *chancre-plague*, if it were not best, for many palpable reasons, not to adopt such a conclusion too hastily. For, because one disease agrees with another in its external *form*, we have no right to jump at the conclusion that these two diseases are identical in *essence*; and the question might be asked, and has been asked by the opponents of Homœopathy, whether the two diseases may not have originated in different causes.

It is indeed true that, if certain symptoms are observed exclusively of a certain malady, these symptoms serve as diagnostic or pathognomonic signs of this disease, by means of which we recognize this latter as a disease sui generis, that can no longer be confounded with any other; but, in order that this fact may likewise be asserted of the above-described symptoms of secondary syphilis, we shall have, in the first place, to show that they neither can nor do occur in any other disease in the same manner, not even by accident. Yea, in order to meet all objections at the very outset, we shall have to show that these symptoms belong to the syphilitic disease *per se*, and are not superinduced, as some assert, by accidentally aggravating causes, such as: inflammation, a vicious mode of living, improper use of drugs, and the like. Let us examine all these points, and inquire how far syphilis is or is not an *unitary, idiopathic disease*.

Sec. 153.—The Idiopathic Character of Syphilitic Phenomena.

"There is no syphilis, and hence no syphilitic phenomena!" so say all the adherents of the Physiological School founded by Broussais some fifty years ago, and adopted even by some German homœopaths. Physiological physicians deny the existence of idiopathic diseases, and of pathology generally, in so far, at any rate, as they view all morbid phenomena as abnormal physiological processes occasioned by accidental inflammatory irritations. According to these physicians, all the so-called scrofulous, syphilitic, scorbutic, rhachitic, cancerous and other special affections of the skin, mucous membranes, glands, bones, etc., are nothing but the natural consequences of simple inflammations, which, according as they affect individuals of a lymphatic, leucophlegmatic, acrimonious or other temperament, or invade one or the other particular organ, adopt this or that particular course, and a more or less modified form, according to the influences that act upon the patient. As a proof of the correctness of their theories, they quote certain facts, by virtue of which an act of coïtion that is supposed to be contagious, but, in reality, only occasions an inflammatory irritation through the acrid nature of certain secretions, produces, according to the constitutional differences of individuals, gonorrhœa in one, chancre in another, or buboes and mucous tubercles in a third; the subsequent benignant or malignant character of these products depending entirely upon the individual constitution of the patient, upon his mode of life, or the treatment that is being pursued in the case; and from these general views they draw the inference that, even if there are *venereal* or non-venereal products, characterized by a copper-brown redness, a rounded form, or more or less depressed and callous ulcers, these phenomena can be accounted for by the individuality of the patient, and by other accidental influences, and that, in order to explain them, it is not necessary that we should lug in the doctrine of an idiopathic disease, or even of a specific morbific principle. Against this theory, which, at first sight, seems quite plausible, there could not be any objection, if what are called idiopathic diseases were not made up of precisely such symptoms as do not depend upon individual peculiarities and accidental conditions, but, under all conditions, manifest themselves with the same signs, and in the same manner; thus determining, among organic alterations, swellings, ulcers and inflammations of a like form, certain fixed, not individual nor accidental differences, founded in the specific nature of these alterations; in other words, *essentially distinct kinds or species thereof*. For the very reason that certain *specific pathognomonic signs* which always manifest themselves *alike* among different individuals, and among a multitude of the most varied influences, induce us to distinguish not only scrofulous, cancerous, scorbutic, but likewise rheumatic, catarrhal, arthritic and other ulcers, swellings, inflammations, eruptions, etc., as so many *special kinds* of these organic alterations—for that very reason we have to regard *syphilitic alterations*, on account of the signs that are specifically peculiar to them, and to no other form of disease, as a species of morbid phenomena, whose concordance, agreement or identity with certain chancres, more particularly with the Hunterian variety, induce us to rank them in this category of syphilitic products. Inasmuch as every fixed special disease must necessarily have a fixed cause, that is, a cause that is permanently the same or *specific*, it seems fair to assert that, as long as no other disease can be pointed out to which those phenomena belong as specific characteristic signs, the specific cause of these phenomena must be the very cause that makes a Hunterian chancre to always appear under the most diversified circumstances, and upon individuals of the most varied constitutional peculiarities, with characteristic signs that are always the same, and peculiar to it alone.

Sec. 154.—The Venereal Nature of Syphilis.

This unequivocal idiopathicity of its symptoms, which distinguishes it from every other disease, is admitted by many of those who reject its venereal nature. They assert, however, that syphilis did not assume this venereal nature until, after the great epidemic of the fifteenth century, all venereal diseases were treated with Mercury. After this period, all the phenomena that were attributed to to the so-called secondary syphilis, so far from being venereal, were on the contrary purely mercurial products occasioned by the insane abuse of this metal. In this respect it is indeed true that, previous to that terrible epidemic, the history of the ancients never makes the least mention of our modern syphilis, and that the indiscreet use of Mercury, first introduced in that epidemic, may cause phenomena which an unpractised eye might easily confound with such as originate in venereal sources. Nevertheless, as has been seen in the two former paragraphs, there exist on the one hand essential diagnostic signs, and, on the other hand, even the most declared opponents admit that these phenomena likewise occur among patients who had never made the least use of this metal.

Hence, if secondary syphilis, whose unity as a disease *sui generis* can, after what has been said, no longer be doubted, is to be accepted as a non-venereal disease, the advocates of this doctrine will have to show in the first place, that notwithstanding syphilis was first described in the middle ages as an idiopathic disease, it had existed from time immemorial without having been recognized as a specific malady; or, if they are not able to accomplish this, to show that beside Mercury another non-venereal morbific cause had become operative at that period, which likewise had power to produce a disease resembling secondary syphilis. In this respect some contend that the so-called primary syphilis, and venereal products, which, indeed, are not denied, were known to the ancients as well as to us, and that the absolute silence of ancient authors regarding secondary symptoms, shows that not one of these symptoms had ever been produced by the disease, and hence, that the modern existence of secondary symptoms, if at all proven, must be traced to any other, perhaps as yet unknown, rather than to a venereal cause. This assertion is met by the counter-assertion that the ancients did not know all the secondary phenomena of modern times; that the phenomenon which constitutes the main subject of discussion, namely, the true chancre, afterwards called Hunterian, had only first been observed towards the end of the fifteenth century, and that, if the non-existence of secondary venereal products was to be proved, the discussion would have to be conducted, not with reference to all the phenomena that are designated as secondary, but exclusively with reference to the above-mentioned chancre. In order to ascertain which of these two assertions is correct, it might be sufficient to rely exclusively upon the facts by which the derivation of secondary phenomena from this chancre is as good as proven; but inasmuch as those who assert that this chancre was likewise known to the ancients, might, as a counter-proof of our own assertions, resort to the statement that the existence of secondary phenomena as emanating from the Hunterian chancre was unknown to antiquity, we deem it incumbent upon us to ascertain the exact bearing of the arguments drawn from ancient authors. For this purpose, we shall avail ourselves of "*Rosenbaum's History of Syphilis among the Ancients*" (Halle, 1839), where we find a complete collection of the passages bearing upon this subject in ancient authors, and where we can see with our own eyes how far the ancients were acquainted with syphilis and how far they were not. Let us therefore critically examine the different passages in Rosenbaum's work, that may shed light on the history of syphilis, in order to determine whether they justify the assertion that secondary syphilis has a venereal origin, notwithstanding that the ancients were entirely ignorant of this fact.

II. SYPHILIS OF THE ANCIENTS.

Sec. 155.—Biblical Forms of Syphilis.

Modern writers on syphilis have been divided in opinion upon the true origin and the different forms of syphilis, since the origin of this disease. Many trace it back to the first beginning of the human race; some pretend to discover traces of this disease in the oldest writings, not only in the writings of the Greeks and Romans, but even in the books of Moses and the book of Job. On the other hand, there are authors who are of opinion that syphilis is a modern disease, whose origin is to be found in the fifteenth century, when it was developed either in consequence of a degenerate modification of the ancient lepra, or was transmitted to us from the newly-discovered continent of America. It is not an easy task to determine which of these different views is correct, so much more as every author bases his opinions upon facts that cannot well be verified at the present time. We will endeavor to examine these facts as carefully as possible, and commence our examination with the Biblical record, containing statements that may indeed bear some analogy to syphilitic phenomena, and upon which those who trace the origin of syphilis back to the earliest period of the human race, depend for their theories. As regards Job's disease, which is looked upon by many as syphilitic pustules, entailed upon him as a punishment for carnal transgressions, it may be said that, even admitting that the history of Job is a real fact instead of being a poem, the passages supposed to relate to syphilis are too vague to infer from them any thing very definite regarding the nature of Job's disease, which, if any thing, should be considered as lepra rather than syphilis, the scales of which never become, like those of lepra, sufficiently numerous to invite the sufferer to scrape himself with pieces of tile, as Job had to do.

The case is different as regards the ordinance given by Moses in Leviticus xv. 16, on account of a "*discharge from the urethra*," by which, undoubtedly, an infectious gonorrhœa must have been meant. However, if those who advocate the doctrine that chancre existed at that early period, see in this ordinance a confirmation of their belief, those, on the contrary, who regard chancre-syphilis and gonorrhœa as two distinct diseases, find in this ordinance a proof of the correctness of their own statements; for, if chancres had existed at that time, Moses would undoubtedly have spoken of ulcers on the sexual organs. It is likewise certain that the Baal-Peor plague described in the 4th book of Moses, xxxi. 16, and transmitted to the Israelites by the daughters of the Midianites, which was so malignant that twenty-four thousand of them died in a very short time, was "*an infectious disease of the sexual organs;*" but it is not certain whether this disease was our modern syphilitic chancre, or some other analogous plague; unless we should deem it proper to infer from this case the existence of several forms of an infectious virus, which we shall consider more fully in the next chapter. Concerning the disease of David, which this poet mentions in Psalms vi. and xxxviii., which some likewise regard as a description of syphilis, it is not certain, since the historical books of the Bible do not make any mention of this disease, whether these two Psalms may not be regarded as a sort of echo of analogous passages from the book of Job, concerning which we have already expressed our opinion.

Sec. 156.—Venereal Diseases of the Greeks and Romans.

Here we find from time immemorial *ulcers*, and even a sort of *excrescences*, described on the sexual organs. Hippocrates, for instance, in his book, "*de aëre, aquis et locis*," speaks of ulcers that break out on the sexual organs; likewise Celsus, who recommends extirpation with the knife of obstinate and incurable *cancerous ulcers* (cancer, not chancre) around the glans; Aetius mentions ulcers on the glans of such a malignant character, that amputation of the penis may be rendered necessary thereby, and which he designates by the name of *ulcera depascentia;* finally, Actuarius and others, who describe, under the name of *thymi*, small excrescences on the glans, prepuce, at the meatus urinarius, and anus; and likewise *rhagades* on the male parts, the anus, and pudendum.

Plinius the Younger relates the case of a woman who threw herself into the water on account of her husband being affected with putrid ulcers on the sexual parts; the Jewish historian Josephus speaks of the private parts of Herod, that had become putrid, and likewise of a corrosive ulcer on the private organs of the blasphemer Apion, which destroyed his life. Palladius mentions the case of Heron, who, while drunk, had connection with an actress, in consequence of which he became affected with an anthrax on the glans, that caused the parts to rot and drop off. If we add to these facts certain allusions to be found in the satirical poems of Juvenal and Martial, we may have to concede the antediluvian age of syphilis to those who regard every contagious ulcer on the sexual organs, or every infectious discharge from the urethra, as a symptom of syphilis. But the above-mentioned facts are too vague and too insufficient to justify the inference that the pretended syphilis of those days is identical with the modern syphilitic chancre. With the exception of the case related by Palladius, not one of the above-mentioned authors ascribes his cases to infectious intercourse, but to a libidinous life generally. Even Palladius regards the case of Heron as a punishment inflicted by God, which he would not have done, if infectious diseases had prevailed among the Greeks and Romans, who certainly were not very abstemious. We omit the many passages from Suetonius, quoted by authors in support of their opinions, and having reference to the nævi and brush-marks found on the Emperor Augustus; the acne rosacea, baldheadedness, and cicatrices caused by the use of blisters, related by Tacitus, of the emperor Tiberius; and Eusebius' case, of a chronic abscess and fistulous ulcers of the Emperor Galerius Maximus; if cases like these, or the ulcers and glandular abscesses of which these authors make mention, had been of a venereal nature, syphilis either cannot have been as universal or as infectious as it has been for the last four centuries, or else it must have been just as common at that time as it is at the present. In the latter case, however, both the Greek and Roman authors would have left us a much more circumstantial description of the disease than mere vague and imperfect descriptions of isolated cases which, moreover, have to be interpreted with a great deal of generous liberality, if the evidence they are supposed to furnish is to be accepted as authoritative.

Sec. 157.—The Venereal Diseases of the Middle Ages.

Here we have, in the first place, the writings of the Arabians, among whom John Mezue, in the eighth century, writes of a purulent discharge from the urethra, with burning when urinating; Rhazes reports of Machumet, the son of Alchases, that he was affected with a disease of the glans, that must gradually invade the whole of it, since the patient was already discharging pus with the urine; finally, Avicenna mentions certain ulcers on the penis which, if they should spread, might cause a rotting of the penis, and render the amputation of this organ necessary. Among the Europæan physicians of the Arabian school, Michael Scott speaks of women whose discharge infects young people, so that their penis becomes diseased, or they become affected with lepra, and that the children born of such parents are born with corrupt humors. Garrioponti's description comes still nearer, partially at least, our modern syphilis; he speaks not only of purulent discharges from the urethra, but likewise of condylomata and other similar excrescences. William of Salicet even makes mention of buboes showing themselves on persons who had connection with impure women, or whose penis was diseased; this author, who lived in the thirteenth century, when speaking of white pustules, rhagades, and other infectious products on the penis or prepuce, regards them as the consequences of impure coït. Lanfranc, a disciple of the former, speaks of buboes arising after ulcers on the penis, and likewise of excrescences on the prepuce and glans, which, if getting worse, may become converted into cancerous ulcers; in one passage, he states that connection with an impure woman may cause a cancerous ulcer (cancer) that may render the amputation of the penis necessary. Gordon, who wrote some time after the former, mentions, as consequences of an impure coït, cancerous ulcers, abscesses, and pruritus, adding, however, that these phenomena may likewise arise from other causes, such as from a fall, blow, etc., but, at the same time, states, that when caused by impure intercourse, these phenomena are much more difficult to cure. Similar remarks are found in the writings of other physicians of the thirteenth and fourteenth centuries, more particularly in those of John of Gallisden, Guy de Chauliac, Valescus de Tarenta, of Montpelier, Pedro de Argelata, etc. One of the most remarkable works is that of William Beckett, surgeon of London, where we find a collection of every printed or written document bearing upon the remote age of syphilis; what is most remarkable in this work, is the number of cases that are said to have been caused by intercourse with leprous women, on which account, the reporters of those cases warn most seriously against all sexual connection with women thus diseased. In this work, Beckett alludes more particularly to a disease which he calls arsura (burning urine), which, according to him, consists in a sort of soreness of the urethra (a sort of gonorrhœa), regarding which, he alludes to a petition to Henry VIII., of England, wherein the petitioner complains that the disease is chiefly spread by the priests, who, having become BURNT by intercourse with leprous women, transmit the disease to other women. This statement of the disease being transmitted by men to women is remarkable in this respect, that all other reports speak of the disease as having been transmitted by women, whose "unfathomed fountain," unless kept clean, "may contain infectious impurities or corruption."

Sec. 158.—Remarks on the preceding paragraph.

Putting all this testimony from authors of the Middle Ages regarding the phenomena on the sexual organs together, and considering that these authors ascribe all these morbid phenomena to intercourse with impure women, whose internal sexual organs contained impure humors, we cannot avoid the conclusion that the sexual disorders described by the above-named authors, were of a truly venereal character. In the next chapter, where we shall speak of the different venereal diseases and contagia, we shall endeavor to shed light on the question whether the phenomena related by those authors are identical with our modern chancre-syphilis. For the present, it may suffice to direct attention to the fact how little attention, in comparison with the authors of the 16th century, their predecessors attached to a more circumstantial description of their ulcers, pustules, excrescences, and phlegmata; and how these disorders were not only derived from impure intercourse, but likewise from other causes, among which Valescus de Tarenta mentions "unclean pantaloons," an "acridity beneath the prepuce;" and Lanfranc mentions "ulcers on the legs," as a frequent cause of "buboes." What seems to be more strange, is, that in spite of the "corrosive ulcers," of which all make mention, and which seem to have been known to the Greeks and Romans, not one author seems to have directed attention to the consecutive phenomena that these ulcers may be followed by in the mouth and throat, and which would not have escaped the attention of those early authors any more than that of the physicians of the 16th century, more particularly since many of these consecutive phenomena, in the present chancre-syphilis, do not manifest themselves at such a remote period after the primary symptoms, but that every observer must be struck by their internal pathological connection. It is true that Rosenbaum quotes Aretæus' description of a kind of ulcers in the throat that might be mistaken for phagedænic chancres in the throat, if Aretæus did not explicitly state that these "aphthæ," which, on account of their lead-colored, white ulcers with their thick scurfs, resemble our modern diphtheritis, occurred principally among children. If we add to this complete omission of all mention of consecutive phenomena, that, as some modern authors will have it, even at this day, some venereal ulcers (such as phagedænic, and more especially gangrenous ulcers) but rarely occasion any consecutive phenomena—at least not in the degree as Hunterian chancres—we are certainly justified, if not in denying the identity of yonder ancient phenomena with the products of our modern chancre-syphilis, at least in asserting that this identity is not by any means made out by the nature of the facts; more particularly, since a good many of the corrosive ulcers described by ancient authors might have been a root of phagedænic or serpiginous tetter, being one of the consequences or manifestations of lepra, which raged in the 15th or 16th century in the South of Europe, as well as in France and Italy. What decides the matter, is the testimony of John de Vigo, living in the 16th century, who, after contrasting both the former venereal diseases and the phenomena of modern syphilis with each other, distinguishes both forms from each other; which is likewise done by Fallopius, and, among other characteristic signs of recent chancres, which he terms *Caroti*, not only mentions their lardaceous base and callous edges, but likewise mentions their livid, dark copper color, that sometimes merges into a blackish tint.

Sec. 159.—Appearance of Syphilis as an Epidemic.

According to the testimony of all authors living at that time, epidemic syphilis broke out in the last years of the 15th century. According to some, cases of this plague broke already out in the year 1492 in Italy and Spain, until in 1494—more particularly during the invasion of Italy by the French—the well-known epidemic syphilis broke out, which soon spread from Italy over France and Spain, and likewise over England, as far as Westphalia, Pomerania, Prussia, and Saxony, and, on its passage, derived its name from the country it had visited last. In France, for instance, it was called the *Napolitan sickness;* in Holland, the *Spanish pox;* in Germany, it was called the *Franzosen*, and in Poland, the *German disease.* It likewise derived its name from its locality. When attacking women, in whom it was chiefly located on the pudendum, it was called *pudendagra;* among men, in whom the face and chin were more strikingly affected, it was called *mentagra*, etc., until at a later period, on account of its being chiefly transmitted by sexual coït, it was generally termed *venereal disease.* All then living physicians and authors testify, that this was a new disease that had not been known heretofore. They endeavored in vain to find a proper name for it among the then known diseases; some regarding it as a variety of lepra; others of elephantiasis, others again as a malignant form of small-pox (variolæ aluhumatæ). Finally, not knowing what to call it, they applied to it the name of the saints whom the people invoked to help them; for instance, *morbus St. Rochi*, etc. Whether this plague was a specific venereal disease, or a combination of the tolerably general lepra and the former venereal diseases, and, by the creative power of circumstances, had become an *idiopathic*, henceforth *self-existing* disease, is not clearly made out by the documents that have been left to us by the authors of that period. It is true, that as described by them, this disease was a characteristically *pustulous disease*, distinguished by the breaking out of large, ugly, purulent pocks, and accompanied by horrid bone-pains; and more particularly communicated by intercourse with women who were attacked by the disease. Those authors, however, do not state, and yet it would have been of great importance for us to know, whether these pustules first broke out on the pudendum, or in the face, or on the whole body; nor do they state whether the first signs of a recent infection were first seen on the sexual organs. If this was not the case, and if, according to the universal testimony of contemporaries, the infection was caught by simply touching the epidermis, or by inhaling the breath of an infected individual, such a cause must have operated much more powerfully during the act of coïtion, which, if true, would not by any means justify the idea that this plague was venereal. In addition to this we have a right to argue, that, if this plague had been, strictly speaking, a venereal disease, the sexual organs ought to have shown the first symptoms of a recent infection, whereas, as Grünbeck justly observes, they only became affected incidentally, in consequence of the general spreading of the pustules over the surface of the body. It is only in the case of women that the pudendum seems to have been principally affected, as we may judge from the name pudendagra. Nevertheless, if this had been a general characteristic, instead of being an accidental occurrence, males likewise would have perceived the first signs of the infection on their private parts, for the reason, that the syphilitic virus first affects these parts, when coming in contact with them, as their favorite site. Hence it is incredible that modern authors of repute, even such a man as Schœnlein, can take the statements of the writers of that epoch for granted, and, without any further critical examination, simply because the disease has been handed down to us under the name of *Morbus venereus*, assign to it a place in their text-books as epidemic syphilis.

Sec. 160.—Development of Chancrous Syphilis.

Whatever similarity of *form* may have existed between that epidemic and more recent syphilitic phenomena, it is evident that it may likewise have been a malignant smallpox epidemic. If so, the infection must have necessarily been more rapidly communicated during the act of coïtion, where the two parties are placed in the most immediate contact with each other. This, however, does not authorize the inference that the disease was venereal, any more than we would be authorized to call the itch a venereal disease, for the simple reason that it is more readily caught during sexual proximity, or by sleeping in the same bed with an infected person. Nevertheless, there are other circumstances prevailing in the history of this epidemic, that must have exerted an undoubted influence upon the subsequent form of the syphilitic disease. If we read, for instance, what Fernel, who wrote not long after that epidemic, says of the diagnostic differences between morbus gallicus and the venereal disease, which, according to him, is no longer characterized by ulcers, buboes and purulent discharges, but by *secondary phenomena*, such as: *pustules, pains, falling off of the hair*, etc.; and if we add to these statements the contrast mentioned in § 158, which had never been before made by any author previous to that epidemic, and which De Vigo established between the more ancient ulcers and those that were known at his time, in the 16th century, of which he says that they had a lardaceous base, and callous, livid, and almost blackish (dark copper-brown) edges; we witness, subsequent to this epidemic, the sudden appearance of a new *venereal form*, resembling in all essential particulars our modern *chancre-syphilis*, and which drove the lepra that had been prevailing until then out of Europe, as if by magic. If this fact were to be thrust before us, as an argument in favor of the remote origin of syphilis, back to the time of Job and Moses, the true character of the disease never having been recognized, but mistaken for lepra: all we have to reply to a suggestion of this kind is, that, when a disease not only changes its name, but at the same time its whole character, as when a chrysalis becomes transformed into a butterfly, we regard this process at least as a metamorphosis, if nothing more. At all events, whatever may have been the pathological nature of that remarkable epidemic, it is certain that, at a period when the world was shaken by the mighty invention of a Guttenberg, and the old creeds and institutions began to totter to their foundations, the nations of Europe were visited by a terrible febrile convulsion, that swallowed up one of the most ancient plagues, as by a volcanic eruption, and substituted in its place a new and desolating disease. In the next chapter we shall see in what manner a correct appreciation of the historic origin of our modern syphilis influences the solution of the question concerning the unity or plurality of the different venereal viruses; in order that this point may be settled so much more fully, we shall have to premise a few words concerning the circumstances and forms under which the new disease was brought into life.

III. ORIGIN AND FIRST FORMS OF THE SYPHILITIC CHANCRE OR CHANCRE-SYPHILIS.

Sec. 161.—American Origin.

Although we cannot consider the so-called epidemic syphilis of the last years of the 15th century as a venereal disease *in itself*, nevertheless we have to view it as the fountain-head of our modern syphilis. In this respect, whatever has reference to the originating causes and the phenomenal forms of that epidemic, must be as valuable to us as the ulterior history of syphilis itself. Unfortunately, however, the writers of that period differ concerning the true causes of that epidemic so much, that nothing remains for us to do except to present all their conflicting opinions, and afterwards to subject them to a critical examination, with a view of determining their relative degree of correctness and credibility. Among these opinions, the most important is the one which traces the epidemic to the discovery of the American continent. According to this view, which was first started by the Spaniard Oviedo, and afterwards repeated by Schmaus, Crato, Fernelius, Lowe, Freind, Hoffmann, Astruc, Robertson, Van Swieten and Girtanner, Christopher Columbus, on his return from his first voyage, on the 13th of January, 1493, is said to have brought this disease to Europe by his crew, who were affected with it; it is stated that the ship on board of which he was brought home as a prisoner, after several voyages to America, numbered two hundred syphilitic patients among her crew. It is not certain, however, whether the germs of this disease had not already been planted before the crew shipped on their voyage, though Branavola, Roderick Diaz, Fallopius and other authors of that period, inform us that the disease had been hitherto unknown in Europe, and, according to the uniform testimony of every one who visited St. Domingo shortly after the discovery of that island, had been indigenous among the natives long before this event happened. This is likewise Oviedo's opinion, whereas Astruc, who likewise advocates the American origin of syphilis, asserts that the disease arose from an acridity of the menstrual blood, caused by a mixture of the heated blood of Southern Italy and Southern America, out of which the syphilitic virus was born. Girtanner, who likewise believes in the story of the American origin of syphilis, has another hypothesis concerning this origin. According to his opinion, the chancre-virus has emanated from ulcers caused by certain insects in South America, known by the name of "*Tschiken*" (pulex penetrans). The extremely voluptuous American women, in order to excite in their naturally cold husbands a desire for sexual intercourse, are said to have given them all sorts of stimulating beverages; and, while their husbands were asleep, to have placed upon their penis certain poisonous insects acting like Cantharides, by whose irritating action the organ swelled up and caused an irresistible desire for coïtion. The wound caused by such a sting is said to have in many cases become converted into a malignant ulcer, with a lardaceous base, and hard, callous edges, resembling our modern chancres; the purulent matter running out of the male urethra, is supposed to have been transmitted into the vagina, where it caused chancre, that henceforth perpetuated itself as an idiopathic, self-existing disease.

Whether this hypothesis is well founded or not, Oviedo, who is the real author of the colonization theory of syphilis, asserts most positively that the desolating plague of syphilis was transferred from the West Indian islands to Spain, whence the Spanish armies carried it to Italy in 1495. From these countries it was carried further, to Naples and France, by the Italian women, who had become infected by the French and Spanish soldiers; and finally, it was spread over the whole of Europe by the German and Dutch troops who, during the war between Francis I. and Charles V., served in the army of the latter.

Sec. 162.—The so-called Maranian origin of Syphilis.

However evident the truth of Oviedo's proposition may seem to be, and however willing European Courts may have been to transfer the responsibility of this whole plague from their own shoulders to those of the poor aborigines of America, nothing is less founded in historical truth than these very assertions promulgated by Oviedo. For, not to mention the fact that up to the year 1518 (twenty-six years after the appearance of the epidemic), in spite of every exertion to discover the first origin of this malady, nobody before Oviedo had imagined to derive it from the discovery of America; which, if this new disease had been brought over from America by the crews of Columbus, would have created as much excitement as the discovery of America itself: all the documents of that period show, in a clear and unmistakable manner, that this epidemic already raged in Naples in 1494, or, perhaps, even in 1492, previous to Columbus' first voyage of discovery; yet the Spanish soldiers did not reach Naples till 1495. John Nauclerus, who died in 1500, and hence must have been a contemporary witness of that dreadful epidemic, states that, of the 400,000 Jews, who in 1492 had been driven out of Spain, under the name of the *Mariani*, a large number, abandoned to misery and want, came to Italy, where Pope Alexander VI. permitted them to settle before the gates of Rome, and where upwards of 30,000 of their number perished of the epidemic that prevailed among them. This plague, which, according to some authors, seems to have been a pestilential, petechial typhus, attended with the breaking out of large pustules resembling those of small-pox, soon spread, not only in Rome (in consequence of the Mariani entering the city in secret), but, as John Salicet, of Tubingen, informs us, travelled, in 1497 to 1500, almost through every country in Europe. Considering that an act of Parliament was issued in Paris, in 1496, where mention is made of a large pox (*grosse vérole*), that had already prevailed *for two years;* considering further the report of an Oldenburg monk, who states that this plague had spread over Westphalia, in the year 1494; and the testimony of Fulgas, who states that this plague had already been known two years before the arrival of Charles VIII., in the year 1492; and, finally, considering that Elias Capreolus speaks of the general spread of this plague, as having taken place in the years 1493 and 1494, it is evident that Oviedo's assertions are utterly unfounded. However, taking it for granted that this plague was brought by the Mariani to Italy, whence it spread over the whole of Europe, it is not by any means certain that it was of a syphilitic nature, and, if it was not, that the syphilitic disease was, after all, brought to Europe by the Spanish crews of Columbus. Indeed, this is not impossible; only, if this thing had taken place in the manner in which Oviedo relates it, it would seem strange that the colonization of this plague from America to Europe, should have remained unnoticed until 1496, even by Oviedo, who, however, was in Barcelona at the same time that Columbus happened to be there. It is only in the year 1496 that mention was first made of the syphilitic disease of the Spanish crews who had returned from America. Hence, the first reliable testimony that we possess of the modern syphilis, is the passage quoted in Section 160, from Fernelius, where chancres are spoken of as something distinct from the great French plague; from which we infer that the phenomena of modern syphilis were first observed subsequent to the time when that epidemic was raging.

Sec. 163.—Probable causes of the Syphilitic Chancre, or Chancre-Syphilis.

Not satisfied with either the American or Maranian tradition concerning the origin of syphilis, some undertook to trace this disease to the influence of planets and stars; some to a suspicion that the Spaniards had eaten human flesh; some, again—and this tradition is deserving of some notice—to a prostitute who is said to have lived among the leprous women, and whose private parts had been affected with a malignant ulcer, of a peculiar kind, the virus from which first attacked the males, who transmitted it to their women, after which the disease spread more and more, as is the case even now. This mode of explanation is, indeed, very simple, and would be perfectly acceptable if we could only show in what manner this leprous ulcer first attained the power of producing in other individuals a disease of an entirely different character.

The opinion that the modern syphilis is derived from the ancient lepra, is not, by any means, uncommon. Vendelin, Bichat, and Lichtenberg, and many other physicians have entertained this opinion, not without cause; for though in defence of this opinion we have to assume that the character of the ancient lepra had to become totally changed, in order that this plague might take the form of the modern syphilitic disease; yet, on the other hand, we should not overlook the circumstance, that among the symptoms of the famous syphilitic epidemic of the fifteenth century, there were many symptoms of the former lepra and elephantiasis, which diseases were well known to the physicians of that age; and that the lepra, to whose symptoms some of our syphilidæ bear some resemblance, disappeared from Europe when that epidemic, some of whose symptoms call to mind some of our syphilidæ, even as, at its first appearance, they may have called to mind some of the pathognomonic features of lepra, disappeared from the European continent. This disappearance of the lepra was so sudden, that the 21,000 lepra-houses which had been erected outside the gates of cities in France, a country of much smaller extent at that time than at the present, were closed in the year 1526, scarcely thirty years after the chancre-syphilis had developed itself into an independent disease, with fixed pathognomonic forms. The same thing was done on the west coast of Italy, in some parts of Spain, as well as in England and Scotland. The fact that some lepra-cases still occur, and that both diseases exist simultaneously in some parts of the world, is no argument against the supposed metamorphosis of lepra; nor does it argue against the fact that yonder famous epidemic, which was neither lepra nor syphilis, nor a pure form of typhus, but had some of the features of all these three plagues, may have constituted the process of transformation, by means of which, out of the struggle of the most diversified pathological elements (former venereal phenomena, lepra, and recent typhus), a new idiopathic disease, combining the hitherto scattered venereal phenomena in one unit, developed itself, and took the place of an old, more or less exhausted, morbid process. Adding to this, the external circumstances favorable to the production of a pathological event as great as it was incredible—such, for instance, as the meeting of large hosts, from every country, encamped for a long time in a climate to which they were unused, and sustained by unwholesome and unwonted supplies of nourishment; considering, moreover, the atmospheric influences, the noxious emanations from thousands of cadavers, excesses and licentiousness of every kind; and, finally, the wild passions let loose by the war, the non-advent of such a plague as the modern syphilis would have seemed a source of astonishment, rather than that its advent should excite our wonder.

Sec. 164.— The Formative Period of Syphilis.

Whatever opinion be entertained concerning the pathological character of that epidemic, it is an established fact that: 1) subsequent to this epidemic, a new form of the venereal malady, our chancre-syphilis, made its appearance, of which nothing was known prior to the raging of that same epidemic; and that, 2) the lepra, since then, has almost entirely disappeared from Europe. This does not, indeed, show that the epidemic in question had any thing to do with syphilis; a relationship of this kind might be accepted as a probable thing, if it were certain that our modern syphilis had not existed previous to the arrival of European soldiers in America, and that, if it was brought over from America, its existence remained unnoticed during the prevalence of the epidemic, with which the syphilitic malady either coalesced, or by which the latter remained suspended for the time being. What most of our manuals teach of the original appearance of syphilis, as a cutaneous disease, and of the gasiform, pneumatic nature of the syphilitic miasm communicating the infection by the mere breath of the patients, must be considered as mere hypothesis, so far as our modern syphilis is concerned, until it is definitively settled that the epidemic in question was nothing else than an acute form of syphilis. For, even if we take it for granted that our syphilis was born of that epidemic, and that it was not a previously-existing disease, which only manifested itself after the disappearance of the epidemic, for the simple reason that it had remained suspended by the latter, and had existed in a masked form during its continuance, the peculiar conduct of that epidemic does not yet account for the independent idiopathicity of the syphilitic disease itself, since the pathognomonic features of that epidemic might still be derived from the *variolous typhus*, which gave birth to syphilis, perhaps, at the very moment when it lost its own pathological characteristics. In addition to all this, nothing is more uncertain, according to every writer of that age, than the different degrees which the syphilitic disease passed through from the time of that epidemic until it reached the present development of its diversified, but yet fixed, and at all times and places, identical forms. The only author who alludes to this point, Astruc, does not furnish any satisfactory clue to this problem. The *seven periods* in which he divides the course of syphilis as so many transition-stages to the present chronic form of this disease, can only be regarded as a substitutive explanation of the real facts. Even Fernelius, who was a contemporary witness of that epidemic, and who regards the subsequent chancre-syphilis as a gradual weakening and the precursor of a final and complete effacement of that epidemic, is unable to account for the connection of these two diseases, or for the passage of the one into the other, but contents himself with stating that the now prevalent (in the year 1540) "*lues venerea*" did no longer, like the former "morbus gallicus," infect people by the air, but solely by sexual connection, or by nursing infants at diseased breasts, or that the disease might be communicated to midwives by the contact of infected sexual organs, or by the mouth of diseased nurslings, or by the spittle of infected persons when kissing, or, finally, by the insertion of the poison in parts denuded of their epidermis; and that, when the disease broke out, it manifested itself by ulcers on the infected parts, by buboes, and discharges, and afterwards, after the whole organism was pervaded by the poison, by pustules on the skin, pains, etc. This shows that, even a few years subsequent to the prevalence of that epidemic, our modern syphilis was born full-fledged, even as Minerva was born armed cap-a-pie out of Jupiter's brain, without it being possible to show the different stages through which this disease gradually marched onward to its present stage. Let us examine the opinions of other writers on this subject; first, however, let us cast a glance at the symptoms of that epidemic themselves.

Sec. 165.—Forms of the so-called Epidemic Syphilis.

The first and worst characteristic of this epidemic was its *volatile contagium*, which, according to the testimony of all contemporary writers, not only infected persons by simple contact, but likewise by the air, and, consequently, more especially during the act of coïtion. Of the malady itself, Petrus Pintar reports to Pope Alexander VI.: "The prevailing epidemic is characterized by a variety of symptoms, more particularly by keen and excessively violent pains. Some do not have any pains, in the place of which they are attacked by *pustules* of various shapes and sizes, being very numerous on some individuals, and on others more scanty. Sometimes the pustules break out only in the face, or on the head, while the other parts of the body remain free; in other cases they are only seen on the abdomen; most frequently they break out on the thighs and legs, but may likewise spread over the whole body." The same author, who regarded this disease as a species of smallpox (variola), continues in another place: The *general* symptoms of this disease are the same as those of any other case of smallpox: languor, restless sleep, a general feeling of heaviness, accelerated pulse, rough and husky voice, dryness of the mouth and tongue, sore throat and pains in the chest. Particular symptoms are: At first a few small vesicles of the size of punctures with needles, more particularly on the chin, glans, in the hairs of the pudendum (this symptom likewise occurs in smallpox—Jahr), sometimes also in the face, on the forehead or limbs; but rarely all at once in all these localities. Gradually these vesicles increase in size, even to that of split peas, until they finally grow as large as the palm of the hand. On most patients these pustules are very dry, sometimes, however, they discharge more or less of a purulent matter; sometimes they form scales; but in all cases they are accompanied by the most violent and agonizing pains, more especially in the upper and lower extremities. At the same time, most patients have an appetite that frequently increases to canine hunger." He states, moreover, that there is little danger if the pustules come out properly and mature rapidly, if pain and fever are wanting, and the patients preserve their courage and appetite. "On the contrary," writes this author, "if the pustules are scanty, dry, prominent, like warts; if the skin shows deep rhagades, the throat is inflamed, the breath foul and the voice feeble, and as if extinct, death is unavoidable." Beside direct infection by contact and living together, he indicates want of cleanliness and the influence of strong heat of the sun as existing causes of this disease. Bartholomæus Steber calls these pustules hideous; he says that they ulcerate, differ in shape, density, color, in venomous character, and in regard to the accompanying pains. Grünbeck, who regards the disease as *mentagra*, furnishes the following description of it: "Some patients were attacked on the head and chin with a horridly-disgusting, dirty and blackish crust, which, with the sole exception of the eyes, gradually spread over the whole face, neck, head, chest, and pubes, so that the poor sufferers, abandoned by their companions in the open field, where they were exposed to the burning rays of the sun, called for no other relief than a speedy death. Others, driven to despair by the pain, tried to tear off this crust, which was harder than the bark of trees, with their nails; others, again, had their whole bodies covered with innumerable quantities of warts and pustules. On many patients there appeared in the face, on the ears, or in the nostrils, a sort of thick, rough pustules, that assumed the shape of elongated horns, secreted a fetid, purulent fluid, and had the appearance of protruding teeth.

The pains accompanying this eruption are sometimes so violent, that the patients are deprived of their sleep for forty, sixty, and even a hundred nights together, after which the pains likewise assail the head. Others experience in their shoulders an indescribable feeling of stinging and weight; others, again, experience the same pain in the elbows, knees, even in all the limbs and joints at the same time, so that they are unable either to walk or to stand, and have to abandon every kind of work." Grünbeck, moreover, states, that the disease commenced with languor and debility of the limbs, after which the pustules break out with intense fever; he adds, that, whenever these pustules or tumors burst open, they sometimes become converted into frightful phagedænic sores.

Sec. 166.—The Forms of Syphilis subsequent to this Epidemic.

On reviewing this picture of the epidemic, it is indeed impossible not to recognize among its features some that resemble more or less our modern syphilidæ. On the other hand, some of its features might cause us to liken it to smallpox (the pustules of which I have seen in my own practice spread even over the penis, prepuce and glans); others again to lepra; and, on account of the peculiar bone-pains of which Grünbeck speaks, we might even liken it to the modern trichinæ-disease. What is most remarkable is that, previous to Oviedo's fable of the colonization of syphilis from America to Europe, nobody thought of seeing in this epidemic a venereal plague, and that Fernelius, probably with a view of refuting Oviedo's explanation, made every effort, in the year 1542, to warn against syphilis being confounded with the former epidemic, which he designated as *morbus gallicus*, and to distinguish the two diseases, which seem to have coexisted in his time, from each other by distinct diagnostic signs. If Schœnlein, who describes this epidemic, without any further proofs, as an acute epidemic, afterwards proceeds to divide the historical development of our modern chancre-plague into two periods, the first of which extends to the year 1550, and is distinguished by the volatile nature of the contagium; his opinion is at once refuted in the most positive manner by the previously-expressed statement of Fernelius. His other observation, that the second period commenced with the appearance of gonorrhœa, is likewise untenable. We have shown, § 156–158, that gonorrhœa, of which he says that it transformed the volatile into a fixed contagium, as well as venereal diseases generally, except the modern chancre, has existed at all times. It is true that soon after that epidemic, or even during its decline, a *new* and hitherto unknown form of gonorrhæa made its appearance, which Borgarucci termed *gonorrhœa gallica*, and of which he says that a diagnostic sign of this new disease was the property "of not being curable by local treatment alone." That this gonorrhœa did not first make its appearance in the year 1550 may be learned from Paracelsus, who taught in Basle in the year 1527, and spoke of this gonorrhœa as *gonorrhœa francigena*. In the next chapter we shall revert to this gonorrhœa, which has given rise to so much dispute concerning the syphilitic and non-syphilitic nature of gonorrhœa; for the present it may suffice to state that this gonorrhœa, which might even yet be called *blennorrhagia gallica*, was a *new* phenomenon.

What Astruc, when speaking of his seven transition-periods of the acute epidemic to our modern syphilis, says of his second period immediately succeeding the epidemic, namely: that this second period has been distinguished by the appearance of condylomata, these condylomata cannot be regarded as a new product, but have to be looked upon as the reappearance of an old symptom that had been known already for centuries; provided always that Astruc does not understand by such condylomata the fungoid growths occurring in the second stage of the Hunterian chancre; these growths, of whose self-existing contagium we shall speak in the next chapter, are likewise to be regarded as pathological products essentially distinct from idiopathic figwarts. The same remark applies to Astruc's subsequent periods, in the third of which he locates the falling off of the hair, and the appearance of leucorrhœa, in the fourth gonorrhœa, in the fifth the supervention of buzzing in the ears, and in the two last the appearance of the much-discussed and the much-denied *mother-vesicle* (chancre-matrix). Arranging together such pathological facts as had become manifest subsequent to yonder epidemic, and of which nothing had been known before, we have: 1) *callous, lardaceous ulcers*, transmitting the infection by immediate contact with the mucous membrane, or with some other part denuded of its epidermis (chancre); 2) *secondary phenomena* (upon the skin, in the bones, mucous membranes, etc.); in one word, the whole of our modern chancre-plague (to which Frascatori first applied the name *syphilis*), whose products, if they had been known to the older writers, would certainly have been recognized by them as connected with the primary syphilitic ulcers, and would not have been confounded with lepra.

Whether syphilis and all truly venereal phenomena depend, as most authors believe, upon a specific virus, or whether these products, as some assert, can develop themselves *spontaneously* out of the simplest inflammations, is a subject that shall be examined more particularly in the next chapter.

SECOND CHAPTER.

OF VENEREAL CONTAGIA.

I. OF THE SYPHILITIC VIRUS GENERALLY.

Sec. 167.—Disputed Points.

THERE is probably no point in the domain of Medicine, concerning which so much has been argued *pro* and *con*, as concerning the existence or non-existence of the syphilitic contagium. Whereas some, starting from the fact that syphilis and its demonstrable infections exist, regard the existence of the syphilitic contagium as an *axiom* that should be accepted without any further proof; others, on the contrary, who deny the existence of syphilis as a specific, idiopathic disease, endeavor to show the non-existence of a syphilitic contagium by the absolute impossibility to trace it in the syphilitic pus; and, since chemical analysis must necessarily fail of discovering such a virus, the chemical physiologists have come to the same conclusion regarding the existence of a syphilitic contagium, that they have come to regarding our homœopathic attenuations: "Where there is not any thing, nothing can result; where there is no syphilitic contagium, there cannot be any syphilis." In spite of all this, syphilis has continued to rage without bothering about the chemists any more than do our attenuations, and, like these, has continued to hide its secret from the microscopical eye of the most practised investigator. It is only by the process of inoculation that it manifested to those who had eyes to see, not only its contagious nature, but likewise its existence, without, however, shedding a single ray of light on the nature of its contagium, for the reason that the pus obtained from the products of inoculation showed nothing different from any other non-contagious pus. Those who reject the existence of syphilis as an idiopathic disease, and who account for its manifestations upon the ground that an individual morbid disposition is excited into activity by the acrid properties of an inflammatory purulent secretion, are no more convinced now than they were before the experiment of inoculation had been instituted; whereas the other party put the difficulty of an explanation further off, saying that the contagium was not the virus itself, but only its vehicle; for that which they were unable to prove remained, after all, for the present at least, the contagium itself. In this way the dispute has been continued to the present time, nor is it likely ever to be terminated, since one party seeks that which does not exist, and the other party is unwilling to admit that something may exist where there is apparently nothing to be found. Truth, in this case, does not lie in the middle, but on both sides, since the syphilitic contagium exists just as certainly as it does not exist, and, on account of its non-existence, can never be demonstrated. Who has ever been able to demonstrate either chemically or microscopically warmth, the force of attraction, electricity, the power of the magnet, the germinating force of a grain of seed, and other mechanical or organic motor-principles, as specially existing entities, and separable from the bodies whose properties they are? Yet all these things exist, not as particular substances, but no less really as the inherent properties of the things to which they belong; for we see or feel warming, attracting, electrical, magnetic, germinating and other bodies, although neither a separate caloric, nor a separate attractive, magnetic, electrical or germinating principle exists; and, in chemical respects, a magnetic iron, for instance, resembles a non-magnetic as perfectly as contagious pus resembles non-contagious. As in the case of the magnetic needle the magnetic iron constitutes the attracting substance, so do, in the case of contagia, the infectious secretions and exhalations of the patient constitute the contagion-transmitting substances. This faculty of transmitting the contagion is just as immaterial a property as the attractive force of the load-stone, or as any other properties that are inherent in different bodies, and the existence of which can only be inferred from their manifestations, but should be accepted as a self-evident truth wherever these manifestations take place.

Sec. 168.—Objections of the Opponents.

The main point in discussing the question of the real existence of a venereal contagium, is therefore not to demonstrate its material existence, but to first prove the existence of syphilis itself, as well as its inherent faculty to transmit the infection by a product of its own kind; for we may regard this faculty as the *conditio sine qua non* of its own existence, and as a means of inferring this very existence from that faculty. These two points are the very facts that are denied by the opponents of the idiopathicity of venereal diseases. They base their denial not only upon the frequent non-occurrence of the syphilitic products after inoculation; but, in order to show that the individual disposition is the sole cause of all so-called venereal phenomena, they refer to the circumstance that, according to a number of facts, all these phenomena can be demonstrably occasioned by a non-contagious sexual connection. According to their assertions, it suffices that even the healthiest woman, who had not the least sign of a venereal infection, may have her catamenia, or an acrid leucorrhœa, or may be unclean, or that the husband may have practised the act of coïtion with too much fire, in order that a simple inflammation may be occasioned, which, through a somewhat heating and irregular mode of life, may give rise: 1) to gonorrhœa, which, when neglected, may cause, 2) a chancre; in scrofulous individuals, 3) a bubo, and finally, in scorbutic or otherwise diseased individuals, 4) all the symptoms that are generally designated as *secondary syphilis*. This view seems to have been entertained by the ancients, who, previous to the well-known great epidemic, were acquainted with *sordes, fœdidates, immunditIes*, as causes of venereal phenomena, but were unacquainted with a *virus* in the modern acceptation of this term. According to Cazenave, this expression has never been used with reference to sexual phenomena by any author, except Vulgarius, who lived in the 13th century, who, however, applies this expression to the consequences of a licentious life generally, rather than to any particular disease, in the following satirical verse concerning Pope Bonifacius VIII.:

"Hic vir decanus est, qui viri specie,
Non vir, sed *virus* est, virosa facie."

However, whatever opinions the ancients may have entertained concerning the phenomena on the sexual organs, the truth is, that, at the present time, be it in consequence of a more thorough knowledge of these diseases, or of the appearance of an entirely new morbific cause, a whole series of phenomena is known which modern phathologists describe as a distinct and accurately defined class, to which, in contra-distinction to other diseases of the sexual organs, they apply exclusively the term *venereal*, and which are distinguished from other phenomena of these organs by the property of being able to transmit an infection of a like nature to other individuals by a specific contagium inherent in the products of this same infection. Let, therefore, the inexperienced in medicine continue to believe that even the soundest woman may communicate a chancre, or a gonorrhœa, running a definite course, as the result of too much fire during the act of coïtion, and let the woman try ever so hard to make the simple believe that the discharge was caused by an acrid menstrual blood, or by leucorrhœa: a scientific physician, if he means to make similar assertions, has to prove, if not that the most harmless embrace is succeeded by phenomena on the sexual organs, at least that a non-infectious act of coïtion is capable of developing in the sexual sphere all the phenomena of which pathologists assert that they can only be produced by means of an infectious contact. In order to conduct this argument, it will be necessary to show that these phenomena can develop themselves spontaneously, and that, where this spontaneous development has taken place, the resulting phenomena are entitled to the exclusive appellation of venereal. Let us therefore inquire how far these two points will stand the test of critical inquiry and analysis.

Sec. 169.—Spontaneous Appearance of Venereal Products.

Considered from a purely theoretical standpoint, such a spontaneous manifestation may not be impossible *per se;* for there is no reason why that which, at one time, originated spontaneously, should not again originate in a similar manner. If, at the present day, we behold only infusoria starting into life spontaneously, yet no one would dare to assert that at some future period we may not witness the spontaneous birth, from a conjuncture of adequate circumstances, not only of cattle, elephants, and rhinoceroses, but even of human races. Why should not new diseases develop themselves so much more readily? May we not say that cholera is a spontaneously developed disease? Do we not see cases of sporadic cholera manifest themselves, day after day, which, though they have nothing in common with epidemic cholera as a specifically idiopathic disease, yet seem to suggest by their very name, the possibility that epidemic cholera may develop itself as a spontaneous plague? Why, then, not syphilitic phenomena? A spontaneous manifestation of these phenomena may not be impossible; but it is not probable, more especially as regards the syphilitic phenomena of which we are writing, and which have not only the name, but the essence in common with those to which we have applied the name of *specifically-venereal.* For, on surveying the whole history of creation, we indeed see whole genera and species of plants, animals, and diseases, start into existence under the influence of adequate circumstances; but from the moment that a whole race is born, its single individuals are afterwards perpetuated by the act of generation, but no longer by the original circumstances that gave birth to the race. If, therefore, the assertion is to be insisted upon, that, in order to contract a venereal disease, it is not necessary to have intercourse with an infected individual, but that so-called venereal symptoms may arise from intercourse with the healthiest woman, in consequence of the irritation produced by acrid menstrual blood or an acrid leucorrhœal discharge, or even by a want of cleanliness on the part of the woman, or by too much ardor during the act of coïtion: we shall insist, in the first place, upon evidence that the phenomena occasioned by the aforesaid causes, are identical with those which pathologists designate as venereal; and that the woman herself had no previous sign of contagion on her person. On looking over the history of the cases which the advocates of this theory adduce as proofs of its correctness, we find, however, that they have taken it for granted, without making any further examination, that the assertions of the women regarding all freedom from infectious symptoms, were true, and that they never imagined that the infected individual might have had connection ten, twenty, thirty, or even forty days ago, with some diseased woman, who communicated to him infectious germs that did not begin to sprout until some time after he had cohabited with her successor. What is apt to occasion an additional amount of confusion is, that the opponents of the infection-theory resort to the most deadening uniformity in classifying the different phenomena in the sexual sphere; be they simple or complex, the most harmless and accidental ulcer, as well as the most malignant chancre, are arranged by them under the vague appellation of *venereal.* Under cover of such a vague terminology, we may not only make the assertion that venereal phenomena may be superinduced by the most harmlesss, or perhaps by a somewhat heating act of coïtion, but that a number of such phenomena may disappear spontaneously without any interference on the part of art. In trying to apply this theory to *specific venereal* diseases, such as chancre, figwarts, etc., the aspect of the case changes, and any one who chooses, may convince himself that Fernelius was right, when, in the year 1542, he wrote of syphilis: "*Hœc lues nulli adnascitur, nisi contagio qui se polluerit.*"

Sec. 170.—Pseudo-venereal Phenomena.

We do not mean to deny that any one of the above-mentioned causes, such as an acrid leucorrhœa, uncleanliness of the female parts, unusual ardor during the act of coïtion, etc., may cause a variety of abnormal phenomena in the sexual sphere, not only discharges, but even ulcers of a greater or less extent, which, under certain circumstances, in consequence of an herpetic, scorbutic, or scrofulous diathesis, may even become very obstinate, and, through a purely consensual continuation of the irritation, may even cause a swelling of the inguinal glands. This, however, would not justify the inference that even the healthiest woman may communicate during the act of coïtion gonorrhœa, chancre, buboes; between these venereal products and the former harmless consequences of ordinary intercourse there may exist an analogy of form, but not by any means an identity of essence. An ordinary discharge is no more like a specifically-contagious gonorrhœa than a syphilitic chancre is like a common, non-contagious ulcer, or a syphilitic bubo like an ordinary swelling of the inguinal glands. Even inflammations of the prepuce and glans, with or without balanorrhœa, phimosis, or paraphimosis, may take place without being syphilitic, and will run an entirely different course from the latter. If we regarded nothing but the general name which all these phenomena have in common, we might indeed start the doctrine that there is no syphilitic product which might not be equally caused by a non-contagious principle of communication. A due regard for the pathological essence of these products will soon convince us of the impossibility of such an occurrence. Nothing seems more absurd than the statement still to be found in pathological and therapeutic manuals: that a prostitute, having cancer of the womb, had communicated to one of her lovers a most malignant chancre and to another a virulent gonorrhœa. No more than a patient with variola can infect others with measles or scarlatina, can a carcinomatous patient communicate syphilis, or *vice versa*, can a syphilitic patient communicate carcinoma. Specific causes can only have corresponding specific effects. If the cancerous girl in question had real cancer, she may have infected her lovers with cancerous, but not syphilitic ulcers; if these ulcers were really syphilitic, in one taking the form of chancre on the penis, in another that of a malignant ulcer in the urethra, the supposed cancer of the womb must have been a syphilitic sore. By means of a number of experimental investigations which Ricord has instituted for the last few years with unparalleled industry and sagacity, he has demonstrated beyond all possibility of cavil that the principle of like producing only its like is so true that special syphilitic products can only reproduce products of a like kind; that a chancre, for instance, can never produce *primary mucous tubercles* or primary condylomata, but will always produce chancre, and *vice versa*, that tubercles and figwarts can only produce their like, but no chancre. The same thing might be said of gonorrhœa; this, however, would lead us to the subject of unity or plurality of the venereal contagium, to which we shall devote a special chapter.

II. DIFFERENT VENEREAL CONTAGIA.

Sec. 171.—General Views.

Although we have discussed this subject when treating of gonorrhœa, as much as the special therapeutics of this disease rendered necessary, yet we have to refer to it again in the present place in order to explain our views concerning it as completely as possible in connection with the whole range of venereal phenomena. Beside the question of the *specific* character of venereal diseases, the question of the unity or plurality of the venereal contagium has led to endless disputes and distressing confusion. Ricord's experimental discoveries, regarding the products which different primary phenomena are capable of producing as primary, protopathic results, might have satisfied the disputants that, where different seeds bear different kinds of fruit, the different seeds may have been analogous, but cannot have been identical; they all may belong to one family, but each seed must possess its own, independent properties. Systematic prejudices or other causes interfered: some, who were *a priori* advocates of the specific character of miasmatic diseases, were not satisfied with merely distinguishing the contagium of gonorrhœa from that of chancre, but went so far as to claim even a specific miasm for figwarts. Hahnemann belongs to this number. Others, again, who did not relish the idea of having to acknowledge at least *one* specific disease, mixed up gonorrhœa, chancre, and figwarts, as accidental manifestations of one and the same pathological activity. Experiments and observations were not wanting; but inasmuch as, in making these examinations, experimenters frequently confounded with each other analogous forms that had not been sufficiently discriminated hitherto, and hence ascribed to all of them results that perhaps only belonged to one of them exclusively, it follows as a necessary consequence that these observations, despite the care with which they were made, must have been more or less contradictory. In addition to this, it frequently happened that among individuals who had already been infected several times, the last infection was charged with consequences that really were manifestations of a previously-existing constitutional syphilis. A multitude of, in themselves, invaluable observations, instituted by Ricord, Hernandez, Cazenave, Baumès, Bell, Sawray, and other French and English authors, may be referred to as evidences of the illogical conclusions drawn from them; nor can we have any difficulty, by carefully examining their observations and discriminating the *different* forms of venereal diseases *of the same name*, in deducing the truth from the contradictory conclusions of observers. In this respect, it seems so much more necessary to subject the statements of *French* and *English* practitioners to a rigid examination, since most of our *German* manuals seem to be based upon them, and many erroneous propositions, by Ricord, Cazenave, Sawray, and others, are copied even by Schœnlein with so little critical acumen, and with so much dogmatism of style, that it seems

20

as though the Professors had only intended to say to their students: "It is so, write this down among your notes!" Let us examine the different doctrines bearing on this subject.

Sec. 172.—Chemical Equality of the Different Secretions.

Putting all things together which the advocates of the absolute unity of the different venereal contagia have asserted in favor of their theory, we may sum up their doctrines in the following three propositions: 1) *The absolute chemical equality of the various different contagious secretions;* 2) *the undeniable fact, that products of different kinds have emanated from the same contagium;* and, 3) *sameness of the secondary and constitutional consequences resulting from the most diversified forms.* The first of these three propositions has been advocated with most zeal by Berzelius and the partisans of chemical medicine, and has been transferred to every pathological manual as an irrefutable theorem, without any one taking the least trouble to inquire more particularly into the tenability of such a proposition. After what we have stated, § 167, that the infectious principle is, properly speaking, nothing but a property inherent in certain secretions and exhalations, of an immaterial nature, and beyond the boundaries of experimental demonstration, it is evident that chemists who are not even capable, without physical experimentation, of distinguishing a Leyden battery charged with electricity from one that is not charged, have no claim to authoritative dictation, when the question is to invesdetigate the presence and nature of properties that can only be determined by pathogenetic provings. It would be impossible to conceive that Berzelius, Liebig, or Dumas, should have undertaken to determine the medicinal powers of drugs by chemical analysis, if we did not know that chemistry and logic are not always inseparable companions, and if, in our own school, physicians who pride themselves in a knowledge of chemistry and the microscope, had not undertaken to issue their mandate, that those who believe in any thing higher that the twelfth attenuation are ridiculous fools. This is not the place to inquire how certain properties, *medicinal properties*, for instance, can be grafted upon other non-medicinal agents, such as alcohol; what is certain is, that physics, with its *movement-theories*, by which the properties of all substances may, perhaps, be made to appear *movement-principles*, in future will do much more for physiology, pathogenesis, and pharmaco-dynamics, than chemistry has done, which itself has to borrow of physics more than one proposition, whenever it endeavors to account for many of its processes. If the different contagious secretions were examined with the microscope, certain movements or currents might perhaps be discovered, which, if they did not remain hidden in pus as much as unexcited electricity does in certain substances, might, perhaps, by their different directions, shed light upon the different natures of the contagia. Until now, nothing has been determined in this direction; except, perhaps, that Doctor Donné, of Paris, has discovered certain infusoria in the secretions of some chancres, which animalcules, however, have not been shown to constitute a necessary requisite for the production of contagion, since the pus, after the animalcules are killed by vinegar, remains as efficient for the purpose of inoculation as before. Even if the presence of these animalcules should constitute the rule, and their absence the exception; or even if we should be able to show that these animalcules, though not containing the infectious principle in themselves, should yet result from the living movement-principles of the latter; and even if we should be able to demonstrate further, that each special specific form of this infectious principle produces a special kind of these animalcules—a long time would certainly elapse before such a discovery would decide the question of the unity or plurality of venereal contagia. Those who desire to have light on this question, will have to depend upon other facts beside those furnished by an analytical examination of the pus.

Sec. 173.—Equality of the Results of Contagion.

If the advocates of the unity of the venereal contagium rest their theory upon the fact that women who were affected with chancre have communicated gonorrhœa instead of chancre, and *vice versa;* if women who had a suspicious-looking gonorrhœa have communicated chancre instead of gonorrhœa, we have to accept their conclusions, for the additional reason that every physician, whose opportunities for observation are sufficiently numerous, has seen statements like the above substantiated by facts from his own practice. In reply to these observations, Ricord, Hernandez, Bell, Baumès, etc., answer, that they must necessarily be erroneous;

that whenever they had inoculated a chancre, a chancre was the result, and that the inoculation of the simple and uncomplicated gonorrhæal virus never resulted in any thing whatsoever; and that, whenever the inoculation of the gonorrhœal virus resulted in a chancre, a careful examination of the female organs always revealed the existence of some hidden chancre. The correctness of these facts has not been denied; nevertheless, the opposing party argue, in reply, that the advocates of the plurality of contagia admit the existence of cases where inoculation does not readily succeed, and that, where the inoculation of the gonorrhœal virus does not cause a chancre, this is no argument against the syphilitic nature even of the most simple gonorrhœa, and that such cases most likely belong to the number of those where inoculation had no effect. Castelnau, of Paris, even mentions a case where, in spite of the total absence of all chancrous symptoms, the inoculation of the gonorrhœal pus resulted in a chancre. Cazenave even remarks, that chancres in the male urethra are very rare, and that, if women become affected with chancre through contact with gonorrhœal matter, this is not always owing to a masked chancre, but in all cases to the chancrous nature of the gonorrhœal contagium. Cazenave, however, overlooks the fact, that the number of hidden chancres or mucous tubercles in the urethra, is much less than the number of chancres communicated by simple gonorrhœal matter. In my own practice, I have met with three cases of gonorrhœa, which I treated for four weeks unsuccessfully with all sorts of remedies, and which finally disappeared all at once, in consequence of a metastatic transfer of the inflammation, in one case to the testes, in another, to the right knee, and in a third, to the inguinal glands; immediately after which, a simple, soft chancre showed itself in the urethra of each of these three patients, which, until then, had remained hidden from observation, in consequence of the swelling of the meatus urinarius, and which, in one of these cases, soon became converted into a phagedænic ulcer. Considering, however, that women are not near as often infected with chancre by the gonorrhœal matter of males as authors would have us believe, at any rate, no more frequently than we meet with chancres in the male urethra; considering, furthermore, that men are much more frequently infected with chancre by women who were supposed to have a simple gonorrhœal discharge, but in whose case the chancres, if any exist, remain much more easily hidden from view; we shall have to admit that the facts with which the advocates of the unity of the venereal contagium seek to combat the arguments of their opponents are not sufficient to invalidate the objections which Ricord and his adherents have raised against the conclusions of the former.

Sec. 174.—Further Proofs of the Unity of the Venereal Contagium.

Beside the facts just mentioned, there are other so-called proofs of the unity of the venereal contagium, which, however silly they may seem, have to be mentioned in this place, were it for no other reason than that they are found in pathological manuals, and are even promulgated by medical authorities, as demonstrated matters of fact. A Dutch physician asserts that, if a patient who has a chancre on the penis keeps this organ too warm, he becomes attacked with gonorrhœa. It is strange that not one of the manuals, which enumerate this absurdity among their reasons in favor of the unity of the venereal contagium, makes the least effort to inquire into the correctness of the statement. Another equally discreditable assertion is the following in a well-known German publication: "Physicians who have been employed in brothels have observed that syphilitic women, who had connection with several men in rapid succession, communicated a chancre to the first, a simple gonorrhœa to the second and third, a still lighter form of gonorrhœa to the fourth and fifth, and left the sixth and seventh untainted." If all these statements and observations were correct, the whole matter would be at once decided, the identity of the venereal contagium would be proven, and we might admit, with Schœnlein, that there only exists a quantitative difference between the gonorrhœal and the syphilitic matter, in so far as the gonorrhœal matter contains the minimum, and syphilitic matter the maximum of the venereal contagium. Upon tracing the above statement to its origin, we find that its correctness is not by any means backed up by the experience of a number of physicians, but that the author of this statement is the surgeon Vigarous, who relates the following: "Six young men who were intimate with each other, partook of a rather liberal supper, after which they had connection with a prostitute one after the other; she infected the whole of them, the first and fourth, who applied to me first, with chancre and buboes; the second and third with gonorrhœa, and the other two, one with a chancre and the other with a bubo." Does this story, which has been thoughtlessly copied from one writer by another, contain one word about the gradual weakening of the infectious matter, until it had lost all its poisonous properties? Who does not see that before accepting this statement as thoughtlessly as pathological authors have done, and building upon it pathological theories, the nature of these two discharges ought to have been critically examined, in order to find out whether there was not something hidden underneath them? And who knows whether each of these young people had not had connection with some other woman, one, two, or three weeks previous? History does not furnish a single ray of light upon these points; of what avail, then, can such a case be toward a correct and scientific diagnosis?

Sec. 175.—Secondary Products of the same kind.

Let us leave all these hypothetical statements to those who are anxious to hunt after shadows instead of grasping realities, and let us consider by what more palpable reasons the identity of the venereal contagia has been sought to be proved, namely, *that gonorrhœa has been known to produce the same secondary phenomena as chancre.* Authors, however, go too far if they mention dolores osteocopi, strictures of the urethra, and priapism, as such phenomena. We say nothing against the dolores osteocopi; but strictures of the urethra after chancre! Is it not an established fact, that these strictures sometimes occur twenty years after the disappearance of gonorrhœa? It would be wrong to charge a stricture upon a chancre, for no better reason than because chancre happened to be the last infectious product. Or are we to understand by chancres the accidental œdema of the urethral lining membrane which often occurs simultaneously with chancre in the urethra, and then disappears again together with the cure of the chancre? Or, perhaps, the spasmodic contractions of the urethra, which, as well as priapism, may take place during every somewhat intense inflammation of the penis or urethra, as a purely consensual phenomenon? In such a case, we should have to consider the poison of Cantharides as absolutely identical with that of gonorrhœa and chancre. The case is different in regard to the truly secondary and constitutional symptoms of syphilis, such as the dolores osteocopi, and various syphilidæ, even chancres in the throat, which have not only been known to occur after chancres, but likewise after gonorrhoea, although very rarely after the latter, as is even admitted by Doctor Cazenave, the most zealous advocate of this theory. We might have added, that most of these rare cases occur among females. In my own practice, I have only seen consequences of this kind occur tolerably frequently after the gonorrhœa of females, but never among males. Putting together: 1) the experimental inoculations (§ 173) and observations instituted by the advocates of the plurality of venereal contagia; 2) my own cases of masked chancres in the anterior portion of the urethra; 3) the ease with which such masked chancres may remain unnoticed in the case of women—it is evident that the few cases mentioned by the advocates of the unity of the venereal contagium, cannot be reckoned among the cases of gonorrhœa with hidden chancres and mucous tubercles, unless the facts of the case should render this arrangement compulsory. Why should so few cases of gonorrhœa be succeeded by secondary syphilitic phenomena, whereas the majority of cases of gonorrhœa, even when merely suppressed by local agents, have no such result? Is it not because in those few cases the gonorrhœal discharge was associated with another principle not by any means essential to the nature of the former, hence no essentially pathognomonic sign of gonorrhœa? Now, if the *essential* signs of simple gonorrhœa are distinct from those of the syphilitic chancre, the contagia producing the one and the other must be so likewise; and the advocates of the unity of the venereal contagium, who admit that the cases where gonorrhœa has produced the same secondary products as the syphilitic chancre are but rare, might content themselves with the above inferences, if there did not exist other valid reasons in favor of the plurality of the venereal contagia.

Sec. 176.—Reasons for the Plurality of the Venereal Contagia.

After having seen, in the preceding paragraphs, that the facts adduced by the advocates of the identity of the venereal contagia are rather against them than in their favor, let us now examine the facts alleged by the advocates of the plurality of these contagia, in support of their own theories. Here these gentlemen begin the controversy by putting forward the undeniable fact, that a chancre never gets well without the interference of art, but that gonorrhœa admits of a spontaneous cure. This fact is denied by the opposing party only in so far as this, that there are likewise many cases of gonorrhœa that do not get well of themselves, and that, on the other hand, there are many chancres that get well without the interference of art; all of which is undeniably true. If we inquire further what kinds of gonorrhœa do not get well without the interference of art, and what kinds of chancre, on the contrary, do get well spontaneously, we answer: "A chancre that will never get well without the use of specifically-appropriate agents, and which, if left to itself, would, after cicatrization, run into other and different forms, is the Hunterian chancre; and a gonorrhœa that will never get well without artificial means, is one that arises from the presence of a masked Hunterian chancre, or of mucous tubercles, unless we choose to regard as a cure the metastatic changes which the latter might occasion." Whether among the other chancres there are some that are capable of a spontaneous cure, we will not stop to inquire; nor will we stop to inquire whether there are other kinds of gonorrhœa that do not get well without treatment; one thing is certain, that a gonorrhœa which heals spontaneously, in no case originates in a Hunterian chancre or in mucous tubercles. This ground is sufficient for further argument. For if the fact is established that the Hunterian chancre cannot heal of itself, without passing into other forms, or breaking out in other localities, it is evident that every gonorrhœa which gets well without exhibiting any of the symptoms of a metamorphosed syphilitic product, is one that has no sort of affinity to chancre, and, therefore, must owe its existence to some other totally different virus. Reviewing in our minds what we have said in § 155–166 of the syphilis of the ancients, of the great European epidemic, and of the transformation of the venereal diseases occurring subsequently to this epidemic, we find: 1) that as far back as the Greeks and Romans, not only ulcers but gonorrhœal discharges were known which had this peculiarity, that their disappearance was not followed by general, constitutional affections; 2) that either during, or, at any rate, shortly after that epidemic, according to the uniform testimony of all contemporary writers, a new and hitherto unknown form of the venereal disease made its appearance, which De Vigo (§ 160) describes as distinguished by lardaceous ulcers, with hard and callous, livid (copper-brown red) edges, and Fernelius (§ 164) as a disease pervading the whole organism, and afterwards breaking out in cutaneous pustules and other (secondary) phenomena, by which the disease, he says, was distinguished from any other formerly existing plague. § 166, we have seen that, soon after that period, a new form of gonorrhœa broke out together with this syphilitic plague, which was denominated *blennorrhagia gallica*, and of which Bargarucci says that, in contradistinction to the hitherto known gonorrhœa, it was neither curable by local treatment nor without treatment. This gonorrhœa was nothing else than the modern contagious "*blennorrhagie*" of the French, associated with syphilitic chancre, a disease that, even at this day, is much more frequent in France than in any other country.

Sec. 177.—Sycosis, Figwart Disease.

A discriminating examination of the facts before us, of an apparently contradictory nature, a superficial apprehension of which might lead to the most erroneous conclusions, together with a knowledge of the historical development of the venereal diseases, show that, at the present time, we are acquainted with at least two venereal contagia: 1) an ancient contagium producing a gonorrhœa, that, after passing through its inflammatory period, runs its course to a spontaneous cure; and 2) a new contagium producing the chronic, copper-colored syphilitic chancre, or chancre-syphilis, with all its general consequences; this disease never gets well without proper treatment, and is likewise capable of producing a symptomatic gonorrhœa, very different from the ancient, idiopathic gonorrhœal discharges. In the first division of this work, we have stated (§ 16) that this symptomatic gonorrhœa is distinguished from the idiopathic (simple) gonorrhœa by its more torpid form, or its less marked symptoms of inflammation; to which we add an observation by Cazenave, "that it is not always the most acute gonorrhœas that superinduce secondary symptoms of a constitutional syphilis, but that this result sometimes follows the mildest forms of gonorrhœa." Hahnemann likewise appears to have considered his so-called figwart-gonorrhœa, which he evidently regarded as a purely symptomatic phenomenon, as not very inflammatory; the question now simply is, whether this Hahnemannian figwart-gonorrhœa is identical with our presently described symptomatic syphilitic gonorrhœa, or, as is

Hahnemann's opinion, belongs to a third so-called sycosic contagium. Looking, with a view of solving this much-disputed question, at the historical and pathological facts that might be interpreted in favor of a third contagium, we find 1) that figwarts seem to have existed already about the time of Juvenal and Martialis, at any rate, long before the great epidemic and the appearance of the syphilitic chancre, and that hence they could not have depended upon the latter; 2) that figwarts, even if they break out as primary or protopathic symptoms, yet, according to the testimony of Ricord and his disciples, never produce a chancre; but that, 3), according to the observations of Baumès, of Lyons, and several other physicians, they are infectious, and capable of reproducing their like, or a gonorrhœa, with which they are very frequently associated. These undeniable facts are, on the other hand, met by other observations that are equally undeniable, according to which the chancre, in its fungoid stage, has not only passed into evidently cock's-comb shaped excrescences and other condylomata, but likewise into humid tubercles, which most German physicians confound with figwarts, and which have first been definitely demonstrated by Lagneau, of Paris, some 30 or 40 years ago. There are few physicians, having opportunities for observation, that have not witnessed similar transformations. Moreover, mucous tubercles, even if their contagium never produces chancres, but always their like, are, like chancre, capable of superinducing all the signs of secondary syphilis. If we would assert that the equality of form existing between the idiopathic figwarts, and the consecutive figwarts breaking out subsequently to chancre, does not argue in favor of their essential identity, the previously-mentioned secondary results would demonstrate this essential identity of the chancre and figwarts in an irrefutable manner. Furthermore, inasmuch as, according to the observations of Reynaud and other French physicians, a chancre, after having passed into its fungoid stage, very often ceases to reproduce chancres, but, when transmitting its contagium, produces mucous tubercles, it follows that our modern figwart-contagium, despite its apparent idiopathic character, appears to be really nothing more than a syphilitic contagium, altered in form, but not changed in essence.

Sec. 178.—Hahnemann's Sycosic Gonorrhœa.

Whether all excrescences that appear on the sexual organs, and are generally termed figwarts, are of a contagious nature, or whether there may not likewise exist among these excrescences some that are not contagious and originate in some harmless cause (see § 75), is a question, which, after the doubts that many physicians have expressed concerning the contagious nature of these condylomata generally, and considering the fact that figwarts have existed long before the appearance of modern syphilis, may safely be answered in the affirmative. What is certain, however, is that when the figwarts are associated with gonorrhœa, they contain the syphilitic virus in the modfied form of the sycosic. It is to be regretted that Hahnemann did not term this gonorrhœa a *mucoso-tubercular gonorrhœa,* since it is these humid or mucous tubercles in which the above-mentioned (§166) *blennorrhagia gallica* originates, which is still very frequent in France, and was unknown previous to the year 1540. Ricord, speaking of these tubercles, says that they sometimes engender those suspicious forms of gonorrhœa or balanorrhœa, the suppression of which is frequently succeeded by constitutional syphilis. That Hahnemann, speaking of his sycosic gonorrhœa, meant nothing else than these mucous tubercles, is evident from the fact, that he locates the spread of this disease in Germany between the years 1809 to 1814, during which period these tubercles were imported from France into Germany; but likewise from the fact that he describes his figwarts (see Chronic Diseases, I., pages 108 and 109) almost in the very same terms used by the French physicians in describing their *tubercules muqueux.* He says that they are very seldom dry and wart-shaped, but more frequently *soft, spongy, sensitive, flat elevations, from which a fetid moisture oozes out.* Nor was Hahnemann quite wrong in connecting this gonorrhœa with a contagium *sui generis;* for, although this contagium is derived from that of chancre, yet it is a *modified chancre-virus,* which, as such, is indeed capable of producing all the secondary consequences of chancre, but never chancre itself. In addition to this characteristic, this gonorrhœa with its mucous tubercles, as well as the fungoid chancre, requires for its cure more frequently *Nitri acidum,* than Mercurius; hence the very same antidote that is required for that stage of chancre in which the modified contagium has originated, and still originates to this day whenever a chancre of this fungoid form, instead of causing chancre, infects the individual with fungoid products. That the sycosic gonorrhœa which we have just now described is identical with the above-mentioned chancre-gonorrhœa, or syphilitic gonorrhœa (§§ 170–175), in so far as both are admitted products of the chancre, if not according to their form, at least according to their essence, does not apply to the simple inflammatory idiopathic gonorrhœa, which, although originating in impure coït, and hence of a venereal nature, yet differs essentially from the former kinds of gonorrhœa and from all syphilitic products even so far as this, that its chief remedy is *Cannabis*, which has never yet shown the least curative action against any of the symptoms of syphilis. Considering, moreover, the pathological conduct of certain cases of gonorrhœa, which, although ever so violent and capable of originating orchitis and abscesses of the prostate, yet never produce a single symptom that has any of the characteristic signs of syphilis, such as its inflammations, abscesses, swellings, ulcers, we must admit that there are kinds of gonorrhœa which, although of venereal origin, yet do not in any respect belong to the province of the ordinary chancrous syphilis. If this is admitted, we are irresistibly led to conclude, that we have indeed two *venereal contagia*, but only one syphilitic contagium, embracing within its range the so-called *sycosis;* hence two *essentially distinct venereal gonorrhœas*, namely, a simple, idiopathic gonorrhœa, which is indeed venereal, but not syphilitic; and a symptomatic gonorrhœa, of an undoubted syphilitic character.

III. CONDITIONS OF VENEREAL INFECTION.

Sec. 179.—General Remarks.

After the conclusions at which we arrived at the termination of the preceding chapter, we shall have no difficulty in comprehending that the much more harmless, almost local contagium of the idiopathic gonorrhœa, whose sphere of action seems to be confined to the sexual and urinary organs, has engaged the attention of physicians much less than the syphilitic virus which pervades the whole organism during the whole lifetime of the patient. For this reason most writers on syphilis have, since this disease has been known, busied themselves more particularly with the chemical nature of the syphilitic contagium, trying to find out whether it is an acid, or an alkali, etc. All have agreed that it must be of a *corrosive* nature, since syphilis spreads about with so much violence and rapidity; Broussais' Physiological School, that rejects every kind of virus, goes so far as to proclaim all the primary phenomena of syphilis a purely local, *chemico-physiological* result of an *accidental acridity*, by which the parts that come in contact with it, are corroded neither more nor less than by any other corrosive substance. However, inasmuch as this view, which had already been entertained by others before Broussais, has been refuted by the course of the infectious products, and it was found that the disease seemed to have a parasitical life of its own, other physicians have undertaken to explain the contagium as an organic germ, of a vegetable or animal nature. We have already shown, § 172, that Dr. Donné, of Paris, has discovered small infusoria in the matter of certain chancres, not uniformly present, however, in every chancre, and not even absolutely indispensable to secure the contagious nature of the pus, since this pus has remained equally efficient for purposes of inoculation, even after the animalcules had been destroyed by vinegar. Whatever peculiar constituent may hereafter be discovered in the venereal pus, be it a salt, an alkali, or an acid, may perhaps secure a more perfect distinction of the venereal from any other infectious matter, but will shed no more light upon its physiological or pathogenetic properties, than the chemical analysis of any other substance will shed light upon its special medicinal properties; for the reason, that the effect which the immaterial contagium, contained in any substance, produces in consequence of stimulating the organism to morbid or abnormal movements, is not a chemical, but a dynamic property (see § 167), that is, a property, which, like warmth, magnetism, the germinating force, and other mechanical or organic movement-principles, can only be recognized by its manifestations. As Chemistry and Physics are related to each other, the former being the science of matter, the latter the science of the movements or the moving properties of matter: so are Anatomy and Physiology related to each other, the former teaching a knowledge of the dead material tissues and organs of the body, the latter a knowledge of the living movements of these organs. If we desire to acquire a knowledge of the specifically morbific properties of a contagium, by which we understand properties that transform the normal living movements into abnormal movements; and if we desire to observe what pathological movements such a contagium can impress upon the organism, either permanently or only temporarily: neither Chemistry nor Anatomy will furnish the desired information, but we shall have to apply to one of the *movement-sciences*, more especially to the Physiology of Diseases, that is, to Pathology exclusively; it is in the domain of Pathology alone that we can find out what effects such a contagium produces, when brought in contact with the living organism. Let us enter upon the same road, and inquire, above all things, through what substances, and in what way, this morbific movement-principle can be forced upon the organism.

Sec. 180.—Carriers of the Contagium.

Even to this day, many pathological manuals, even Schœnlein's, teach, as an article of faith, that the contagium when first appearing in 1491–1540, was of a *volatile* nature; that it selected the air as a carrier, and communicated the infection through the agency of this gas. This story might be repeated as a traditional romance, but it is too little substantiated to be taught as a scientific theorem. The history of this tradition shows that it originated in a desire to make the common people understand that even princes, abbots, prelates, monks, and nuns could be attacked with the reigning epidemic. Nothing, according to these apologists of the privileged classes, was easier than that the disease could be contracted by touching the hands, clothes, or any other piece of property of an infected person; that it spread most readily in places where large crowds congregated—in churches, for instance; that the breath of the faithful communicated it in the confessional to their confessors; and that the pestiferous air might transmit the disease from the place of an infected person to a distant locality. "The French disease," writes Victorius, in the year 1551, "spreads without any intercourse of a man with a woman, or a woman with a man. I have known honorable nuns who, notwithstanding that they were carefully guarded, and protected by iron bars, were attacked with this disease by the atmospheric air, and the foul condition of their humors." But supposing that this was no attempt to explain suspicious facts in a comprehensible manner, and that a disease which spread in this manner was no variolous typhus, but our modern syphilis, it is certain that, at the present time, the disease is no longer communicated by the air, nor by the mediate contact of the clothes, or other pieces of property of an infected person, but only by the *immediate* contact of the infectious matter with a spot that is specifically susceptible of its influence. According to some, this carrier is the *pus*, or the morbid secretion from a syphilitic ulcer, or some other syphilitic product; whereas, others maintain that the infection can be communicated by touching a spot that is simply inflamed, and, without secreting any thing, is already tainted with the venereal poison; or that the communication may even take place by means of remaining syphilitic indurations that have ceased to secrete any thing. Some even go so far as to contend that the naked body of a syphilitic person can communicate the infection by simply touching the naked body of some other person. That nurslings can be infected by the milk of nurses who have constitutional syphilis, even without any ulcers on the mammæ, is a fact to which we shall advert in a subsequent paragraph, as well as to the infection being communicated to persons who lie naked in the same bed with individuals affected with constitutional syphilis. As regards becoming infected with primary products: I know of cases where gonorrhœa was communicated even before any discharge had become perceptible from the male urethra; or chancre, from a badly-healed cicatrix, where no secretion was any longer visible, and nothing more remained of the disease than a coppery color of the affected locality; but I have always found, in such cases, that a careful examination of the parts still showed, if not a decided secretion of matter, at least a scarcely perceptible exhalation. In case the infection was communicated by the spittle, I have always found that there were chancres in the mouth. Facts like these induce me to be of the opinion that those who regard the secretions from the affected parts as the true carriers of the contagium, are correct.

Sec. 181.—Of the Parts susceptible of the Infection.

On looking over those localities and tissues of the body where symptoms of syphilitic contagion are seen, we find that, not by any means, are all these parts equally sensitive to the syphilitic contagium, and that it is particularly the *mucous membranes* that possess this sensitiveness to the highest degree. Whether this sensitiveness is graduated according to the nature of the organs —existing in the highest degree in the sexual organs, less in the rectum, still less in the mouth, nose, lips, eyes, etc., and not at all in the stomach—is a question of much more difficult solution than the authors of many compendia imagine. If the genitals are much more frequently affected than other parts, this does not show their greater sensitiveness, but is owing to the fact that these parts are brought in contact with the syphilitic contagium much more frequently than other parts. The ready communication of the infection to the buccal mucous lining, through poisonous kisses, would seem to show that this membrane, of itself, is just as liable to becoming infected as the sexual organs; the mucous lining of the stomach might, perhaps, be found equally sensitive, if it were possible to establish a much more direct contact between it and the contagious matter, than is done by means of the pills prepared for the purpose of conducting these experiments. As regards the mucous lining of the rectum, I have seen several cases of primary condylomata, chancres, and figwarts in this organ, that evidently originated in unnatural gratification of the sexual passion. Notwithstanding I have seen several cases of this kind, I have, on the other hand, met with cases where the direct contact of the idiopathic gonorrhœal virus with the lining membrane of the rectum remained without any result whatsoever. I have felt disposed to infer from this circumstance, that this virus can only infect the lining membrane of the urinary organs, and that of the eyes. In regard to the external skin, in a state of perfect integrity, I do not altogether share the assertions of authors, that it is inaccessible to the action of the venereal contagium. I have seen cases where the friction of the diseased penis against the thigh, and the axilla of a woman, induced in one case a syphilitic ulcer, and in the other a bubo. Lagneau, of Paris, likewise speaks of a chancre at the umbilicus, that originated in a similar manner. It is possible that, in these cases, the epidermis had become more or less inflamed, and had assumed a form somewhat resembling that of a mucous membrane; but the known cases of ulcers on the thigh and scrotum, after these parts had been bathed for some time during sleep with the discharge from a diseased penis, are likewise facts. Massa speaks of a young man who touched the chancrous pudendum of a woman with his fingers, after which his hand became swollen, and covered with syphilitic ulcers. The Paris "Journal de Médecine," of the year 1759, relates the case of an accoucheur, whose hand and fingers were perfectly uninjured, and who became infected with syphilis, in consequence of attending upon a syphilitic woman, and, in his ignorance of the character of the infection, communicated it to his own wife. Such cases are, however, very rare, and a closer inspection might, perhaps, show that the epidermis was more or less broken in every case. It is a well-established fact, that open sores in the skin, and inflamed portions of skin, like erysipelas, are more susceptible of infection than the mucous membranes themselves, and that the syphilitic disease, in such cases, is more dangerous, and runs a much more rapid course.

Sec. 182.—Of the channels through which the Poison is introduced into the Body.

It is scarcely necessary to repeat that the act of coïtion is the most frequently travelled road by which the venereal contagium is introduced into the body. It is likewise known, that direct contact with the diseased organ, be it the sexual parts, the anus, mouth, or tongue, is another frequent channel of communication. What is still questionable, is, whether the infection can be caught from an otherwise perfectly sound woman, who had connection with a diseased individual immediately previous. Widemann, a contemporary of the great epidemic, not only deems this possible, but warns his readers against having anything to do with a woman who had connection with an infected individual shortly before. Later physicians have doubted the possibility of such an infection, without, however, adducing any convincing proofs in favor of their doubts. Supposing even that the contagium had at once been removed from the pudendum by absorption, and that the woman had washed herself immediately after connection, a small portion of infectious matter may yet have remained adhering to the parts. That this is possible, has been shown me by the following case: A young man had connection with a woman, immediately after which he washed himself, and on the same day had connection with a healthy girl. A fortnight after, both this girl and himself had chancres. An examination showed that the other girl was diseased. If a chancre exists on the lips, in the mouth, or throat, the syphilitic disease may be communicated through a kiss, in consequence of the spittle becoming united with the secretion from the chancre. For this purpose, it is not necessary that the tongue should be inserted into the mouth of the infected individual, the simple contact of the lips is sufficient to effect contagion in such cases. The communication of the infection is very much facilitated by the fact that the syphilitic disease had become localized in a small pustule in the corner of the mouth, which often escapes the patient's own notice, and may have been the means of imparting the disease to more than one individual, without the patient himself being aware of the existence of the pustule. Examples of this kind are not unfrequent. Muritanus relates a case where every nun of Sarenta became infected by kissing a little girl whom an infected stranger had first kissed on the mouth. Nursing at the mammæ constitutes another channel through which the infection is frequently communicated. Syphilitic infants may infect their nurses, and nurses with syphilitic nipples may infect their nurslings, and the disease may spread in this way over a large circle. Portal relates a case where an infant that had been brought from Paris to Montmorency infected its nurse, the nurse infected her husband, the husband gave the disease to another woman, until the whole town had caught the infection. Vercelloni, Disbon, and other physicians relate similar cases. Van Swieten relates a case where a woman, whose business consisted in drawing the milk out of the breasts of recently-confined women, continued it even after she had a chancre on her tongue; the consequence was, that first a number of women and afterwards their husbands, and even their children caught the disease, and many of them died. In a similar manner the disease may be spread by using tobacco-pipes, drinking-vessels, wind-instruments, and the like, to which the pus from chancres on the lips, tongue, etc., is adhering; and more particularly by the insertion of syphilitic teeth, by which means a great deal of mischief has already been done.

Sec. 183.—Unusual Channels of Communicating the Infection.

The above-described channels of communicating the infection

are the most natural and most common; beside these, there are other modes of communication, among which *inoculation*, or the insertion of the poison under the epidermis for purposes of experimentation, or the unconscious transfer of the contagium to open sores, deserves particular mention. In this category belong the not unfrequent cases of mid-wives and accoucheurs who are infected with the disease, when attending upon syphilitic women, if there is the least sore on the fingers or hands; or the cases of surgeons, if they cut themselves when operating on infected parts; in this way many persons may become infected without having the least suspicion of the taint. Van Swieten, for instance, relates the case of several peasants in Moravia, who, according to Schenk's statements, caught syphilis in consequence of being cupped with cups that had been used shortly before on an individual infected with the disease. Daguerre reports that a miller who undertook to *cure* people, infected them with syphilis by his lancet, which he never cleaned with any thing else than his saliva. The bite of syphilitic patients has likewise transmitted the disease in consequence of the infected spittle being inserted into the wound. Whether this poison can be communicated by the uninjured epidermis, is another question. We have mentioned, § 181, the case of an obstetrician who, although his skin was perfectly sound, was nevertheless infected by waiting upon a syphilitic woman in confinement. Cazenave relates of a young hospital-physician that, a few days after examining several syphilitic women, he was attacked with a syphilitic eruption on his hands, the skin of which was intact. Such cases may occur; but if we consider how little trifling injuries of the skin, punctures with needles and the like, are heeded, more particularly after they seem entirely healed, and the scurf, if there was any, has become detached, and if we, moreover, consider the large number of cases where physicians appointed to watch over the inmates of brothels come in daily contact with the syphilitic contagium without ever experiencing the least traces of an infectious disease upon their own persons, we certainly are bound to accept all such reports with a great deal of caution and allowance. The same remark applies in a much higher degree to cases in which the infection is said to have been communicated by sleeping in the same bed with infected persons; by wearing their pantaloons or other garments, or by resorting to public water-closets. Such cases may likewise occur, inasmuch as a portion of infectious matter may have accidentally come in contact with a susceptible part of the body; for instance, when sleeping with an individual affected with chancre, the chancrous secretion may touch the sexual organs, lips, nose, or eyes of the non-infected individual, or the tip of the glans may touch a spot in the water-closet, where a portion of gonorrhœal matter, from one who had visited this closet shortly before, had remained adhering; or recent traces of syphilitic secretions may remain adhering to the bed-clothes and come in contact with the mucous lining of other non-infected individuals. But, in all such cases, infection takes place in consequence of a direct contact of the contagium with the exposed part, and it will have to be admitted that, in order to secure such a result, an extraordinary coincidence of circumstances is required to take place. Indeed, it is not in this sense that communication of the infection by the skin is understood; those who advocate it mean, that persons who are thoroughly syphilitic can communicate the disease by their general secretions; for instance, by the saliva, sweat, by the imperceptible exhalations of the body, by their breath, and even by the bed-clothes and garments to which these secretions adhere. We shall examine this point in the next paragraph.

Sec. 184.—Limits of the Liability to Syphilitic Contagion.

Although it is generally admitted at the present day that syphilitic primary products, such as chancre, figwarts, gonorrhœa, etc., can only be occasioned by direct contact of the morbid secretion with a spot that is susceptible to the action or influence of the contagium, yet there are not only lay-persons, but likewise physicians, who believe that the fluids of a patient may become so thoroughly poisoned by constitutional syphilis, that the disease may not only be communicated by contact with his person or clothes, but even by the air that has become impregnated with his breath, at least within a certain proximity, as when sleeping with him in the same bed. Without appealing, in examining this question, to the authority of our greatest writers on syphilis, such as Hunter, Babington, Cazenave, Ricord, Lagneau, etc., who, backed by a large number of the most careful observations, deny the possibility of the disease being communicated through these channels, I am prepared to state from personal experience that, in the numerous cases where persons whose constitutions were thoroughly saturated with the syphilitic disease slept for months with perfectly sound individuals, primary products were never caused in any other way except by a direct contact of the infectious matter with the lips, mouth, or other equally susceptible localities. Whenever the eruptions on the lips, affections of the mouth, or chancres in the throat, were known to be of a secondary, not primary nature, I have never known kisses or any other contact of the mouths or tongues cause any appearance of syphilitic disease. This has been so uniformly true that, whenever primary symptoms resulted from any such causes, I have always felt certain that there were primary products present in the mouth, whereupon, an examination of the parts always resulted in confirming my suspicion. If an observation of this kind, however, is to hold good, the *consecutive* phenomena have to be carefully distinguished from exclusively secondary products, and not both be mixed up together in one class, as is still done by a number of our physicians; the *consecutive* phenomena on the sexual organs, such as *mucous tubercles*, *condylomata*, etc., are always contagious; the truly secondary phenomena are not, or rather never, contagious. Now, if secondary phenomena themselves do not transmit the contagion, even when two bodies are placed in the most direct and most intimate contact with each other, how then are the sweat, saliva, clothing, etc. of such patients to acquire the power of infecting other individuals? What may have given rise to the supposition that these objects can become capable of communicating the disease, is probably the circumstance that syphilitic secretions do not lose their infectious power, even after they have become dried up for some time, and that this power again becomes active, after the fashion of certain infusoria, as soon as the fluidity of the secretion is restored. Thus, lint, to which old syphilitic matter is still adhering, may infect a person by being placed upon a recent wound. A pocket-handkerchief, with which a syphilitic patient had wiped his chancre, may communicate the infection to a sound person, if he should use it for the purpose of blowing his nose, and the secretions from the nose should have liquefied the solidified chancrous pus.

In the same way, pantaloons or bed-clothes may communicate the infection, in consequence of the dried-up chancrous matter becoming softened by the warm sweat of the patient and coming in contact with some susceptible part of his body. We have not yet found out how long such dried-up contagious matter may retain its infectious power; it is generally known, however, that the idio-electrical bodies, such as glass, wool, silk, etc., retain this power much longer than electrical conductors, such as metals, coal, etc. The infectious power of the contagium is likewise very soon extinguished either by a high degree of warmth, 25° to 50° R., or by intense cold; whereas, with a moderate degree of temperature, it may continue for years. According to some, the contagium, at the period when it emanates from the producing agent, loses all its infectious power for a few moments, especially when several acts of infectious coïtion have taken place in rapid succession, one after the other; this point, however, it may not be very easy to prove.

Sec. 185.—Circumstances by which the Power to transmit the Infection is either diminished or increased.

It is a well-known fact that there are individuals who cannot expose themselves in the least to venereal infection without either having a chancre or gonorrhœa; whereas others, even prostitutes who abandon themselves with unbridled recklessness to the most libidinous intercourse with the other sex, remain perfectly free from venereal taint, even like animals, no species of which has as yet been known to be susceptible of the venereal diseases of the human family. Again, of several persons who have connection with the same syphilitic woman, one becomes tainted, the other, even if generally very susceptible, may remain free from all contagion. These different degrees of susceptibility have been sought to be accounted for in different ways, more especially by the circumstance that both parties, the woman as well as the lover, observe the most perfect cleanliness after the act. Every frequenter of brothels, who has never yet been caught, imagines that his apparent immunity is owing to the circumstance that, after having connection, he makes it a point to always wash himself thoroughly. A want of cleanliness may evidently contribute a great deal toward aggravating existing ulcers or other products to a very high degree; but it is a sad and pernicious mistake to suppose that the contagium can be removed by washing the parts immediately after connection. We know from thousands of cases that, in spite of the most thorough washing, the contagium can be absorbed by the organism even during the act of coïtion, and develop all the ill effects of the poison. Another error is committed by Hunter, when he teaches that all danger of contagion is removed by washing off the traces of morbid secretion immediately previous to having connection; the secretion of matter going on all the time, it is replaced just as fast as it is removed by washing. What has been said of the parts becoming blunted by frequent attacks is equally disproved by facts. A former inspector of the public health has assured me that there are prostitutes who, six months after having been discharged from the public dispensatories, have to be returned to these institutions, on account of again having become diseased, and that they spend the best part of ten or fifteen years under medical treatment. Whether the susceptibility to disease is increased by a first attack, is not made out by such facts as we have reported. Nor is it sure whether mental emotions, or the use of spirituous beverages, increase the susceptibility; the many cases of infection occurring during a debauch most likely occur in consequence of the parties being utterly unaware of what they are doing, or with whom they have connection. The same doubt exists regarding what many books teach of the influence of climate, temperament, and social position and circumstances, on the susceptibility of venereal contagion. It is true that the people of the North, persons of phlegmatic temperaments and in opulent circumstances, are less liable to attacks than the people of the South, or persons of sanguineous temperaments, or the working classes; but this is not owing to a less degree of susceptibility inherent in the former, but to the fact that they do not expose themselves with the same indiscriminate recklessness as the latter. What is, however, a more absurd opinion than any, is, that the intensity of the contagium diminishes in proportion as the act of coïtion is repeated more frequently, and that the forms of the communicated infection consequently grow milder. The contagium always remains the same, producing, as the case may be, gonorrhœa, chancre, or consecutive products; and the subsequent intensity of the phenomena is so little dependent on the quantitative degree of infectious power inherent in the original matter, that an individual affected with a whole crop of chancres and buboes may only communicate a small, not very malignant chancre; whereas another individual, with a scarcely perceptible ulcer, may communicate the worst form of phagedænic chancre. It is only the species (gonorrhœa, chancre, mucous tubercle) that is determined and communicated by the act of coïtion; all the rest depends upon the nature of the soil where the seed is planted, the same as in the vegetable world.

IV. HEREDITARY SYPHILIS.

Sec. 186.—General Remark.

Although we have stated and plainly shown in the preceding article that secondary syphilis can neither be transmitted by the spittle, or the sweat, or the imperceptible perspiration of the patient, the case is different as regards the transmission of secondary symptoms in an indirect way, by the father's seed during the act of coïtion, by the mother's blood during pregnancy, or by the nurse's milk while feeding the baby at the breast. This mode of transmitting the syphilitic disease, which may take place even if no visible trace of the disease exists, is one of the most mysterious processes of communication; but should not be confounded with the manner in which the disease is communicated to the infant by syphilitic nipples, or by chancres, or tubercles in the vagina, with which the child may come in contact during its passage into the world; nor should it be confounded with the case where the father or mother is infected with primary syphilitic ulcers during the act of generation, and the embryo becomes tainted at the very moment of conception (congenital syphilis). These three kinds of communication, the last-mentioned, as well as the two former, are *direct* modes of transmitting the contagium; the mode of transmission of which we are treating in this paragraph, and which results in the production of hereditary syphilis, takes place without any apparent influence of a developed contagium, and constitutes, so to say, a progressive unfolding of the parental constitution that had become morbidly altered by a formerly contracted syphilitic disease, and which is transmitted to the offspring, in the same way as the scrofulous, tuberculous, arthritic, cancerous, and other hereditary dispositions, diseases, or diatheses. It is uncertain whether ancient authors were acquainted with this mode of transmission of syphilitic constitutions. It is not probable, however, that they were, since, in using the term hereditary syphilis, they evidently meant a syphilis acquired by direct contact with some primary syphilitic product, such as chancres in the vagina, etc. Fabre, for instance, remarks, that syphilis can be inherited, if, during the act of generation, either the father or the mother is affected with syphilitic ulcers; or Van Swieten says, that the syphilis of the infant may be caused by the syphilitic products with which the mother becomes tainted either during the act of generation or during her pregnancy. An essential distinction between these two modes of transmission of the disease consists in the fact that, when tainted with congenital syphilis, the child shows traces of the disease immediately after birth, or is still-born, or dies soon after it is born, especially if the mother, during her pregnancy, did not undergo a thorough anti-syphilitic treatment. In hereditary syphilis, on the contrary, the child is often born with every sign of good health, and the syphilitic symptoms, such as all sorts of exanthems, exostoses, affections of the mucous membranes, suspicious ulcers, etc., only develop themselves at a later period, sometimes not till years have elapsed, scarcely ever before three or six months after birth. How this transmission of the syphilitic disease takes place without the fœtus becoming tainted with a new infection; whether, in such cases, the blood of the mother, or the semen, or the nurse's milk constitutes the carrier of a tainted contagium, or of a specifically-abnormal movement-principle, which, without being able to infect healthy persons, can communicate itself to the fecundated germ (or the nursling by the nurse's milk), and, as soon as the organism after birth enters its own sphere of independent development, continues the abnormally-excited movements of the infantile organism in the same direction as they had been going on in the organism of the father or mother; will, most likely, remain as much of a secret as the transmission of all other intellectual and moral qualities from the parents to the children.

Sec. 187.—Conditions necessary for the Hereditary Transmission of Syphilis.

It has been generally accepted as a fact, that the mother, if she had been cured of syphilis a short time previous to the birth of the child, or was still affected with secondary syphilitic phenomena, may give birth to a child tainted with the disease; an indispensable requisite to effect this result was supposed to be, that the mother must still exhibit unmistakable symptoms of the syphilitic disease. That this, however, is not necessary, and that the disease can be transmitted by a mother in the apparent enjoyment of perfect health, even years after every vestige of the infection had apparently been wiped out, is shown by a case related by Vassal, of France, where a woman who had had syphilis, of which she seemed to have been radically cured, had two children by a second husband, both of whom were born and died with unmistakable signs of syphilis. Her husband died of typhus, and never had shown the least symptom of syphilitic taint. What seemed still more remarkable was, that this same woman again gave birth to three syphilitic children by a third husband, whom she married soon after the death of his predecessor, whereas she herself continued to enjoy the most blooming health, and not one of her husbands ever showed the least symptom of syphilitic taint. Another remarkable circumstance in this case is, that the second of these children infected its nurse with syphilis. That the syphilitic disease may not only be inherited from the mother, but likewise from the father, and that the mother may be predisposed by a syphilitic husband, for all time, for giving birth to syphilitic children, though she herself may never exhibit a single sign of any syphilitic taint, is authenticated by a remarkable case related by Vidal, of Paris, where a woman, after having had a child that soon after its birth died with all the symptoms of hereditary syphilis, by a man who was infected with chronic syphilis of long standing, four years after this event gave birth to a syphilitic child by a perfectly sound man, without a single syphilitic symptom having ever broken out on her own person. Another mystery, or, at any rate, a fact in the generative sphere that has not yet been accounted for, is the following: If a *perfectly white* slut is impregnated for the first time by a black dog, some of her young will be white, some black, some spotted white and black; if, afterwards, she is impregnated by a totally white dog, the color of her first mate will reappear in more or less striking spots. The male impresses upon the female a type that shows itself in the subsequent offspring of the same mother. Cazenave relates several similar cases where mothers, who seemed perfectly free from all syphilitic taint, gave birth to syphilitic children, some of whom infected even their nurses. One of these cases is remarkable for the fact, that a woman who had become infected during her pregnancy, but had been perfectly cured, gave birth to a perfectly healthy child, all of whose other children, however, were born syphilitic. If Cazenave, however, infers from these cases that the mother always remains sound as long as the husband is only affected with constitutional syphilis, I recall, in reply, the reader's attention to a case from my own practice, § 103, where the mother had never become tainted during the time that she lived with her constitutionally-syphilitic husband, but who, during the last month of her pregnancy, and more particularly after having been confined of a dead child, broke out with a secondary exanthem, of the form of *lichen*, over her whole body, more particularly over her arms and legs. These cases, where the capacity of the father of directly transmitting the disease had become roused again into activity, after it had been slumbering for a long time, and where, in one case, a mother was infected by her dead fœtus, and, in the other, two nurses, by infants that were syphilitic at birth, and had been conceived under the influence of a latent syphilis, are exceedingly remarkable, and, for the present, meet with something analogous only in certain plants, whose latent poison only develops itself during their stage of flowering and fructification.

Sec. 188.—Syphilis inherited from Nurses.

In the preceding paragraph we have spoken of latent syphilis being communicated through father and mother. Syphilitic infection can likewise be communicated by the milk of a nurse. Such cases likewise come in the category of hereditary syphilis; for here too the disease is communicated by a latent contagium, not by means of the open and demonstrable action of the syphilitic virus, as is the case when the nurse has syphilitic nipples or chancrous ulcers on the mammæ. These cases of syphilis that are inherited from nurses, are probably much more numerous than is generally supposed; indeed, most of the cases of syphilis, where the disease is transmitted by nurses, most likely belong to this category. I only know of two of such cases, where the disease had undoubtedly been communicated by the milk from a nurse's breast; one of these cases is recorded in Bertin's "Treatise on the Syphilis of Pregnant Women and New-born Infants," and the other case occurred in my own practice. Bertin's case is that of a perfectly sound farmer's wife, who had never had syphilis any more than her husband, and whose perfectly healthy child was attacked with chancrous ulcers on the labia five months after her birth, of the nature of which the surgeon who had been consulted on the subject was ignorant, and which he dried up with lead-water, shortly after which, buboes and syphilitic pustules on the thighs and legs made their appearance. Until then the child's parents had enjoyed perfect health; five months after the child had been taken sick, the nipples of the mother, who continued to nurse the child, were attacked with syphilitic rhagades; afterwards other syphilitic symptoms broke out in other localities. Upon inquiry, it was found that an aunt sometimes tended the child, and that this aunt was affected with constitutional syphilis. In order to quiet the child, she not only put it very frequently to her own breast, but warmed the water, with which she was in the habit of washing the child's private parts, in her own mouth. Although this case does not show whether the aunt had syphilitic ulcers in her mouth, and it may be supposed that she had not, for the reason that, if the contrary had been the case, the reporter would undoubtedly have made mention of them, this case derives additional confirmation from another case, which I have watched myself even to the minutest details. It was the case of the child of a young German here in Paris, who, having been educated in the strictest principles, only frequented religious societies, and, at the age of twenty-four years, in a state of perfect moral and physical soundness, married a young girl of seventeen, equally free from all physical and moral taints. She gave birth to a robust and lovely girl, who, on account of her parents' teaching music in town through the day, had to be intrusted to a nurse, whom I examined with the greatest care, nipples, breast, skin, etc., and pronounced perfectly sound and free from all possible taint. In spite of all this care, syphilitic pustules broke out two months afterwards on the thighs and nates of the child. Upon further inquiry into the circumstances of the nurse's family, who was still perfectly free from any appearance of disease, it was found that her child, soon after birth, had died of an inflammation of the throat, which the physician of the village had pronounced *diphtheritic*, and that her husband was still affected with symptoms of an inveterate chronic syphilis, more particularly with ephelides on the breast and on other parts of his body, which we have described in another division of this work as scattered, exceedingly chronic spots, resembling liver-spots, from which they are distinguished, however, by their circular, definitely-circumscribed borders. The nurse was dismissed, and the child, having taken *Mercurius* 3, half a grain every four days, was soon freed, and remained free, from every symptom of disease.

Sec. 189.—Diagnostic Signs of Hereditary Syphilis.

We have already stated, at the beginning of this article, that congenital syphilis shows itself at the birth of the child, whereas hereditary syphilis breaks out at a later period. As regards the time of its appearance, authors do not agree; some, like Fabre, Rosen, etc., assume that it may slumber in the body for years, and may not betray its existence until the age of pubescence. Generally, however, the disease begins to show itself in about eighteen or twenty months after birth, but may break out already in a few months. Most frequently the disease first manifests itself during the period of teething, in which case the manifestations never are of the order of *primary*, but invariably of that of *secondary* phenomena. In most cases it is an exanthem, more particularly *roseola syphilitica*, that constitutes the beginning of the series, after which the affections of the mucous membranes make their appearance, first and most frequently in the nose and throat. These affections are speedily followed by other ulcers and caries of bones, until death soon after relieves the sufferer from all earthly woe. This termination is the more frequent the younger the child; if the disease does not break out until the child is two years old, the prognosis is not so unfavorable. The constitution of such patients is always suffering in a remarkably characteristic manner. Such children are almost always the victims of a deeply-searching marasmus, as if the organic tissues were being decomposed even during the lifetime of the sufferers; their skin is livid, lifeless, and dry, like parchment, and an appearance of old age and decay imparts to them an expression of cachexia, such as is witnessed in the case of older syphilitic individuals. Such children may die already in the mother's womb; if this happens, no sign of syphilis is seen on the bodies of such still-born children any more than on those of other children that are still-born from any other cause; whereas, if the syphilitic disease is acquired during the act of generation, syphilitic signs are never wanting, even on the skin of still-born children, and are always the same that show themselves in congenital syphilis a few days after birth, and belong more or less to the *primary* period of syphilis. In most cases of this kind, we find the sexual parts of such children studded with mucous tubercles, or syphilitic exanthems are found upon the skin, more particularly ecthyma (see § 102), or the syphilitic pemphigus (see § 98). Except pemphigus, which is one of the most dangerous forms of secondary syphilis in the case of new-born children, all their other syphilitic affections are much more easily cured when acquired at birth or during the act of generation than when hereditary. We repeat, not all children who are tainted with hereditary syphilis die prematurely; some grow up to manhood before a single symptom of syphilis manifests itself in their frames. It is difficult to decide what is the cause of the diversity of the degrees of intensity and danger manifested by such hereditary dispositions; some of these differences may perhaps originate in the circumstances that will be dwelt upon more fully in the next chapter, when surveying the course of development which syphilis takes from the first moment of infection to its definite and full manifestation.

THIRD CHAPTER.

GENERAL DEVELOPMENT, COURSE, AND TERMINATION OF SYPHILIS.

I. DEVELOPMENT OF SYPHILIS.

Sec. 190.—Period of Germination.

Every unprejudiced observer must admit that between the moment of the infectious contact and the appearance of the first protopathic phenomena, a longer or shorter interval elapses, during which the absorbed poison prepares the subsequent manifestation of the disease; this interval has been designated as *the period of incubation or germination.* It is true that some physicians—even Ricord, of Paris, relying upon his experiments in inoculation,—deny this period of incubation, and maintain that, so far from being absorbed by the organism, the contagium, on the contrary, remains adhering to the locality where it is applied, and where, as its first effect, it produces an ulcer, which is only when fully developed succeeded by the absorption and diffusion of the poison in the organism. In order to give still more weight to this view, he alleges, as a proof of its correctness, the fact, that in all cases where a chancre produced by inoculation is cauterized a few days after its first appearance, or at any rate previous to the setting in of the characteristic induration of its base, the inoculated individual remains perfectly free from all subsequent secondary phenomena, even if no internal treatment had been pursued, and that secondary affections only manifest themselves in case the cauterization takes place after the base has already become indurated. Although facts cannot be contradicted, yet the conclusions drawn from these facts may differ, according as the import of the facts is viewed in a different light by one party or the other; and this is likewise the case in regard to the conclusions which Ricord has drawn from his experiments of inoculation. In the first place, his experiments, which he always instituted on patients who were already attacked with syphilis, do not prove any thing regarding the cases where *healthy* persons become infected; for, if it be at all true that a certain interval has to elapse between the initial infection and the production of the first primary or protopathic symptom of the disease, this interval was not required in the case of individuals who were already diseased, and in whom the protopathic manifestation of the disease might, therefore, have taken place much more speedily. Indeed, in Ricord's cases, it usually takes place in one or two days. Most generally the primary symptom was developed on or before the third day. The conclusion which he draws from the speedy appearance of chancre, that a chancre can be removed by cauterizing without the least danger, as long as the poison has not yet been absorbed by the organism, is likewise erroneous. This conclusion is likewise based upon an equally incorrect application of the observed facts to conditions such as occur in the natural course of syphilis. If he had operated on healthy persons, and, while they remained under his supervision, had not seen cauterization followed by buboes, mucous tubercles, or other consecutive phenomena, how could he know that a general infection, which had already begun previous to the appearance of the primary product of inoculation, would not sooner or later manifest its existence by secondary phenomena? Operating as he did upon individuals who, on account of other syphilitic affections, were subjected to internal treatment, how could he know that the non-appearance of secondary phenomena, even for a period of years, was not owing to this internal treatment, instead of attributing it to the innocuousness of the inoculation-sore that was only four or five days old? Be this, however, as it may, Ricord's assertion is contrary to daily observation, according to which a period of six days, or two or three weeks, has to elapse from the moment that the infection is first communicated to the period when the first primary product of the syphilitic disease manifests itself upon the sexual organs.

Sec. 191.—Pathological Processes during the Period of Germination.

This period of incubation being once admitted as a fact, the question then occurs, what changes the locally-applied contagium effects in the organism in order to predispose it for the development of such an exceedingly chronic disease that never again becomes extinct of itself? This subject has been a bone of contention among physicians until our time. All admit, that the contagium is absorbed; but whither it travels, or where it finally becomes located, whether in the liver, the bile, the fat, as was asserted by the partisans of Galen, or whether in the fluids, the blood, or even in the lymphatic glands—nobody is prepared to indicate, with positive certainty, any more than whether it is conducted any where in particular; or whether, according to Ricord and his adherents, it does not rather, like a grain of seed planted in the soil, remain hidden under the epithelium of the mucous membrane, or under the subjacent cellular tissue, until the germ succeeds in piercing its coverings. This last mode of explanation, however acceptable it may appear to Berzelius, Liebig, and the chemists generally, who do not understand any thing of the living processes of the organism, might perhaps seem more tenable than it really is, if we could be made to understand why the organism, which so readily absorbs through its epidermis semiliquid substances, such as mercurial ointments, should desist from its laws of absorption in favor of the syphilitic contagium, and should decline to absorb this totally fluid substance through the mucous membranes, which are possessed of an extraordinary degree of absorptive power. No, indeed, the poison is *absorbed;* and that it attacks the whole organism and disharmonizes the unity of its vital processes, even before a trace of the primary syphilitic products is perceptible, is not only shown by the excited feelings with which sensitive patients, even without being aware of the least sign of infection, are sometimes troubled from the moment that the infection takes place, to the very period when primary symptoms are on the point of breaking out—this mental excitement being moreover associated with a feeling of malaise, and of general languor and weariness,—but is likewise shown by the febrile motions which sometimes precede the breaking out of primary symptoms, and are either overlooked by the patient, or attributed to some other cause. Castelnau, in his annals of the cutaneous diseases, relates two very remarkable instances of this kind. The first case was that of a journeyman mason, in whom this fever was attended with malaise, violent pains in the small of the back, and loss of appetite, and became so violent that he had to leave off work and go to bed; three days after which, a small swelling showed itself in the left groin, which increased in the following days to the size of a pigeon's egg, the fever, together with the other ailments, abating all the while, until the bubo remained without any other symptoms. The other case was that of a prostitute, who was attacked with a small chancre at the inferior commissure, and at the same time with fever; this chancre was first succeeded by buboes, afterwards with abscesses on the cheeks and neck, during which the fever continued with equal violence until the abscesses had healed. By dint of making inquiries whenever I had a chance, I have found out, in spite of the great carelessness of most patients, who never apply to a physician until they are compelled to do so, that this fever is not at all uncommon, but consists, in most cases, in a certain characteristic feeling of languor and weariness, attended with more or less chilliness, which in some individuals increases to a shaking chill, and is frequently felt only on the day before the primary product breaks out. Whether the contagium is absorbed rapidly or slowly, the fact is, that it is absorbed just as surely as the organism perceives signs of a general disturbance previous to the breaking out of the local symptoms.

Sec. 192.—Breaking Out of the Local Symptoms.

It is well known that, in most cases, the first symptoms generally make their appearance at the spot where the infection has been communicated. This fact is so generally recognized, that those who regard chancres, protopathic buboes, etc., as purely local symptoms, rely more particularly upon this circumstance to prove the correctness of their theory. But the case here is the same as in many other contagious diseases, where the general organic reaction against the poison that had been forced upon the tissues first embodies itself in a visible form at the very spot whence the shock first emanated. In hydrophobia, for instance, where, at the moment when, after a sometimes considerably protracted period of incubation, the general disease breaks out, the wound which the animal had inflicted with its teeth, and which had become cicatrized a long time previous, breaks open anew, becomes aggravated, and finally inflames. The same process takes place in inoculation of the smallpox, when the pustules prefer the spot where the matter had been originally inserted, for their first appearance, but, as Blache and Aubry relate, may likewise show themselves over the whole body. This circumstance may likewise occur when the syphilitic contagium is introduced in open wounds, as is shown in the case § 99, of the second division of this work, where a chancrous eruption over the whole body emanated from such a cause. Who knows whether many of the pustulous syphilitic exanthems, that have been regarded as secondary phenomena heretofore, do not constitute protopathic primary symptoms, spreading all over at once, in consequence of a renewed infection? At all events, it is not true that the consequences of a *natural* infection show themselves *immediately* at the original spot of communication; I cannot imagine upon what grounds certain German writers base their assertion, that the first local symptoms generally break out forty-eight hours to four days after the infection had first been communicated. This is a theory which, like the fable of the "*crystalline vesicle*," that is said to be always present and only to remain unnoticed occasionally, may be accepted and believed by those who only know of venereal diseases from books; but any one who has seen a sufficient number of syphilitic cases, is aware that, in most cases of natural chancres that had not been produced by inoculation, the first germs never show themselves forty-eight hours, or four days, after infection; but *usually* from the seventh to the fourteenth day, and frequently not until three or four weeks have elapsed. No less incorrect is the assertion, that in the first twenty-four hours after infection, signs of a general reaction become apparent, such as: considerable determination of the blood, turgescence, increased turgor vitalis, increased redness, and alteration of the secretory activity. The fact is that, during the whole period, from the moment of infection to the period of the breaking out of the disease, which breaking out is generally completed within twenty-four hours, absolutely nothing is noticed in most cases at the spot of communication, whether the breaking out takes place seven or twenty-eight days, or even later, subsequent to the infection taking place. It is difficult to determine why, in one case, the disease should break out sooner, in another case later. This period may even vary in the same individual that had caught the infection several times. In spite of the greatest excesses that may be committed during this period, it may last longer than if the patient remains perfectly free from physical or moral excitement. All that can be asserted in regard to the various typical or fundamental forms in which the venereal disease may appear, we have observed from the earliest period to the present time: 1) *Idiopathic gonorrhœa;* 2) the various forms of *chancre;* 3) *Condylomata* (mucous tubercles and figwarts). Whether the syphilitic contagium, as some assert, can remain latent in the body for years, without showing any manifest signs of existence, after the fashion of the hydrophobic virus, is a question that it may be very difficult to decide. If a person is bitten by a mad dog, the whole town knows of it; and every body can state the time, how long it will take for the disease to break out. But, if a man gets bitten by a rabid girl, he is not apt to publish it to the world; and, if the thing should become known, nobody can tell whether the trouble originated in an old offence, or in a recent trespass.

Sec. 193.—Development of the Various Forms.

If Cazenave and other French physicians assert that the form in which the venereal disease may manifest itself, after the infection has taken place, depends exclusively upon the individual disposition of the patient, and upon other accidental circumstances, a statement of this kind is undoubtedly correct, in so far as a certain form of chancre, for instance, need not necessarily produce a like form, but may bring forth a simple Hunterian, or phagedænic chancre, no matter what the original chancre-form may have been. But, if these authors go so far as to assert that, no matter what sort of venereal contagium may have originated the disease, this disease may assume any imaginable form, chancre, mucous tubercle, or protopathic bubo, and that these diversified results are altogether determined by the constitutional individuality of the patient, and by the various influences to which he may be exposed, the falsity of such an assertion must be apparent, even from what we have said in §§ 176, 177, concerning the plurality of the venereal contagia, and can only be accounted for by assuming a want of a correctly discriminating diagnostic acumen. We might as well take it for granted that cherry, pear, or peach trees can grow out of an appleseed, and that a result of this kind depends altogether upon the nature of the soil in which the seed is planted, and upon the circumambient influences under which the unfolding and growth of the seed take place. Inasmuch, however, as our definitions might become mixed up, and consequently might be opposed by *apparent* facts, we will here again present a cursory view of the conditions under which the different venereal typical forms can accomplish and complete their growth, and ultimate shape and realization.

1) *Chancre-forms.*—These can at all times, and under any circumstances, only grow from chancre, not even from condylomata and their accompanying sycosic gonorrhœa, for the reason that condylomatous forms that have acquired an independent existence, although born of chancre, yet constitute a lower degree and inferior variety of the chancre-form, in so far as they belong to a modified or altered stage of the growth of chancre, and hence cannot possibly reproduce their prototype of a higher order.

2) *Condylomata.*—These growths, which may assume the form of mucous tubercles (tubercula mucosa seu humida), and that of figwarts (condylomata, excrescentiæ), may, in accordance with their different natures, spring from two different modes of contagion:

a) by *direct* infection, with existing mucous tubercles or figwarts, and the symptomatic gonorrhœa accompanying these forms; and

b) by infection from chancre in its fungoid, condylamatous stage, but never by infection from a chancre in its first, ulcerous stage.

3) *Gonorrhœa.*—According as it is either symptomatic or idiopathic, it may proceed from one, or from several different modes of infection, namely:

a) The simple *idiopathic* or local gonorrhœa, depending upon a contagium of its own, can neither come from chancrous nor condylomatous infection, but can only be caused by its own specific virus.

b) *Symptomatic gonorrhœa.*—This form of gonorrhœa, which is always associated with mucous tubercles, figwarts, or latent chancres, can never be developed from truly idiopathic gonorrhœa, but may readily result from an infection caused by any of the other forms—chancres, mucous tubercles, or figwarts, in which case it will never appear alone, but always in company with one of the above-mentioned phenomena.

4) *Protopathic bubo.*—This may succeed an infection by the virus of chancre, as well as by that of mucous tubercles or figwarts, but never an infection by simple gonorrhœal virus, which can only produce a consensual swelling of the inguinal glands.

5) *Secondary phenomena* may not only appear after chancres, mucous tubercles, and figwarts, but likewise in consequence of symptomatic, but never as a consequence of purely idiopathic gonorrhœa.

What special form each particular chancre, mucous tubercle, and secondary exanthem, may assume with respect to its malignant nature, further spread, or other differences, depends upon the individual disposition of the infected person, as well as upon accidental circumstances that may either promote or impede the further development of the form conceived of the infection, and concerning which we shall make all needful remarks, after having previously considered the general course of syphilis.

II. COURSE AND PERIODS OF SYPHILIS.

Sec. 194.—The Different Periods generally.

We have already stated more than once in other places, that it is not by its symptoms, each considered by itself, but by the connection of these symptoms among themselves, that syphilis constitutes a unitary, progressively-unfolding *chronic malady*, that does not get well spontaneously, and the phenomena of which, as they appear from time to time in the organism, constitute symptomatic manifestations. At the same time, we have distinguished among these symptoms such products as belong to the initial appearance of this malady, from those that only manifest themselves after the disappearance of these initial symptoms, and constitute, as it were, a new phase in the course of the disease. However, after having described in the first and second divisions of this work the different primary and secondary phenomena, each with as much careful detail as possible, we still have to consider the internal connection of these symptoms, and of their successive development, in a regular series, from the unfolding of the first germ to the most perfect pervasion of the whole organism with constitutional syphilis. Let us now examine, with more particular care, how this polypous monster takes root in the organism from the first moment of its existence, and in what order, and through what metamorphoses, it continues to spread and ramify, until it has dipped its thousand stings into every fibre of the organic tissues. We have seen that even the frequently mentioned mucous tubercles and figwarts, notwithstanding their apparent idiopathicity and inherent capacity for reproduction, are nothing else than sprouts of the chancre from which the syphilitic disease generally emanates, so that we may commence our subject with a consideration of the chancre as the true and sole root of all syphilitic mischief, so much more as the idiopathic gonorrhœa, that has been so often unjustly charged with the sins of its malicious neighbor, after all, only does a small amount of mischief in the organism, and need not occupy our attention in this place. It must have been seen, from what we have stated in previous chapters, that the first thing the chancre seeks to accomplish, immediately after its initial localization, is to create a more or less œdematous, swollen base of cartilaginous hardness, where it forms a cup-shaped excavation surrounded by callous edges, whence it can not only spread its devastating disorganizations, but likewise throw out roots for new vegetations. This is the first destructive period of chancre, which, however, does not last long, so that, unless it should have become converted into a phagedænic sore, the chancre takes root after the fourth, or, at the latest, after the sixth week, so far as to expand into a fungoid growth, with manifold ramifications. In this second or fungoid stage, it not only passes from its destructive form into that of a condylamatous expanse, but even throws out at the same time new sprouts in the neighboring tissues, which, in the shape of mucous tubercles and figwarts, even after the extinction or cicatrization of the original form, continue infectious, and capable of reproducing in healthy individuals, if not the original type, at least the fungoid form of chancre. This stage of development likewise passes by, and another period sets in, when these infectious forms cease to make their appearance, but the fully-developed polypus sprouts in every direction through the various tissues of the organism. This third period initiates a second epoch in the life of syphilis, essentially distinct from that of the chancrous period, when we no longer speak of chancre or its primary products, but of constitutional syphilis, the offspring of the former. It is to these two epochs of the *unfolding* and the *unfolded* general syphilis, to which the name of primary and secondary has been applied, each one of which we shall now proceed to consider more particularly with reference to their special characteristics.

Sec. 195.—Special Characteristics of Primary Syphilis.

What constitutes the pathological distinction between the primary and secondary periods of syphilis, is the circumstance that in the former their still exists a struggle between the polypous monster and the organism that has become disharmonized, but not yet overwhelmed by its pestiferous breath. In this struggle, the monster, on the one hand, seeks to extend its influence, and, on the other hand, the organism, incapable of overwhelming the hostile thing, seeks to limit its activity as much as possible to the locality where the infection had first been perceived, or, at any rate, to keep the hostile effort within local bounds. For this reason it is that the first primary symptoms always make their appearance at the original spot of communication. If this should not be the case, as, for instance, when protopathic buboes break out, the primary symptoms still remain local symptoms, and never appear very far from the original spot of communication. What these primary local manifestations of the syphilitic disease are, we know from the preceding paragraphs: 1) the different forms of chancres; 2) *mucous tubercles and figwarts:* 3) the *symptomatic gonorrhœa* depending on these products; and 4) the *bubo*, which, according to circumstances, may either be a primary (protopathic) or a consecutive (deuteropathic) manifestation. These are the forms that belong exclusively to primary syphilis; if they show themselves any where else than on the sexual organs, for instance, the chancres and mucous tubercles on the lips, in the mouth and throat, and in the corners of the mouth, or around the anus, we might safely conclude that they result from a direct insertion of the virus in these parts, if we had not to take into consideration another circumstance that not only can, but frequently and unfortunately does, exercise a mortifying influence upon the natural course of primary syphilis. This influence is the hand of man, which often interferes with the natural course of this disease in the most criminal and reckless manner, and, instead of destroying the hydra itself, contents itself, whenever this monster shows one of its heads, with chopping it off, not considering that, where one head is chopped off, several others at once grow up in its place. This is true as regards the chancres, mucous tubercles, or buboes; if they are only removed from their local site by external means, instead of being met by specific internal antidotes, the same primary symptoms usually are not slow to break out in an analogous form, like chancres or mucous tubercles, in some other locality, more particularly on the mucous membrane of the throat or mouth, or around the anus, on the scrotum, etc. These phenomena, which have been termed "secondary chancre," "secondary mucous tubercles," are, however, far from being symptoms of secondary syphilis, but, by their pathological nature, belong no less than the consecutive bubo to the primary epoch of syphilis, during which the reacting organism still endeavors to localize the syphilitic disease. In proof of this, these products, whenever they appear in this manner, are always the almost immediate consequence of chancres or mucous tubercles that had been removed by cauterization; as such, they are consecutive, not secondary products of syphilis, and just as capable of communicating the disease as their suppressed primary prototypes. Hence, we have two kinds of primary symptoms, that are not only essentially distinct from each other, but have likewise to be carefully distinguished from the really secondary phenomena; *a*) the *primary* local symptoms that always make their appearance at the original spot of communication; and *b*) the *consecutive* phenomena breaking out in other localities after the primary symptoms had been suppressed by improper management, and still constituting to some extent purely local symptoms. In this respect, we say, that chancre, buboes, mucous tubercles, figwarts, and gonorrhœa, whether they appear as primary or consecutive phenomena, at the original spot of communication or in some other locality, still appertain to the primary epoch of syphilis, where the disease had not yet become constitutional; although some of them, for instance some kinds of figwarts, if they have once broken out, continue in the secondary period for years; but in this period can never break out anew, unless a new infection has taken place.

Sec. 196.—Special Symptoms of Secondary Syphilis.

As regards this period in the ulterior course of syphilis, its chief sign is the appearance of new phenomena that never show themselves as primary symptoms after infection, either on the skin, or on the mucous membranes, in the osseous system, or in other tissues. In this period of the disease, the syphilitic products no longer appear single and localized, as is still the case with the consecutive phenomena, but they either show themselves like exanthems, on various portions of the skin, or likewise in other tissues in company with other syphilitic products, thus evidencing a general overpowering of the organism by the sypilitic disease. That this period begins, as some assert, after the chancre has disappeared, or has become cicatrized, is just as incorrect as the notion that whatever symptom shows itself after the disappearance of the primary phenomena, must necessarily constitute a secondary manifestation. What alone distinguishes and separates these two periods from each other, is the isolated, absolutely local reappearance of the phenomena in one, and the simultaneous, more or less general appearance of diversified phenomena in the other period. Let the consecutive buboes, chancres in the throat, mucous tubercles, etc., of which we have spoken in the preceding paragraph, break out ever so remotely after the complete disappearance of the primary products, and let them continue for years in a condition of fungoid growth; nevertheless, if no other symptoms supervene on the skin, or in other tissues, the primary period continues until such symptoms occur. The reverse of this is likewise true, if such symptoms break out while the chancre is still existing in its integrity at the original spot of communication. Let this chancre be ever so recent, and ever so remote from the stage of fungoid growth; from the moment that these other symptoms show themselves simultaneously with the chancre upon the skin, on the mucous membranes, or in the osseous system, syphilis enters upon the secondary period of its existence. Moreover, inasmuch, as we have stated at the beginning of this paragraph, as the essential characteristic of this secondary period not only consists in manifesting itself by more general phenomena, but more particularly in this, that being a true metamorphosis of the disease, it no longer occasions, after the fashion of the primary period of syphilis, local transpositions of the primary symptoms, but manifests itself by new forms that had not been existing hitherto, and never appear as the immediate results of infection, we conclude that whenever such a form, even isolated, manifests itself upon the skin, the mucous membranes, or in other tissues, it is a sure sign that secondary syphilis has set in. This altered form, deviating more or less from the fundamental types of the primary period, is, in the end, the only permanently remaining characteristic of secondary syphilis; for although, during the evolution of this period, the universality of secondary syphilitic action throughout the whole organism is distinctly recognized either by the simultaneous appearance of several of these forms, or by the supervention of these forms during the existence of primary phenomena; nevertheless, in the further course of this period, a moment of time arrives when the first tumult of syphilitic action appears diminished; the primary symptoms, which still existed at the commencement of this period, have either been removed by the hand of art, or have remained stationary as stunted remnants of the disease, and the continual presence of syphilis in the organism is no longer manifested by the prevalence of general products, but by the development of local phenomena which, like the corona veneris, or the psoriasis palmaris, either continue unchanged for years as the sole visible sign of the disease, or only appear from time to time, generally as local symptoms. It is to this *involution*-period of secondary syphilis that the term constitutional syphilis has been more particularly and not improperly applied, and about which, on account of the importance which attaches to it in the history of syphilis, we shall offer a few additional remarks.

Sec. 197.—Constitutional Syphilis.

As we have shown, the course of syphilis, from the moment of its first appearance to the moment when it seems to have concluded, as it were, a treaty of peace with the organism, presents two essentially distinct phases, in the first of which the disease, after having committed certain primary destructions, changes to a fungoid body, which, in the second period, after having acquired its full growth and characteristic shape, penetrates the whole organism with its ramifications, in the shape of herpes, pustules, and tubercles of every sort, and, from the epidermis to the marrow of the bones, does not leave a single tissue free from its pestilential taint. In the second division of this work, we have more fully considered the products of the fully developed secondary syphilis. Looking at the pathological behavior which each of these forms observes in its course, we cannot fail to notice that a certain system of mutuality or reciprocation seems to exist between incipient condylomatous growths and their ulcerative destruction, so that, whenever the destruction has taken place, cicatrization follows without the assistance of art, by the sole power of Nature. This, however, does not prevent the syphilitic disease from at once reproducing new pustules and tubercles in the place of those that had become cicatrized, and to continue the same system of destruction and restoration with these new formations as with the former. This seems to indicate a continual struggle between the organism and the parasitical growth of syphilis, which the organism is unable to arrest, and can only keep in a state of temporary subjugation, during which the slumbering disease does not become roused as when it made its first debut in the system, but continues to manifest its existence, either by occasionally renewed outbreaks, or by an obstinate preservation of the already existing products. The symptoms of syphilis that manifest themselves during this period, and are much less intense than the symptoms of the prior periods, have been termed by some, among whom we may mention Ricord, of Paris, *tertiary syphilis*. This, however, is incorrect; for in the whole course of syphilis there are only two *reproductive periods*, 1) the period of *conception* and *development* of the original cardinal or typical forms, and 2) the period of the *metamorphosed* primary or fundamental typical forms, together with all the phenomena in the different tissues of the organism belonging to the province of this metamorphosis. These last-mentioned phenomena are, all of them, included in the stage of evolution of secondary syphilis, and a constitutional syphilis is nothing else than a syphilis that has become stationary, and does not unfold any new phenomena, but rather enters upon a new stage of involution. A syphilis of this kind, so far from producing another series of new creations or metamorphoses, only develops such symptoms as are inherent in the development of secondary syphilis. Inasmuch as there is no third period of development in the life of syphilis, there cannot be any tertiary symptoms, and all those apparently tertiary symptoms that might possibly occur during the new process of involution, on the part of the constitutional syphilis, must of necessity belong to secondary syphilis. We might indeed talk, in some respects, if not of tertiary syphilis and tertiary symptoms, of a third or even fourth stage in the general course of syphilis; but even in such a case the phenomena of constitutional syphilis would belong to the secondary period, and to no other syphilitic evolution, as may be readily seen from the following list of the different stages which this disease runs:

FIRST PERIOD.

Primary Syphilis, with local symptoms: PRIMARY PRODUCTS.

1ST STAGE: *Ulcerous condition of the Primary Ulcers:* Primary phenomena.

2D STAGE: *Condylomatous or Fungoid Growths*, and consecutive local phenomena, in the place of the primary ulcers transferred by art from the original spot of communication to other localities: Consecutive phenomena.

SECOND PERIOD.

Secondary Syphilis, with general, new phenomena: SECONDARY PRODUCTS.

1ST STAGE: *Evolution* and appearance of a variety of new forms, being signs of a true metamorphosis of the primary disease: GENERAL SYPHILIS.

2D STAGE: Completed evolution of these phenomena, and retrogression of the general phenomena towards a localization of the same forms: CONSTITUTIONAL SYPHILIS.

Thus we may establish four different kinds of phenomena, 1) *primary*, 2) *consecutive*, 3) *secondary*, and 4) *constitutional*, an arrangement that excludes for the present *tertiary* and *quaternary* products, until a new metamorphosis or evolution of syphilis, succeeding the secondary period, shall have been demonstrated.

Sec. 198.—Remarks on the Symptoms of the Four Stages of Syphilis.

The distinction of the above-mentioned four stages of syphilis is of importance in other respects. The dispute concerning the contagious or non-contagious character of the products of secondary syphilis, that has been raging for a long time, is well known; as far as we ourselves are concerned, it is our opinion (see § 184) that no truly secondary product is contagious. Here, too, we adhere to this opinion, but at the same time reiterate the advice that *consecutive* phenomena, which still appertain to the primary period of chancre, should not be confounded with secondary phenomena originating in a metamorphosis of the chancre. A misapprehension of this kind unfortunately occurs quite frequently, even in "Rueckert's Klinischen Erfahrungen." What has had its being previous to this metamorphosis, and has originated in a purely metastatic transfer of the chancre or mucous tubercles to other parts on the skin, mucous membranes or lymphatic glands—in other words, all truly *primary* (*primitive* as well as *consecutive* prototypical) forms, all chancres, mucous tubercles, figwarts, and buboes, transmit the infection at all times and without fail, no matter whether chancres are seated on the sexual organs or in the throat, or whether the latter are located in the inguinal region or in the axilla, or any where else. This distinction is of particular importance as regards the phenomena appearing in the throat and around the anus, which hitherto, unless they had originated in a direct contact with the infectious matter, have always been numbered among the secondary phenomena, many of which may be nothing but consecutive primary phenomena, transferred to those localities by virtue of a process of metastasis. In order, therefore, to render all misapprehension absolutely impossible, even for those who do not know what is, and what is not, primary or secondary syphilis; and inasmuch as, after what has been said, we can express ourselves more definitely, we will here condense the statement we have enunciated in § 184, in the following two general propositions:

a) All fundamental or prototypical forms, products of the primary action of syphilis—hence all chancres, mucous tubercles, figwarts, and gonorrhœa; in general, all products that can be shown to be immediate results of infection,—transmit the contagion absolutely and at all times, no matter where they are located, and whether they have made their appearance as primitive or consecutive phenomena.

b) All products that owe their origin to the secondary action of syphilis subsequent to a previous metamorphosis of the prototypical forms—hence all tetters, rhagades, pustules, tubercles, and other ulcerations, and in general, all products that cannot be shown to be the immediate results of infection, and can only be produced by a process of metamorphosis,—are incapable of transmitting the infection to healthy persons.

Yet, although the products of secondary syphilis have evidently lost their power of reproduction, yet they still possess the power to perpetuate themselves in the affected organism, by putting forth new sprouts; as well as the power to transmit hereditary syphilis, which power they seem to retain even during the period of involution of constitutional syphilis, since the facts so far known, and those that we have mentioned §§ 186–188, satisfactorily show that syphilis may be transmitted to the offspring even by parents in whom every vestige of a former constitutional syphilis had disappeared from the sphere of phenomenal observation. It is, however, remarkable that during an involution of this character the syphilitic disease will sometimes reappear again in one of its prototypical forms, most frequently under the form of mucous tubercles. It is difficult to decide when this power to transmit the syphilitic disease to the offspring becomes extinct in an individual afflicted with constitutional syphilis, or whether this power ever ceases; we do not even know any thing positively certain regarding the duration of this last-named period.

III. TERMINATIONS OF SYPHILIS.

Sec. 199.—Termination in Recovery.

If many Old-School authors continue to assert, even to this day, that syphilis can get well spontaneously, without the assistance of art, they either mean by such a spontaneous cure the momentary disappearance of a few isolated forms of the disease, or else they blindly copy one from the other, or assert that which they know to be false. It is not only possible, but an established fact, that several syphilitic exanthems, and certain primary ulcers, called "*fugitive chancres*," disappear of themselves after a certain period; even the Hunterian chancre, after having passed from the stage of ulceration into that of fungoid growth, may finally dry up and cicatrize without leaving any thing else behind than a hard, globular, copper-colored elevation at the place where it had been located. But to call this a cure, not only of the chancre, but of the syphilis itself, either implies ignorance of what is to be understood by curing, or ignorance of the syphilis itself. That, after such a disappearance or cicatrization of isolated products, the whole syphilitic process is not extirpated, is not only shown by the fact that, after a shorter or longer period of time subsequent to this disappearance, other forms of the disease break out; but likewise by this other fact that, after a chancre is removed from the sexual organs by cauterization, it soon breaks out again in the throat or in other localities. It would be desirable to determine by experiments—on criminals, for instance, who, being condemned to death, might be pardoned for such a purpose—what becomes of syphilis, if it passes through all its stages without any interference whatsover; for, in order to decide the question whether syphilis, after having reached its constitutional form, finally becomes extinct of itself, the clinical observations that have been made so far, are not sufficient, since in all cases where the disease seems to have been thoroughly eradicated, the resources of art have been more or less instrumental in accomplishing this object. But even if the natural, spontaneous decrease of the signs of syphilis to their final reduction to a latent form, should be a demonstrated fact, the question would still remain open whether syphilis indeed dies out entirely, or whether its root, even after every outward sign has vanished, still remains alive, like a perennial plant, to the very end of organic life, and, under certain circumstances—for instance, after violent emotions, acute fevers, severe injuries, and such like causes—may sprout forth again years after it had left the sphere of phenomenal manifestation: so that it would be nonsense to talk of the disease having terminated in health. Indeed, wherever a radical, rational treatment has not been pursued with a view of destroying the very root of the parasite, great uncertainty regarding the thoroughness of the apparent cure must continue to prevail. Even in cases where a cure with specific antidotes seems to have been achieved, a rest of disease often remains that might be mistaken for syphilis, but very frequently is nothing more than some organic malformation, such as a cicatrix after large wounds, or badly healed fractures, etc., which had remained after the removal of the syphilitic disorganizations, for the reason that the affected organ had so far deviated from its normal condition that it was found impossible to restore it. In this class belong some indolent swellings of bones remaining subsequent to syphilitic caries, or sycosic malformations of the mucous membrane on the prepuce, etc.; or mercurial ulcers may remain in consequence of the treatment that had been pursued, which are no longer syphilitic.

Sec. 200.—Termination in Fatal Cachexia.

The termination of syphilis in death, which was quite common about the time when the disease first made its appearance on the stage of human ailments, occurs but seldom at the present time, at least not directly, as is the case with typhus, smallpox, or other diseases which, having reached the highest degree of intensity, either destroy life by paralyzing the central organs of vital action, or, even after the disease is removed, often leave the patient so weak that he has not got strength enough left to live. Nevertheless, several authors talk even to this day of a general syphilitic cachexia. Although, in most cases that are related of such cachexias, Mercury seems to have played a much more conspicuous part than syphilis, yet Cazenave, of Paris, relates a case that indeed did not terminate fatally, but came very near it. In this case the disease had progressed so far, that the patient was not only covered all over with syphilitic pustules, tubercles, and ulcers, and had sunk into a state of extreme marasmus, with a withering and sallow skin, but was likewise seized with such a violent, colliquative diarrhœa, that death seemed inevitable, and was only prevented by prompt and appropriate treatment. According to other authors it happens, even to this day, that patients, after protracted sufferings, and covered with syphilitic exanthems, deprived of their speech, hearing, smell, and even vision, sink into a state of extreme emaciation, with a lax, dry, sallow skin, and with a peculiar fetor emanating from their bodies, until they are attacked with incurable diarrhœa and hectic fever, that puts an end to their misery, among all the signs of a most perfect decomposition of their fluids. Even if death from syphilis does not always result in this *direct* manner, in consequence of a general progress of the disease, yet it may result in another *indirect* manner. Such fatal terminations may take place, if the existing ulcers, by corroding large vessels, give rise to hæmorrhages that cannot be arrested. Death may likewise be superinduced by the pressure of exostoses on the inner wall of the skull-bones upon the brain, whose functional activity is thereby paralyzed; one of my patients died in Baden-Baden of the consequences of such an exostosis. The same thing may result, if the skull-bones become perforated by syphilitic caries, and the brain itself is injured by the ulcerative process. Cases where syphilitic ulcerations of the larynx can superinduce a fatal ulceration of this organ, as well as cases where death may take place from destruction of the cervical vertebræ, in consequence of chancrous ulcers in the fauces, are well known, and have been mentioned by us in other parts of this work. Less frequent are cases of a fatal destruction of the uterus, caused by ulcers on the neck of this organ. What authors relate of the transformation of syphilis into carcinoma of the womb, may be correct in so far as the syphilitic disease may rouse a cancerous diathesis into activity; nevertheless, syphilis cannot be transformed into cancer; if death should result in such a case, it is caused by cancer, not syphilis. Beside these cases, syphilis, even if it should not attain a high degree of development, may destroy life in consequence of sleep being prevented by agonizing sufferings, or in consequence of extensive suppurations or hectic fever; or, finally, in consequence of the gummata in lungs, liver, heart, and stomach, of which Virchow has given us a description; all such causes may lead to such vast disturbances in the vital functions, that death must necessarily ensue unless help should still be possible.

Sec. 201.—Transition of Syphilis into other Diseases.

There are physicians who not only persist in asserting that syphilis can pass into scrofulosis, even during the life-time of the organism, but likewise in believing that children, born of syphilitic parents, may be born *scrofulous* instead of syphilitic; some even go so far as to assert that scrofulosis is nothing else than hereditary syphilis. A physician who starts such doctrines, neither knows the history of diseases, nor is he acquainted with what is understood by a special disease depending upon some *specific* principle; otherwise he would know that scrofula has been just as frequent as it now is, even prior to all syphilitic manifestations, and that a specific disease cannot be transformed into another specific diathesis, any more than a cat can be changed into a dog. Altogether, even as Hunter correctly observes, syphilis is never *transformed* into, any more than it *coalesces* with, another disease. In herpetic, scorbutic, and scrofulous individuals, the various products of syphilis, and of the natural diathesis, can be seen associated side by side with each other, without a single one of them losing its specific character. The only thing that may take place, and, indeed, does take place, is, that syphilis may, like any other powerful invasion of the organism, rouse a latent, but already existing diathesis from its slumbering state, and that this diathesis, as soon as the syphilitic disease has become somewhat subdued, may seem to take the place of the latter, without any sort of transformation from the latter into the former having taken place to any extent whatsoever. In this sense syphilitic buboes may continue, in the form of scrofulous buboes, in scrofulous subjects; if, in such cases, the syphilitic disease had assumed the essential character of scrofula, no specific remedy for the syphilitic bubo would be required; the syphilitic disease, having been transformed into scrofula, would yield to an anti-scrofulous treatment. As a general rule, the morbid dispositions which syphilis excites into active manifestation, do not break forth until some time after the syphilis is cured; very frequently, however, they become manifest towards the termination of the cure, or perhaps do not owe their awakening to syphilis, but to the insensate masses of Mercury, Iodine, Iodide of Potassium, and other powerful agents with which Old-School physicians sometimes drench their patients, as if they were chemical retorts; it is even possible that many of the so-called sequelæ of syphilis, which likewise occur under improper homœopathic treatment, are caused by excessive doses of Mercurial Iodides, Phosphorus, Nitric acid, etc.; such sequelæ may constitute a sort of pseudo-syphilis, and, in reality, may be nothing else than medicinal diseases. However, in whatsoever manner certain original morbid dispositions become roused, be it by the syphilis itself, or by the tumultuous manner in which this disease is treated, the diseases thus roused into action, such as tubercular suppurations of the lungs, scrofulous glandular swellings, affections of bones, cancerous ulcerations, etc., continue to exist, by virtue of their own specific cause, long after the syphilis had been cured; but, in such a case, will only manifest their own special characteristic properties, and none of those of the syphilitic disease. Even if this disease should not have been entirely eradicated, but should continue to betray its existence by the occasional outbreak of constitutional symptoms, these latter will always appear perfectly distinct from the symptoms of scrofula, and will be clearly recognizable by their own specific forms.

IV. OF THE INFLUENCE WHICH OTHER CIRCUMSTANCES EXERT UPON THE DEVELOPMENT, COURSE, AND TERMINATION OF SYPHILIS.

Sec. 202.—Age, Sex, and Conditions of Life.

Regarding the different circumstances that may exert an influence upon the development and ultimate shape of syphilis, very little is said that can be considered positive. The teachings of pathological manuals, in reference to this matter, are so general and unmeaning, that it would seem as though their authors had preferred filling their columns with insignificant statements and hypothetical inferences rather than to devote their space to something more useful and tangible. Nevertheless, a few sensible remarks concerning these influences can be uttered, were they nothing else than simple criticisms suggested by the aforesaid manuals.

Influence of age.—There is no doubt that syphilis is much worse and more dangerous among children than among adults. The danger is equally great, no matter whether the disease is contracted at birth, or at the moment of conception, or had been transmitted as an hereditary condition. Exostoses, ophthalmic affections, and diseases of the throat, are indeed less frequent among children. Syphilitic exanthems are of more frequent occurrence, more particularly *pemphigus*, which is the most dangerous disease of this class; but even without such an eruption, all such infants sink very readily under a general cachexia. Past the age of pubescence, the danger resulting from syphilitic infection decreases, but increases again in proportion as individuals grow older. If the danger among young people is less, it is not only because the syphilitic disease, among this class of patients, runs a less dangerous course, but likewise because the forms of syphilis to which young people are liable, are in themselves of a milder type than the forms of syphilis which are more exclusively confined to persons of a more advanced age. The more frequent occurrence of secondary syphilis among young people than among old, is not owing to age, but to the fact that young people are more reckless and less mindful of the consequences of neglect or improper treatment than older persons.

Sex.—Among females, the primary as well as the secondary forms of syphilis are much milder than among males. Among the former we find, in Paris at least, proportionally fewer chancres than mucous tubercles and figwarts, together with symptomatic gonorrhœa. I have known young men affected with Hunterian chancre communicate the disease to female friends, in whom it resulted in the breaking out of superficial chancres or syphilitic erosions that soon began to change to fungoid excrescences, associated with a number of small mucous tubercles on the neighboring parts, and with symptomatic gonorrhœa, the whole of which symptoms were rapidly cured with *Cinnabaris.* Nobody can imagine how such excrescences prevail among the young prostitutes of Paris, who fancy themselves attacked only with gonorrhœa; this being a fact, we cannot wonder that the French blennorrhagia so often entails sad consequences upon the patient. This is the reason why the young men in Paris are much more frequently attacked with gonorrhœa and figwarts, than with simple idiopathic gonorrhœa.

Social condition.—If we may judge of the statistical tables arranged by writers on syphilis, the various trades and professions do not exert any visible influence on the shape and course of syphilis; but the social circumstances of the patient, in other respects, do exert such an influence. It is quite natural that secondary syphilis among the poorer classes occurs much more frequently than among the more opulent classes. The latter have the means of taking better care of their health; whereas the privations, the cares, the bad food, the hard work, the unhealthy dwellings, and the poor and scanty living of the working classes, constitute some of the main causes that aggravate the syphilitic disease among the latter.

Sec. 203.—Climate, Seasons, Weather.

If pathological manuals teach the doctrine, that the syphilis of warm climates is less malignant, and generally embodies itself in the shape of some cutaneous affection; whereas in the cold climate, we have more diseases of the mucous membranes and affections of bones—this doctrine is indeed confirmed by a large number of undeniable facts. If Northerners move into a southern climate, their syphilitic ailments decrease perceptibly in a very short period, and soon disappear entirely for some time; on the other hand, if the inhabitants of southern climes move northward, they frequently witness a new outbreak of syphilis, even after it had become all but latent. French soldiers, for instance, who have contracted syphilis in Africa, Naples, Madrid, Algiers, and Mexico, after their return home, become subject to severe aggravations of their complaint, which obstinately resists all the means employed against it. But if our manuals teach that the syphilitic disease is *cured* in the above-mentioned countries without Mercury, by the mere use of sudorifics and purgatives, all we have to say is that this is no cure, but only a reduction of the disease to a latent condition; otherwise it could not break out again after the patient's travel from a warm climate into a colder one. It is likewise wrong to assert, as some of our pathological manuals do, that, if the form of syphilis be milder in warm countries, on the other hand, the inhabitants of those countries are more susceptible to the syphilitic contagium; in proof of which, they assert the fact that one half of the inhabitants of Spain and Italy are affected with syphilis. It is true that syphilis is more frequent in the South than in the North; but this greater frequency is not owing to an increased susceptibility, but to an extraordinary looseness of morals, and to the recklessness with which the people in those countries expose themselves to syphilitic contagion; so that, if all these men and women, with a single syphilitic individual amongst them, were suddenly transferred to the frigid zone, their condition, as regards the spread and violence of the syphilitic disease, would probably be the same as among the natives. Even here in Paris, the ardent and inconsiderate sojourners from warm climates are much more frequently attacked with the syphilitic disease than our cold and more discreetly-indulging natives. The assertion that gonorrhœa is more frequent in warm, and chancre more frequent in cold climates, likewise has to be modified so far as this, that the gonorrhœa of warm climates is not our simple, idiopathic gonorrhœa, but a gonorrhæa depending upon mucous tubercles, of which we have already stated in the preceding paragraph that it is quite common in Paris. It is likewise incorrect to assert that syphilis occurs more frequently in warm than in cold seasons. A statistical table, now lying before us, shows that, of 112 cases of syphilis, 11 to 14 occurred in each of the months of December, January, March, April and June; 7 to 9 in each of the months of February, May, August, October, and November; and only 4 to 5 in July and September. These numbers show conclusively that, in respect to this point, our pathological manuals are entirely mistaken. Of greater importance is undoubtedly the influence of the epidemic genius of certain seasons upon the prevalence of certain forms of syphilis; although, even in this respect, existing statistics do not furnish any definite results, and whatever has to be said on this subject, has to be viewed in the light of theoretic hypothesis, rather than in the light of carefully-verified facts.

Sec. 204.—Individual Morbid Dispositions and other Morbid Influences.

We have already observed in previous chapters, that individuality acts an important part in the diversity prevailing among the different forms of syphilis; in this respect, it is certain that natural morbid dispositions should not be overlooked. We are not prepared to determine whether scrofulous individuals are more frequently affected with gonorrhœa than with chancre; at all events, it is certain that impetiginous forms and affections of the osseous system occur more frequently among scrofulous individuals than among other classes of patients; what is beyond doubt is, that syphilis, if it attacks feeble, sickly, cachectic individuals, is very apt to assume a very malignant character. On the contrary, if vigorous individuals, affected with some chronic malady, are attacked with syphilis, both diseases, instead of combining into one, will be found to run a parallel course; syphilitic affections may coexist side by side with scabies, arthritis, herpetic eruptions, and the like. At this very moment, I am treating a patient for syphilitic roseola, upon whom the remains of an old furfuraceous herpes are distinctly visible. The case is different if acute diseases, like measles, scarlatina, smallpox, typhus, etc., supervene during the course of syphilis. In such a case, the further course of syphilis is generally suspended until the new disease has run its course. This suspension is sometimes carried so far—more particularly on the part of smallpox and typhus—that even chancres, buboes, mucous tubercles, gonorrhœa, exanthems, etc., disappear entirely, while the acute disease is running its course, a fact that has given rise to the idea that typhus and variola have power to destroy the whole syphilitic process in its very germ. This, however, is not the case; the morbid process had only been suspended; even if the suspended primary phenomena do not reappear, the syphilis is not on that account eradicated, but, as I know from personal observation, secondary phenomena break out sooner or later, after the typhus or smallpox has run its course, or even during the period of convalescence; and these secondary phenomena increase in intensity, in proportion as the patient gains in strength. In some cases, these secondary symptoms do not break out till some time after every vestige of the acute disease has entirely vanished. It may even happen that, if such an acute disease breaks out while the organism harbors a masked constitutional syphilis in its tissues, the supervention of an acute disease may occasion an outbreak of the syphilitic disease; any other non-epidemic, but purely accidental disease, may have the same result. A violent catarrhal fever, a considerable derangement of the stomach, a severe mechanical injury attended with wound-fever, a fever-and-ague, in short, any thing that may give rise to some disease, such as violent emotions, intoxication, excessive physical exertions, hard labor, etc., may cause secondary syphilis to leave its latent condition, and to become an active and manifest disease. Whether the prevailing genius of disease contributes something to give shape to the syphilitic malady, in this sense, for instance, that, if catarrhs or sore throats prevail, syphilitic diseases of the mucous membranes are more frequent; or if erysipelatous inflammations prevail, exanthematic forms constitute the ruling manifestations of syphilis; yea, whether, as some pretend, the present increase of syphilitic diseases has its origin in the epidemic scarlatina of 1820 and 1821, we are unable to prove by arguments; these have yet to be furnished by those who have started such a very broad assertion. From a theoretical point of view, this seems, indeed, possible, and even comprehensible; however, what seems *possible* is not, on that account, always *real*, more particularly with regard to syphilis, which runs, anyhow, a very capricious course.

Sec. 205.—Dietetic and Medical Influences.

If some authors, relying on the popular measures against syphilis enacted in the year 1524 by the public authorities; and relying, moreover, upon the apparently favorable results of the starvation-cure, maintain that nothing is more favorable to the development and strengthening of syphilis than an invigorating diet, and strong beverages, and if they quote among the list of these dangerous articles such things as chocolate, ham, roast-veal, etc., we feel bound, in common with all enlightened homœopaths, to oppose such wild theories. So far as I am concerned, I have never seen the least injury result from a wholesome, nourishing diet. I have cured the worst kind of chancre by appropriate homœopathic treatment, more speedily and thoroughly, notwithstanding the patient enjoyed the best kind of food, than the boasted starvation-cure has ever been able to accomplish; for, even if the virulence of the disease should seem somewhat lessened, under the influence of such a proceeding, it returns again in all its original vehemence, in proportion as the patient regains his strength by resuming his former diet. That all excesses in eating and drinking, especially the immoderate use of spirituous beverages, favor the progress of syphilis, is so self-evident, that it seems unnecessary to dwell upon such a point. What, however, cannot be impressed upon the attention of physicians with too much force, is the fact, that large doses of improper medicines, or even of the most appropriate and specifically-curative medicines, promote the spread of syphilitic ulceration. Although this truth has been frequently proclaimed, even by old-school physicians, yet it unfortunately remains unheeded, even by many so-called homœopathic practitioners, who boldly assert the doctrine that Mercury, Iodine, Phosphorus, etc., may be given in large doses, without aggravating the disease, and that all such seeming aggravations are mere natural exacerbations of the malady, that have to be met by still larger quantities of the medicine. What other physicians, of the so-called philosophico-natural school, write of substances friendly to syphilis, and of other substances hostile to syphilis, some of which—like Mercury, Gold, Copper, Arsenic, Lead, Sal-ammoniac, and other preparations of Kali—always exert a *curative* influence; whereas others—such as Iron, the Carbonates, Cinchona, Angustura, substances containing Tannin, and likewise Phosphorus, Sulphur, and other agents having power to destroy the metallic character—exert a hurtful influence, favorable to the promotion of syphilitic growths: such doctrines, beside containing many germs of truth, yet are so replete with baseless theories, that we cannot subscribe to them as indiscriminately as they are authoritatively presented in allopathic treatises. Even the high reputation of the sulphur-baths of Aix-la-Chapelle, as restorers of a masked syphilis, seems to me only partially merited. I have seen patients return from such baths with an apparently restored syphilitic exanthem, which, however, upon closer examination, proved to be a true sulphur-eruption, that had been falsely diagnosed by the allopathic attendant as a syphilitic exanthem. As regards the salts of Chlorine, I am prepared to confirm the universally-received opinion, that the emanations of the sea, and hence sea-voyages, are almost always prejudical to syphilitic patients, and impart, more particularly to primary ulcers, or to bad forms of secondary syphilis, a very malignant and obstinate character. This remark likewise applies to salt diet. If, in the first period of Homœopathy, Hahnemann's disciples interdicted every species of salted or smoked meat, this strictness—although, as a general rule, the dietetic rules of Homœopathy are much less rigid now than they used to be—had better be kept up, so far as the treatment of syphilis is concerned. The exclusion of herrings, dried cod-fish, ham, salt meat, oysters, mussels, and the like, from the table of syphilitic patients, can only redound to their advantage, for the additional reason that these articles of diet do not constitute a strictly wholesome nourishment. Whether, as some assert, syphilitic ulcers are made worse by the use of crabs, and other kinds of shell-fish, or by the use of pork and goose-flesh, I am unable to say; at any rate, no patient will get hurt by abstaining from the use of these articles. We shall discuss these points more fully in the next division of this work, where we shall likewise introduce a few general diagnostic and therapeutic considerations that seem to us deserving of a careful perusal by those who desire to combat syphilis with success.

FOURTH DIVISION.

GENERAL THERAPEUTIC OBSERVATIONS

ON THE

TREATMENT OF SYPHILIS.

CHAPTER FIRST.

GENERAL DIAGNOSTIC REMARKS.

I. MASKED SYPHILIS.

Sec. 206.—General Syphilitic Diagnostic Signs.

We have seen that syphilis, in its secondary period, may manifest itself in a thousand different shapes, and in every tissue of the organism, and may even continue to exist, in a latent form, after every perceptible sign of the disease has disappeared, and the organism seems to be perfectly free from it. Some extraordinary event, severe injury, a dangerous acute disease, a deeply-penetrating emotion, and the like, may again rouse it into action; or, even if it should remain in its latent form, it may be transmitted to the offspring. In the former divisions of this work, we have shown, very fully and satisfactorily, we imagine, in what forms the syphilitic disease chiefly manifests itself, either in its *primary* or *secondary* period; all that remains for us to do on this occasion is, to add some remarks concerning *latent* or *masked* syphilis, which, in its primary period, sometimes assumes the form of gonorrhœa, and, in its secondary period, is destitute of every sign of outward manifestation. As regards the first of these two points, we have already, when speaking of the different forms of gonorrhœa (§16), mentioned the signs by which the symptomatic syphilitic gonorrhœa is distinguished from the simple idiopathic form of this disease, but deem it necessary to revert again to this point, because, in our estimation, nothing can be more hurtful to the patient than that these two kinds of gonorrhœa should be confounded with each other. With physicians who do not suppress the discharge by means of injections, but treat every case of gonorrhœa with internal remedies, the danger is, of course, much less, since, under such treatment, if the discharge is of a syphilitic nature, other diagnostic signs of the syphilitic character of the disease will not fail to make their appearance, as may have been seen in the cases related in § 174. Nevertheless, it behooves every physician to be on his guard in managing a case of gonorrhœa, more particularly when no sign of inflammation seems to be perceptible, and the case belongs in the category of the so-called *gonorrhœa torpida.* The slighter the pain, the less considerable the discharge, the less marked the inflammatory symptoms, the more this apparent mildness of the disease should be distrusted, and the more mindful we should be of the proverb, that "still waters run deep." Nevertheless, these are not the worst cases, for here the physician will have at least one suspicious symptom that appeals to his watchfulness and care. But what about cases where, after the syphilitic disease has been apparently cured, its root is still so deeply planted in the organism, that the disease is transmitted to the offspring; that the milk of nurses thus tainted often communicates to their nurslings the germs of the most hideous and dangerous forms of the syphilitic plague?

How shall the physician, under such circumstances, proceed, in order to become cognizant of the true condition of his patients; and what answer shall he return to those who inquire of him whether they need not fear any relapses; whether it is safe for them to marry, and whether their children will not be born with any syphilitic taint? If no outward sign of disease is any longer present, it is evident that the diagnosis can no longer rest upon pathological phenomena, but has to be determined by therapeutic means. The question, therefore, will be, whether among the different modes of treatment, by means of which the primary or secondary symptoms of the disease had been removed, there is one which, by virtue of its own inherent essence and fixedness, furnishes satisfactory evidence that the root of the disease has been so completely and unmistakably eradicated from the organism, that it cannot possibly germinate anew, and produce another syphilitic monster. It is well known that the different modes of treatment employed against syphilis only secure a superficial removal of the syphilitic phenomena, and preclude the possibility of a thorough eradication of the syphilitic poison; but, supposing that all signs of syphilis have been removed by the most judicious internal treatment, how do we know that the treatment has been sufficient, and by what evidence is this to be determined? If there is any uncertainty regarding the sufficiency of treatment, by what signs can this uncertainty be cleared up? These are questions that we will now proceed to examine more in detail.

Sec. 207.—Evidence of a Sure Cure.

The older French physicians, more especially Louvrier, Lafecteur, and Fabre, adopted the theory that the disease must terminate in some crisis, or in critical evacuations, such as ptyalism, sweat, diarrhœa, or a copious flow of urine; they maintained that, wherever such critical evacuations had not taken place, the cure that had apparently been obtained, could not be depended upon. Hence the mercurial cures of former times, that were carried to the worst extremes of ptyalism; and the use of purgatives for the purpose of securing critical evacuations of the poisonous matter by the bowels, in case they did not occur spontaneously during the inunction-cure. Other physicians sought to obtain critical eliminations by the use of sudorifics, and others again by acting upon the bladder through diuretics. In spite of such critical evacuations, experience showed that a radical cure of the disease could no more be depended upon than if such evacuations did not take place, and it is therefore questionable whether the syphilitic disease cannot be radically cured without such critical changes being secured. I can point to cases in my own practice, where the first signs of an improvement subsequent to the administration of two half-grain doses of the first centesimal trituration of *Mercurius* for obstinate or malignant chancres, were attended with a copious flow of urine for two or three days, or where, in other cases, the improvement was initiated with slight febrile movements about dusk, followed by tolerably profuse night-sweats. In one case, where two inflamed buboes were present at the same time, the coincidence of a critical improvement and a profuse night-sweat was so remarkable that in the very night when the sweat broke out the buboes diminished in size to a considerable extent, and the cure could be fairly dated from this change. If a crisis takes place in every case of cure of the syphilitic disease, it is often so inconsiderable—since the body is not drenched with a barrelful of poison—that most patients, who never watch the symptoms very closely, are not aware of it; at all events, if such critical changes occur subsequently to the exhibition of our small doses, they are not the cause but the consequence of a radical destruction and elimination of the virus. Such changes, brought about as it were by a re-awakening of the reactive energies of the organism, do not prove anything in favor of any artificially-produced critical evacuations. These so-called *crises* do not, therefore, furnish sufficient evidence that the disease has been really cured; if produced by the small doses of Homœopathy, these crises are not sufficiently marked to afford adequate scope for observation; whereas evacuations consequent upon the use of massive quantities of non-specific drugs, have no critical significance whatsoever. It is well known that in 1788, Hahnemann regarded the supervention of a mercurial fever as an indispensable proof that the virus was properly eliminated; and that even as late as 1816, he held that some perceptible mercurial effects were necessary, in order to secure the perfect reliability of a cure; afterwards, however, he abandoned this ground entirely, and taught that, to constitute a perfect cure, it was sufficient that, after the exclusively-internal use of the smallest possible doses of Mercury, the chancre gradually commenced to become cleansed, and to heal spontaneously as it were, without leaving behind a single trace of discoloration of the skin. Indeed, until now, this has remained the safest and most reliable criterium of a radical cure, more particularly if such a change is accompanied by an increased appetite and a heightened buoyancy of feeling and a perception of well-being, as after a severe and protracted malady. If, after a pretended cure, a hard, uneven, badly-colored cicatrix, or a dirty, unnatural color of the skin remains behind, and if the general feeling of health is not such as it should be, and always is, after a severe sickness has been radically overcome by proper treatment, we may rest assured that the cure is not reliable, and that every imaginable kind of trouble may remain in store for the poor sufferer.

Sec. 208.—Syphilitic Reagents.

But it is not always with such specific remedies that a cure of the venereal phenomena is effected in this rational manner; but, even in such a case, after using for a certain period of time more or less adequate or inadequate means of treatment, the most striking primary or secondary phenomena may disappear, and the disease, as we have seen in §§ 196, 197, may enter upon the stage of involution of secondary syphilis, and may assume the *masked form* of which we are here speaking, and where, notwithstanding that every sign of the syphilitic disease has vanished from the sphere of observation, this disease still continues to exist, as it were, in a state of slumber. While the disease exists in this condition, several physicians, in order to become sure what they might have to expect or to fear from it, have proposed the use of certain *syphilitic reagents*, which, when introduced into a body affected with latent syphilis, compel the disease, in a very short time, to show itself in broad daylight. With this view, Swediaur already directed attention to *Iron*, other physicians to the Sulphate and Phosphate of Soda. However, the facts which these authors adduce to support their assertions are not sufficient to shed light on the point in dispute, since the result obtained is confined to the well-known phenomenon that, when ulcers, concerning whose mercurial or syphilitic nature there is a doubt, are painted with solutions of the above-mentioned substances, the ulcers very soon show their true nature, the mercurial ulcers healing very soon after, the syphilitic, on the contrary, becoming very much aggravated. Without entering upon a critical analysis of this statement, which has been introduced into almost every treatise on Pathology, we content ourselves with pointing out the fact, that we do not require a reagent by means of which mercurial and syphilitic ulcers can be distinguished from each other, but one that shall bring the masked syphilis to light again. The physicians of the naturalistic school have named as such reagents: 1) Sulphur, Phosphorus, and most of the Carbonates; 2) China, Angustura, Cascarilla, and other astringents, etc. As regards Sulphur, and more especially the world-renowned Sulphur-baths of Aix-la-Chapelle, we have already expressed our opinion regarding them in § 205; in the same manner we may admit that Phosphorus, the Carbonates and tannin-containing substances, will, by their continued use in excessive quantities, not only cause exanthems, but ulcers of every description; but if one would regard these effects, without any further examination of their diagnostic value and meaning, as signs of a re-awakened syphilis, he would be very much mistaken. Considering how often homœopathic physicians employ Sulphur,

Phosphorus, both kinds of Charcoal, and other similar remedies, with the best success, both for consecutive and secondary syphilitic phenomena, it must be plain to any one how little these purely theoretical conjectures of the Naturalistic School can be depended upon in practice. It is indeed questionable whether masked syphilis can be at all roused from its latent condition by any known substance. I know of but one case from my own practice, where a single dose of *Arsenicum*, three pellets of the thirtieth attenuation, seemed to have an effect of this kind. It was the case of a boy ten years old, whose father, previous to his marriage, had caught a chancre on two different occasions, which had been removed with caustics, and with large doses of the Iodide of Potassium internally. The boy's sister had died of syphilitic pemphigus shortly after her birth. In consequence of a slight injury, a sore broke out on the tibia, which soon degenerated into a suspicious-looking, but not yet distinctly-characterized tetter, for which I administered Arsenicum. Three days after exhibiting this remedy, the whole body became covered with a characteristic, syphilitic, lichenoid exanthem. I cannot say that I attach much diagnostic value to this case.

Sec. 209.—Suspicious Symptoms.

Strictly speaking, a few suspicious signs might perhaps be pointed out. This was likewise the opinion of the older physicians. Although these signs are not definitely characteristic, and do not even occur in every case of masked syphilis, yet they do manifest themselves in some cases, and afterwards confirm their syphilitic character by the fact that, through the operation of certain extraordinary causes, they very frequently assume an evident and unmistakable character of constitutional syphilis. Among these signs we number: A certain pale, faintish-white, or dirty-yellow complexion, with an unclean forehead; occasional breaking out of isolated pimples on the hairy scalp or in the whiskers, not itching, but scurfy; emaciation of the features, with dry coryza and crusty nostrils, or discharge of a fetid, purulent nasal mucus, without any distinct signs of a regular ozœna syphilitica; moreover, frequent attacks of a slight angina, with evening-hoarseness, ill-defined redness, and a varicose condition of the vessels; frequent appearance of erosions on the inner surface of the prepuce, without any definite character, soon disappearing again, never itching, and resembling herpes præputialis ; isolated attacks of bone-pains ; scattered appearance of isolated pustules or indurated pimples, which are scarcely noticed, and disappear again in a short time ; rhagades on the inside of the joints of the hands or fingers ; slight swellings of single bones, scarcely perceptible ; lowness of spirits, sadness. These symptoms do not occur simultaneously, but singly, and are generally so mild that they are overlooked by the patient, and that even the physician, unless he should have his suspicion, is disposed, on account of their ill-defined and imperfect development, to regard them as ordinary symptoms of an arthritic, scrofulous, rheumatic, or catarrhal disposition or diathesis, nntil they finally become more marked, and their true nature can no longer be misapprehended. Many sudden outbreaks of a syphilis that had been forgotten for years, are undoubtedly foreshadowed by such apparently trifling symptoms in the course of years ; their true nature remains unknown ; but, whenever several of them exist together, the physician will do well to keep his eyes wide open, and to institute careful and cautious inquiries into the past history of the patient's ailments. However, such inquiries should not be conducted with an anxious mind, nor should such symptoms lead the physician at once to jump at the conclusion that there is a latent syphilitic taint, except the character of each symptom reveals some undoubted analogy with corresponding syphilitic manifestations. In this respect, grave mistakes are committed by many pathological manuals, which present to their credulous readers even hæmorrhoids, dropsies, gastric ailments, chest and nervous affections, hæmorrhages, paralysis of the feet, steatomata on the neck and chest, occasional glandular swellings, etc., as symptoms of a latent syphilis. Of course, it is possible that all these affections may develop themselves as *consensual affections*, during the course of very violent venereal diseases where special organs have become involved ; of themselves, they cannot be regarded as symptoms of a latent syphilis, for the reason that they do not constitute idiopathic phenomena, either of the primary or secondary period of this disease ; on the contrary, belong to an entirely different range of diseases, and, if they occur in the syphilitic disease at all, constitute purely accidental disturbances. A symptom which, of itself, cannot take upon itself the characteristic appearance of a syphilitic phenomenon, cannot be regarded as a suspicious symptom ; a suspicion of this kind can only be properly entertained when several of these symptoms are present, and there is no other disease to which they could be traced as characteristic manifestations. Of far greater importance to a correct diagnosis are the symptoms occurring in children, including a correct discriminative distinction between mercurial and syphilitic symptoms, on which account we shall consider *infantile* and *mercurial* syphilis in two separate articles.

II. INFANTILE SYPHILIS.

Sec. 210.—General Symptoms.

We have already stated, in §§ 186–189, in what manner children may become affected with syphilis: 1) according to some authors, *at birth* (which we feel disposed to doubt, see § 213), while passing through the vagina and vulva where syphilitic ulcers are seated (*syphilis adnata*); or, 2) in consequence of one of the parents or both having syphilitic symptoms on the sexual parts at the moment of conception (*syphilis congenita*); or, 3) in consequence of father or mother, although apparently in perfect health, being tainted with latent syphilis (*syphilis hereditaria*). On this occasion, we have directed the reader's attention to the general symptoms by which hereditary syphilis is distinguished from congenital syphilis, as well as from that which is acquired at birth; nevertheless, we deem it advisable to once more present a cursory view of the symptoms which characterize infantile syphilis in either of the above-mentioned forms. In general, these symptoms are no other than the various symptoms that have been described in the preceding chapters as belonging to the primary and secondary forms of the venereal diseases; in the first place, however, some of these symptoms are particularly proper to children, and others assume a somewhat altered form when manifesting themselves on children, be this owing to the greater tenderness of their skins, or to other causes. Usually the mucous membranes are attacked first, next the outer integuments, afterwards the lymphatic glands, and, lastly, the bones; sometimes, however, all these different tissues simultaneously. If the mucous membranes are attacked, we see at their openings on the surface of the body either protopathic or consecutive discharges, ulcers, even true chancres, mucous tubercles, fig-warts, and fungoid growths; in the glandular system we have buboes, enlargements, or swellings of various kinds; and in the osseous system we discover exostoses and caries, which, however, occur less frequently than other derangements. According to the results which Diday and Bertin have obtained through observations continued for a long series of years, there have appeared: 1) *chancres* and other *ulcers* about the mouth, on the palate, tongue, shoulder-blades, umbilicus, labia majora, glans, and extremities; 2) *figwarts* and other vegetations, on the tongue, at the inferior commissure, in the vagina; 3) *syphilitic pustules and tubercles* on the head, chin, shoulders, chest, abdomen, labia majora, nates, thighs, and legs, arms, fingers, and toes; 4) *vesicular eruptions* on the neck and legs; 5) *swellings* and *buboes* on the head, neck, shoulders; 6) *discharges* from the nose and vagina.

What deserves especial notice in this kind of syphilis is the peculiar expression of all these children from the moment when these syphilitic phenomena first make their appearance. The skin, especially in the face, loses its transparency, looks dusky as if painted; the more this tint spreads the more marked it becomes. It is especially striking on the lower half of the forehead, on the nose, eyelids, cheeks; it occurs much less frequently on the more depressed portions of the face, for instance, in the inner canthi, the folds in the cheeks, etc. Even if this peculiar tint does not seem to extend over a large surface, yet the whole skin partakes of it more or less; the child becomes pale, of a yellowish hue, and the skin has a peculiar lack-lustre appearance, by which the syphilitic affection of such children, when seen at the breast, at once betrays itself. Sometimes this yellowish tint is so distinct that the skin seems covered with liver-spots; most generally, however, the tint is not very striking, so that it would scarcely be noticed but for the fact, that it is almost always accompanied by the peculiar lack-lustre appearance of the skin. Usually this tint is preceded by a general pallor, and requires from eight to ten days for its full development.

Sec. 211.—Cutaneous Affections.

In the case of syphilitic children, the skin symptoms show themselves first and foremost. Among them we distinguish:

1) The *pemphigus* of new-born infants, which we have described in the second division, and which usually breaks out in the palms of the hands, and on the soles of the feet, and consists of vesicles which, surrounded by a violet-red areola, reveal, after bursting, ulceration of the subjacent integuments.

2) The various *pustules* and *tubercles*, appearing either flattened, salient, tubercular, scurfy, ulcerated, or chancrous, the first-named of which, the so-called flat or mucous tubercles, mostly break out on the scalp, in the face, on the chin, scrotum, at the margin of the anus, on the thighs, hands, and feet; whereas the ulcerous, phagedænic tubercles sometimes cover both extremities.

3) *Chancres.* These are partly protopathic, partly consecutive, and, in their form, deviate but little from the known kinds; for here, too, they either occur as simple or as indurated, elevated, and phagedænic chancres. They occur most frequently at the frænulum of the tongue, on the velum palati, and in the fauces, in the shape of small, round, somewhat prominent vesicles that soon burst; whereas, if they occur on the inner surface of the cheeks, they appear in the shape of small cracks, and on the hands and feet in the shape of true rhagades; those that break out on the scalp and in the face are phagedænic, and soon terminate in fatal gangrene.

4) *Ulcers on the heels.* This is a peculiar affection of syphilitic children, commencing with redness and inflammation of the skin of the heel. This redness increases, the skin ulcerates, and whole patches of the cellular tissue under the coverings of the heel-bone become detached, so that the cushion forming the heel finally drops off entirely.

5) *Thickening of the skin of the palms of the hands and soles of the feet.* This is a species of psoriasis; the skin becomes rough, thick, shrivelled, like that of washerwomen; the affected parts swell up, assume a red or pale yellow color, the skin hardens, and shows more or less deep, sometimes ulcerated rhagades; at a later period scales form, which fall off, and then form anew, until this process stops entirely, and the whole of the indurated epidermis becomes detached. After this is accomplished, the affection

assumes a different form; the old epidermis is replaced by a new one of the thickness of a thin pellicle; feet and hands assume a dark-blue hue, especially around the finger and toe-nails; the nails soften, and trifling ulcerations sometimes break out all around. Next to the above-mentioned peculiar color of the skin, the dry coryza and the rhagades of the lips, this induration of the skin, according to Trousseau and Larègue, constitutes one of the most frequent phenomena of infantile syphilis.

6) *Rhagades on the lips and at the anus.* These cracks show themselves where the mucous membrane unites with the outer skin. They are located in the folds of the membrane, and are so much deeper and broader the further remote they are from the epidermis; their bright red and bleeding bottom, and their brown hue, imparts to the lips a very peculiar appearance. If no pustules have as yet formed in the corners of the mouth, they usually break out in the mesian line of the lips, generally in company with these pustules, and simultaneously with the dusky-black color of the skin; and often become the direct cause of a transmission of the syphilitic disease to the nipples of the nurse.

7) *Syphilitic roseola.* This exanthem resembles measles, but is much darker and exceedingly fugitive; remains only four or five days, but is always the precursor of much more troublesome phenomena, since the copper spots, after becoming more marked, do not delay changing to pustules and afterwards to ulcers.

8) *Figwarts.* These break out very seldom on infants, and, if at all, generally are found located on the mucous membranes. They are likewise seen around the anus, on the outer surface of the labia majora, or between the sexual organs and the thighs.

9) *Erysipelatous exanthems.* The skin is wrinkled, covered with brown-yellow pimples, and erysipelatous spots; here and there the epidermis becomes raised, or it may even become raised over the whole body and suffer destruction; at the same time the face and whole body show the *emaciated appearance of old age*, which is so exceedingly characteristic of the syphilitic affections of children.

Sec. 212.—Affections of the Mucous Membranes, and other Complaints.

Under this head we have, in the first place, to notice, as of the highest importance, an affection that is never wanting in any syphilitic infant, namely:

1) *Syphilitic catarrh*, or *ulceration* of the Schneiderian membrane (ozæna syphilitica).—At the commencement, this affection is like the ordinary dry catarrh of infants, from which, during the first period of its existence, it is not distinguished by any special symptoms. Soon, however, the child commences to lose from its nose a few drops of blood, or bloody mucus. This occurs several times during the day, and may increase to true epistaxis. As the disease progresses, the discharge from the nose becomes more ichorous, corrodes the alæ nasi and the upper lip, where it may occasion ulcerations that become covered with crusts and rhagades. In most cases, the affection remains confined to the Schneiderian membrane; if the ulcerations are not covered with hard crusts, the ichorous secretion is always mixed with blood. This ulceration always commences in the interior of the nostrils, and shows more inclination to spread backwards towards the velum palati and fauces, than forwards towards the outer parts of the nose. If this continues, the nasal bones lose their support, the nose becomes flat and collapses, so that it almost forms a level plane with the cheeks; the breathing becomes more and more snoring and difficult, so that the child is scarcely able to nurse without danger of suffocation, and the secretion from the nose remains ichorous and bloody. The course of these ulcerations is extremely changeable; sometimes they destroy the bones in a few weeks, sometimes in a few months; whereas, in other cases, they stop of themselves in their course, without destroying the bones. In other cases, this ulceration spreads onward to the fauces, and even to the larynx; in which case the voice becomes husky, loses all resonance, and may even be lost entirely, the breathing changing to a mere wheezing, as in croup. These extensive ulcerations are, however, very rare; in most cases they remain confined to the Schneiderian membrane and the cartilages of the nose; they constitute one of those disorders with which infants are most frequently attacked.

2) *Affections of the lymphatic glands.*—Upon the whole, buboes

are very rare in syphilitic infants. If they do occur, they are more frequently simple glandular swellings than inflamed buboes. After breaking, an ichorous matter oozes out like that of consecutive ulcers, in whose company, or subsequently to which, they make their appearance. Sometimes they do not show themselves until long after the disappearance of all other syphilitic symptoms; whereas, in other cases, they occur as protopathic products without being preceded by any other symptoms. Always remaining more or less stationary, they frequently disperse spontaneously, and, upon the whole, are much more indolent than the genuine primary buboes. In general, they resemble scrofulous glandular swellings, with which they might very readily be confounded, if the whole constitution of the child, the presence of other syphilitic symptoms, and a knowledge of the previous circumstances of the child's parents and nurse, did not place the diagnosis beyond all doubt.

3) *Affections of the osseous system.*—Although this system, in syphilitic children, is very seldom invaded before the end of the first year, yet there are cases where periosteal swellings and exostoses occur even during the first months of infantile existence. Bertin relates the case of an infant, 35 days old, whose whole body was covered with pustules and tubercles, and where a periostosis of considerable size was seen on the upper and posterior side of the ulna. In children of five to seven years, I have seen such exostoses on the tibia, as well as on the skull-bones.

4) *Syphilitic cachexia.*—This name is applied to the erysipelatous exanthem described in the preceding paragraph, under No. 9, with which some children are born, and which is, moreover, distinguished by the above-described dusky or yellowish color of the skin, as well as by the most perfect marasmus, and by the appearance of old age, by which this exanthem is always accompanied.

5) *Scrofula.*—If Hufeland and other physicians, as well as homœopathic practitioners who copy them, maintain that hereditary syphilis, in children, often manifests itself under the forms of scrofulosis, such a doctrine is based upon nothing else than the most shocking ignorance of sound and definite perceptions of

pathology. Either syphilis and scrofulosis are idiopathic and distinct diseases, or else they are not. If they are distinct diseases, syphilis cannot produce scrofulosis, any more than a plum-tree can produce cherries; but if every disposition to glandular swellings and osseous affections is to be termed scrofulosis, syphilis cannot be any thing else than scrofulosis; and what becomes, in such a case, of the diagnostic distinction between the two?

Sec. 213.—Diagnosis, Prognosis, and Treatment.

In the third division, in §§ 186–189, we have shown the different ways in which syphilis can be transmitted to children; at the same time, we have stated that congenital syphilis, and the syphilis acquired at birth, generally show their symptoms immediately after birth, and that hereditary or constitutional syphilis does not become manifest until six or eight weeks, and in the larger number of cases, not till months or even years have elapsed. What we desire to add in this place is, that the syphilis adnata of manuals, that is, a kind of syphilis which is transmitted to the child while it passes through the vagina, most likely has no existence. If the mother, at confinement, is affected with venereal symptoms on the sexual organs, in consequence of an infection caught during her pregnancy, the child must have become syphilitic while yet in the womb; this may be considered as perfectly certain, if the child is born with signs of syphilis. However, let us pass this subject over, and let us cast a glance at the diagnosis, prognosis, and treatment of this kind of syphilis.

As regards *diagnosis*, there is not the remotest doubt of the nature of the malady, whenever the above-described pustules are present simultaneously with chancres, resembling those of full-grown persons; or if rhagades on the lips, at the anus, or umbilicus, are seen, or lymphatic swellings in various parts of the body. Moreover, it is well known that scrofulous swellings develop themselves only at a later period. Less sure as a diagnostic sign is erysipelas (*erysipelas neonatorum*), which may likewise exist in otherwise perfectly sound children; but the above-mentioned erysipelatous redness of syphilitic children is quite different from ordinary erysipelas; it resembles the redness which, in full-grown persons, is seen on the velum palati and in the fauces whenever these parts are invaded by the disease. Whether, in certain dubious cases, it is safe to decide whether the nurse has infected her nursling, or whether the infection has proceeded from the latter to the former, it must be evident, after what we have said in § 188, that this point must always remain obscure, unless all doubt can be cleared up by a perfect knowledge of all the previous circumstances bearing upon the case; since it is an established fact that syphilis can be communicated through the milk, even if the mammæ do not show the remotest trace of syphilitic disease. In such a case, the matter can only be cleared up by a most careful investigation of the previous circumstances of the nurse, as well as of those of the parents.

As far as the prognosis is concerned, it is evident that the danger connected with infantile syphilis has been deemed greater than it really is. If such children are at once placed under suitable influences, in hands where their health is well cared for, and where they enjoy the benefit of a perfectly rational treatment, there is no doubt that most of them can be saved. I have preserved more than one child of this class, and have succeeded in freeing their constitutions from every vestige of syphilitic taint. Where such a child has not only to struggle with every species of distress and misery, and the physician is moreover interfered with at every turn of the road by silly and stupid parents, it may perhaps be advisable not to undertake the treatment of such a case. Moreover, some forms of the disease are more dangerous than others; pemphigus for instance, which almost always terminates fatally; likewise chancres on the lips and in the mouth, which may destroy the infant in an indirect way, by interfering with the introduction of food; and lastly, ozæna syphilitica, which may likewise have the same effect. An improper suppression of discharges from the nose and vagina, by the absurd use of astringents and the like, may be followed by a sudden destruction of life. Ophthalmia, if properly managed, is a curable disease, and need not necessarily result in blindness. The same thing may be said of chancres, pustules, swellings, even when located on the skull-bones; all these symptoms generally yield to a truly rational treatment with specific means, provided they are used with care and discretion.

As regards the treatment of this form of syphilis, nothing need be remarked in addition to what has already been stated in the course of this work, concerning the use of the different anti-syphilitica, such as *Mercurius*, *Cinnabaris*, *Nitri acidum*, *Thuja*, etc. One thing is required; the infant must at once be taken from the breast, whether it is nursed by the mother or by a strange woman, and both must be subjected to proper treatment. This is an indispensable precautionary measure; I know from abundant experience that too much leniency in this respect may entail a good deal of mischief.

III. MERCURIAL SYPHILIS.

Sec. 214.—General Observations.

The older physicians already knew, and stated in their writings, that Mercury, if administered in excessive and improperly continued doses, is not only an extremely dangerous remedy of itself, but, unless employed with great precautions, aggravates the syphilitic disease instead of curing it. With some this opinion went so far as to induce them to attribute the phenomena of secondary syphilis exclusively to the employment of Mercury, and consequently to reject the use of this metal in the treatment of syphilis. Between these two extremes our School formerly held a middle position; on the one hand, we have admitted the injury arising from the use of excessive and of too frequently repeated doses of Mercury, whereas, on the other hand, we contend that small and properly administered doses of this agent are indispensable to a successful treatment of the syphilitic disease. It is true that recent critics have undertaken to sneer at the idea that the incautious use of Mercury may involve pernicious consequences; but we do not hesitate, even at the risk of being considered servile imitators of Hahnemann, to make the statement that, if the destructive effects of Mercury do not seem as marked at the present time as they were when it was deemed necessary to give Mercury in sufficiently large doses to excite ptyalism, some of the perceptible effects of this agent are witnessed, even to this day, not only under allopathic, but even under homœopathic treatment. Even from the first trituration, I have noticed the following effects on persons somewhat sensitive to mercurial action: Ulcers that were mostly superficial, though sometimes more deeply penetrating, and lined with a cheesy matter, healing spontaneously in ten or twelve days, but sometimes breaking out again in eighteen months, even if the remedy had been discontinued during this whole period;—aphthæ and milky-white ulcers on the inside of the lips, and similar rhagades on the margin of the tongue, or between the cheek and gums;—superficial flat ulcers on the dorsum of the hand, arising from itching vesicles: these ulcers looked as if they had been gnawed at by insects, became covered with a scurf that frequently fell off and formed anew, and finally disappeared in from twenty-five to thirty days, without leaving a trace of the ulcer;—itching blotches on the legs, resembling mosquito-bites, becoming covered with scurfs after being scratched open, and, after being removed by scratching, showing superficial ulcers on the skin, of the size of split peas; a bloody serum oozed from these ulcers, which, after having become covered with a new scurf, began to itch, and finally dried up;—similar pimples on the hairy scalp, itching and changing to ulcers of the size of a three cent piece to that of a dime; they would dry up in two or three weeks, and, in the course of two years, frequently break out again. A very disagreeable effect of Mercury, which I have only witnessed three or four times, and which came on six, eight or ten months, and, in one case, twelve months after using the metal uninterruptedly for two months, was a highly characteristic *debility with slow fever*, complete loss of appetite, intolerable pains in the limbs, trembling walk, desponding melancholy, and an indescribable feeling of bodily and mental malaise. Let us now pass in review the effects of allopathic doses of Mercury, so that we may at once be able to distinguish them from other symptoms whenever such effects occur.

Sec. 215.—Acute Effects of Mercury.

Any one who wishes to obtain a correct and full knowledge of the poisonous effects of Mercury, will have to consult the excellent works of Dieterich, Hermann, Heim, and Ludolph, of which mention has already been made in the Introduction to this work. Here follow some of the most important facts from these works:

1) *Mercurial fever*, of which we have already spoken. It sometimes sets in with such a violent headache, that one might apprehend the approach of acute typhus; there is chilliness mingled with heat, great dryness of the mouth, with thirst; general

languor, weariness and debility; extreme prostration and sadness; heat and dryness of the skin; red urine, a full and rapid pulse. These symptoms are sometimes, but not always, accompanied by an inclination to vomit, tooth-ache, ear-ache, rheumatic pains in the limbs, and other complaints which, however, are not constant. The fever often terminates critically between the fourth and seventh day, especially if it begins while Mercury is still used by the patient; whereas, if it only breaks out at a later period, three or six months after the use of the metal had been abandoned, the fever is apt to continue twenty-five to thirty days.—In other cases the fever sets in as adynamic fever, with sallow complexion, with a dim and glassy expression of the eyes, which are surrounded with blue margins; coldness of the extremities, nose and face, evening chills, rapid and small pulse, deathlike pallor; the patient lies down in a state of apathy, without strength, etc.; lastly, inclination to vomit, delirium, starting up in bed, as from terror, and even death.

2) *Ptyalism.*—This symptom is so well known that it seems unnecessary to describe it any further. The present treatment of syphilis with Mercury, even in allopathic hands, is modified to such an extent, that ptyalism nowadays never reaches the fearful height to which it was carried in former times, when chronic ulcers of the mouth, necrosis of the teeth and jaw-bones, scorbutic gums, and many other affections, were among the ordinary consequences of this terrible disorder.

3) *Abdominal ptyalism.*—This effect of Mercury is rare, but does occur. It is characterized by frothy, whitish, tenacious, sometimes greenish stools, as many as fifteen in the course of a day; at first they are attended with colicky pains, afterwards they are painless, with a dull burning pain in the region of the pancreas, and a sensation as if something were coming away from this spot. This region is painful when pressed upon. If violent, this symptom may become dangerous to life.

4) *Hydrargyria*, or the mercurial *eczema.*—A febrile exanthem, consisting of small, itching vesicles, crowded together upon a skin having an erysipelatous redness; they are filled with a yellowish lymph, peel off like bran, and are said to occur only after mercurial

frictions. In other cases the skin assumes a scarlet-redness, the vesicles burst, cover the surface of the skin with a viscid, fetid fluid, after which, about the fifth day, the epidermis peels off in large patches, leaving sore places of considerable size.

5) *Mercurial rash.*—A febrile exanthem, which is preceded by anxiety and restlessness, first breaks out on the chest, and, after effecting several partial manifestations every day, for four or five days to come, finally completes its development at the end of this period. The rash is white, and densely crowded together. The fever is of a torpid character, and accompanied by nervous symptoms.

These two exanthems, which, when breaking out after massive doses of quicksilver or after frictions with mercurial ointment, are always acute and attended with fever, may likewise assume a chronic form, after smaller doses of Mercury, as may be seen from the following observations of Hahnemann, and his son Frederick, volume I. of the Materia Medica Pura: Eruption consisting of red, raised spots, with stinging itching; small, transparent vesicles, full of a watery fluid, breaking out on various parts of the body early, before daylight; rounded stigmata, gradually changing to ulcerated spots, which become scurfy; rash over the whole body, especially on the chest, thighs, and on the lower part of the back; measle-shaped rash, with burning and itching; eruption consisting of small, red, raised spots, with stinging and itching; nettle-rash, afterwards changing to red spots. *Erysipelatous inflammations.*

Sec. 216.—Chronic Forms of Mercurial Poisoning.

Under this head, it may suffice to direct attention to the *external* alterations, approximating those of syphilis.

1) *Swellings.*—Among these we not only have inguinal swellings, but likewise swellings of the axillary and parotid glands, of the pancreas, and mesenteric ganglia. What Dieterich relates, after Matthias, of figwarts and ganglia, supposed to have been caused by Mercury, most likely applies to syphilitic rather than a mercurial poisoning. The swelling of the testicles, of which the

same author makes mention in his work, is more likely to have been caused by the gonorrhœa for which the calomel was given, than by the calomel itself.

2) *Chronic eruptions.*—Here we have principally: Eruption on the hairy scalp, with itching, which induces one to scratch; scurfs on the hairy scalp, with itching, and burning after scratching; elevated scurfs, matting the hair together; humid eruption, which eats away the hair, with *itching* of the sore parts; painful blisters on the nose; large tubercle beneath the integuments of the cheek; *red spots* in the face; *pustules* on the chin, of the size of a pea; millet-sized, *ulcerated* eruption on the chin, with yellow crusts underneath; reddish-white herpetic spot on the zygoma; red elevations on the arm, with white-scurfy itching tips, and burning after scatching; large, *round*, *scaly spots* on the forearm and wrist, with burning pain; *tetter* on the forearm, with voluptuous *itching*, *desquamation* of the skin; *peeling off of the dorsum of the hand;* itch-like eruption on the hands, with nocturnal itching, and a raging pain in the forehead; vesicles on the wrists, full of a watery fluid; red papulæ on the dorsum of the hand, with burning when first breaking out; *exfoliation and falling off of the nails;* itching eruption on the thighs, with oozing of a burning water after scratching; *herpes* on the thigh, with voluptuous itching, and peeling off of the epidermis after scratching; gnawing-itching little *ulcers* on the thigh, inviting one to scratch; small, itching pimples on the leg, changing to ulcerated spots, the *epidermis peels off* after the ulcers heal; eruption resembling pustulous scabies on the legs, sexual parts, in the bend of the knee, on the neck and abdomen, very much *raised*, *red*, as if *sore*, humid and *itching; pustules* on the upper and lower limbs, with purulent tips, itching; herpes, with burning when touched; dry, raised, burning-*itching* tetter on the legs, arms, hands, and between the fingers; *ulcerated patches* on the joints of the fingers; deep cracks and rhagades in the hands and fingers.

3) *Ulcers.*—*Phagedænic ulcers; spongy*, bluish, *readily-bleeding* ulcers; ulcers that look as if they had been *gnawed at by insects*, unequal elevations and depressions, great painfulness to contact, and discharge of an acrid, corrosive ichor; *cracks and rhagades* in the lips; *soft*, *red*, *ulcerated patches in the swollen*

upper lip, with discharge of a watery, yellowish, fetid fluid; they bleed when touched, and itch furiously; bluish-white spots and *painful ulcers on the inside of the lower lip;* ulceration of the corners of the mouth; *rhagades in the prepuce*, with swelling of this part, which is covered with a red, fine rash; white vesicles on the glans, *spreading* and *dipping down to the subjacent textures;* small ulcers on the inside of the prepuce, having originated in small vesicles; *round ulcers* beneath the prepuce, with *everted edges*, looking like raw flesh, with a *cheesy bottom*, discharge of a yellowish-white, strong-smelling matter, much bleeding and pain to contact that seems to be felt throughout the whole body; *suppuration between the glans and prepuce*, with redness, swelling and inflammation of the latter.

4) *Affections of the mucous membranes.*—Discharge of greenish mucus from the urethra; discharge of acrid pus from the nose, smelling like old cheese; swelling and cracking of the Schneiderian membrane; scurfy nostrils, they bleed when one blows the nose; (œdematous swelling of the root of the nose); discharge of a yellowish, fetid, bloody pus from the ear; soreness and excoriation of the inner ear; soreness in the *mouth;* round, elevated, white blisters in the mouth; aphthæ, *ulcers*, and *ulcerated patches* on the buccal mucous membrane, with burning and smarting; *ulceration of the margin of the tongue*, becoming indented from the pressure of the teeth; the tongue is hollowed out, ulcerates, with swelling.

5) *Affections of the osseous system.*—Carious ulcers; caries and abscesses in the joints; thickening of the periosteum; swelling of bones; pain of the skull-bones, occipital region; pain of the nasal bone when touching it; *caries of the maxillary and palatine bones;* hard elevation on the right tibia, with shining redness and swelling; fragility of the bones, preceded by rheumatic pains.

Sec. 217.—Diagnosis, Prognosis and Treatment.

We omit the balance of mercurial ailments, such as *tremor*, *laming rheumatism*, *nervous stuttering*, *neuralgia*, *melancholy with complete depression of all bodily and moral energy;* they are well known, and will not escape the attention of the cautious physician in case they should occur under the homœopathic treatment of syphilitic affections with somewhat large doses of Mercury. A few diagnostic, prognostic, and therapeutic remarks on mercurial poisoning may, however, not be out of place.

In regard to *diagnosis*, the difficulty is not so very great, provided we remember that: 1) all *mercurial cutaneous affections* are distinguished from analogous syphilitic pustules, papules, herpes, or ulcers, by the *itching*, which is *never wanting* with *mercurial*, and *scarcely ever present* in *syphilitic* eruptions; and, 2) that *mercurial ulcers* are always more superficial, and that their edges have a bluish-white color; at the same time they have not the rounded, cup-shaped appearance of syphilitic ulcers, nor are their edges as callous or copper-colored as those of the latter. Moreover, mercurial symptoms, provided the metal is discontinued, disappear within ten or thirty days, although they show a disposition to return again. In other respects, the case is with the mercurial disease as with syphilis; a single symptom of the former malady is scarcely ever seen alone, they always appear in company, although, if they are very slight, it requires a practised eye to discover and recognize them.

The *prognosis* depends upon the quantity of Mercury that has been crowded into the body. What must not be overlooked in this disease, is the recurrence of the paroxysms every six months, or even every year; the mercurial symptoms may be entirely subdued during this period, and yet the poison may still be haunting the organic tissues. The worst is, that massive doses of this metal are sometimes given in rapid succession without causing any perceptible ill effects, until the disease breaks out all at once in all its violence, which may happen even six months or a year after the metal had been entirely discontinued. If moderate doses of this drug do not produce a decided improvement of the syphilitic disease within a reasonable period, on the contrary, aggravate it, it would be criminal to continue its use any longer for the purpose, as it is called, "of saturating the organism," in the fancied security that because no perceptible effect of Mercury has as yet shown itself, there cannot be any danger in continuing the desperate game a little longer. If the metal has not been abused to excess, and the effects of its use only break out some time after it had been discontinued, the prognosis is not so very unfavorable, although, on account of the symptoms being liable to break out afresh, the cure is rather slow; on the other hand, if the symptoms break out while the patient is still taking large doses of the drug, the *acuteness* and *violence* of the disorder may result in a speedy destruction of organic life. In this respect, the worst symptoms are those described in § 215, *hydrargyria* and the *mercurial rash.*

The treatment is chiefly conducted with: *Kali jodatum, Aurum, Iodium, Hepar, Nitri acidum, Phosphori acidum, Staphysagria, Mezereum, Phosphorus, Sulphur,* etc. For hydrargyria, of which I have only had one single case in my practice, I found Cinchona entirely useless, whereas *Kali jodatum,* at the rate of *ten* grains to four ounces of water, a tablespoonful every three hours, proved highly beneficial. This is likewise my chief remedy for mercurial *ptyalism,* and for mercurial *debility,* with or without fever, and for which an additional indication is furnished by the complete prostration of all the physical and mental energies of the patient. In chronic mercurial affections, I recommend more particularly, for affections of the *mouth* and gums: *Carbo veget., Hepar, Nitri ac., Dulcamara, Staphysagria;* for mercurial *angina: Argentum, Lachesis, Carbo veg., Hepar, Nitri ac., Lycopodium, Thuja;* for *ulcers: Nitri ac., Hepar, Carbo veg., Ferrum, Silicea, Phosphori ac., Lachesis, Sarsaparilla, Aurum;* for affections of the *bony system: Kali jod., Aurum, Phosphori ac., Calcarea, Staphysagria, Asa fœtida;* for *glandular swellings: Aurum, Dulcamara, Carbo veg., Silicea;* for *pains in the limbs: Guaiacum, Sarsaparilla, Carbo veg., China, Hepar, Nitri ac.;* for *diarrhœa: Plumbum, Nitri ac., Phosphori ac., Hepar;* for nervous *debility* (beside *Kali jodatum*)*: Hepar, Nitri ac., Phosphori acidum, Aurum, Carbo veg., Ferrum;* for excessive *liability to taking cold,* and extreme sensitiveness to changes in the weather: *Carbo veg., Dulcamara, China, Silicea.* Several other remedies might be mentioned; these, however, will be deferred to a special treatise on *mercurial disease.*

SECOND CHAPTER.

GENERAL THERAPEUTIC OBSERVATIONS.

I. PROPHYLACTIC RULES.

Sec. 218.—Various Prophylactic Measures.

MOST writers on syphilis, when speaking of this subject, enter upon a long discussion concerning the measures which the State should enact for the purpose of eradicating this plague, or, at any rate, protecting individuals as much as possible against the infection. Properly speaking, this question does not concern us in a work where we do not profess to deal with the economical aspect of this subject, but with the restoration of individual health. However, inasmuch as almost every writer not only starts this question, but likewise answers it in the queerest manner, and inasmuch as we may not have a chance to refute the many absurdidities that have been proposed in reference to this matter in any other place, we beg the reader's leave to state in a few brief lines all that we may deem proper to suggest concerning it. As regards enacting measures for the absolute eradication of this plague, it seems incomprehensible how sensible men can entertain such an idea —all measures of this kind, be they what they may, are *absolutely unrealizable.* Supposing, for the sake of argument, that, on a given day and at a given hour, every individual inhabitant of a country, rich or poor, young or old, male or female, could be examined by a careful physician, and that those who are found in the least tainted with the disease could be placed under the strictest surveillance of the authorities; and supposing that these examinations, on account of having to make the necessary allowance for the period of incubation, should be continued every day for one or two months: it would likewise become necessary to examine every traveller from a foreign country, and every inhabitant on the frontier, where the people would necessarily pass to and fro, and these examinations would have to be continued every day for at least a couple of months, otherwise the whole scheme might be frustrated, for the reason that one scaly sheep corrupts the whole flock. Does not this show that all measures that might be proposed for the total eradication of syphilis, are purely chimerical, and cannot be executed?—unless every inhabitant of such a State is to be bound, after the fashion of the ancient Jews, to show himself at least once a week to the physician, and to obtain from him a certificate of health, that can be shown to the officially appointed inspector when he makes his domiciliary visit. But even this measure could easily be eluded, and would be eluded by a large number, and the whole plan would thus be rendered abortive. All that the authorities can do, is to exercise a strict surveillance over the health of the inmates of brothels; even this measure, which is the one adopted by the French police, is of questionable propriety. It is true that, upon the whole, a much smaller number of young men are infected by those common prostitutes who are under the surveillance of the police, than by the so-called *grisettes*, who are beyond the pale of such regulations. On the other hand, however, the surveillance of the police has this disadvantage, that young men, relying upon the good effects of such measures, and considering themselves safe beyond all peradventure, abandon themselves to the illicit intercourse with prostitutes without any reserve, not considering that a woman may have caught the infection between one official visit and the next, and that even the practised eye of a physician may have failed to detect every little chancre that may have been concealed in one of the folds of the vaginal membrane. Considering, moreover, that a woman may have had connection with a diseased man a few moments before she receives another customer in perfect health, and that she may give him the disease by means of the least quantity of contagious matter that had remained adhering to her parts from her previous lover, it is evident that the sanitary measures which the government has seen fit to adopt in this respect, have, so far, utterly failed to accomplish the object for which they were intended.

Sec. 219.—Individual Prophylactic Measures.

Without troubling ourselves about the precautionary measures instituted by the State, let us examine the different methods that have been proposed for the use of individuals as proper means to escape the consequences of improper connection with infected women. Not to mention the use of amulets; of saints' images, like that of St. Roche, for instance; or the carrying of Biblical verses on the abdomen, after illicit intercourse with bad women, a custom that was introduced soon after Luther's Reformation: others have proposed to neutralize the efficacy of the poison by washing the parts, immediately after connection, with alkalis, acids, or other chemical substances. As late as the year 1815, a French surgeon, Luna Calderon, pretended to have discovered a sure means of destroying the venereal poison, and without making his discovery public, instituted several public experiments, in the syphilitic hospital. Among other experiments, he inoculated himself with chancrous matter on both sides of the penis. To one of the wounds, he immediately after applied some of his preservative, the consequence of which seemed to have been, that no chancre broke out on this side, whereas, on the other side, a chancre did make its appearance. Independently of the many pathological doubts concerning the correctness of Calderon's observations, which doubts force themselves upon the reader's mind, during the perusal of his little treatise, the title of which is found among the list of publications mentioned at the commencement of this work,—it is certain, even if we do not wish to raise any objections against the manner in which Calderon conducted his experiments, that the poison cannot be destroyed after the act of coïtion has once taken place. During the performance of this act, so much of the virus becomes absorbed, that, even if the quantity remaining adhering after the act could be destroyed, or removed by washing, or by chemical antidotes, the infection of the general organism would not be prevented by such a proceeding. For this reason, others have imagined that, by painting the mucous membrane of the genital organs with oil, fatty substances, etc., it would be rendered inaccessible to the poison, whose absorption could thus be prevented. But, inasmuch as the oil is rubbed off during the act, the infection continued to be caught, until Conton, an Englishman, about the time of Charles II., introduced the use of a membrane, or "safe," which had already been recommended by Fallopius, prior to the year 1520, and which has remained to this day the surest preservative against the disease. Since this contrivance, however, is not always handy, others have conceived the idea to blunt the organism against the poison, by repeated inoculations, inferring, as they did, from certain general propositions dropped by Ricord, that, after repeating the process of inoculation a number of times on the same individual, the product of inoculation finally ceases to appear. Even at this day, there exists a society of physicians in Paris, whose object is to make investigations in this direction by direct experimentation. Whether these gentlemen have obtained any very brilliant results, has not yet been divulged; but every sensible physician may rest assured that these infatuated men resemble the fool who, in order to escape the lightning's stroke, threw himself out of the window. What, now, shall we say of those who fancy that they can secure perfect immunity from the consequences of an impure coït, by swallowing, immediately after connection, a few globules of *Mercurius* 12, or even of a grain of the second trituration? This proceeding might, perhaps, be a preventive, if not against gonorrhœa or figwarts, at least against chancre, if we did not know that those who are under homœopathic treatment for chancre, and take a few doses of *Mercurius*, day after day, often catch a second chancre, in consequence of exposing themselves again before the former ulcer is quite healed. On this account, the best advice we can give to all those who desire to remain free from all contagion, is that contained in the old distich:

> "Quid facies, facies Veneris dum veneris ante?
> Ne sedeas, sed eas, ne pereas per eas!"

II. THE TREATMENT OF SYPHILIS TO THE PRESENT TIME.

Sec. 220.—Original Mode of Treatment.

The first impression which syphilis produced upon the physicians who first watched its devastations in the fifteenth century was a feeling of surprise, mingled with terror. No one was able to bethink himself of a remedy, through whose influence the rapid spread of this terrible disease, which suddenly invaded every tissue of the organism, could be prevented, or even moderated. Every possible remedy that had hitherto been employed against the various ills that flesh is heir to, was tried; sanguineous depletions, purgatives, cleansing potations of every description, the most violent remedies, as well as the most complicated prescriptions—in short, every thing to be found in the Materia Medica, and the formularies of that period, containing the united wisdom of the Arabian and Mauric Schools. It is not positively known how the use of Quicksilver was first introduced; some say that it seems to have been suggested by the immunity which the workmen in the Spanish quicksilver mines seemed to enjoy from the ravages of this disease, or by the remarkable rapidity with which its effects were removed from their systems; others trace the use of this agent to the custom that had been prevalent among the Spaniards, for a long time previous, to employ Mercury as a remedy for all sorts of cutaneous diseases; others, again, attribute its use to the accidental notion of likewise trying Mercury, where so much else had been tried in vain. Be this, however, as it may, it seems certain that the use of this agent first came from Spain, where it had been employed for a long time already against certain forms of lepra; and that its employment must already have been pretty general in the fifteenth century, since a variety of mercurial ointments were already proposed in 1496, by Joseph Grünbeck, of Burkhausen, Secretary to the Emperor Maximilian; in 1497, by John Weidmann; in 1498, by Sebastianus Aquitanus; and in 1499, by Gaspard Torella. These ointments, to which every physician added different ingredients, in accordance with his own taste and judgment, were necessarily composed in so many different ways, and contained Mercury in so many different proportions, that their effect was any thing but uniform, until, finally, Jacob Von Carpi, whom Fallopius wrongly considers as the inventor of the inunction-cure, sought, in the year 1512, to regulate the employment and preparation of these ointments upon definite principles. In 1506 already, the use of the ointments had been associated with mercurial fumigations, for which purpose *Cinnabaris* was chiefly used, until, in the year 1528, Paracelsus, and afterwards Peter Andreas Matthiolus, substituted the internal use of this agent, in the place of external frictions and fumigations. For this purpose, the last named employed the *red precipitate*, which he first washed by distilling it with plantan and oxalic acid; he then dried it by the fire, and prescribed it in doses of five grains each daily. Afterwards, Barbarossa (brother of the celebrated pirate), learned from a Jewish physician the preparation of pills composed of Mercury, turpentine, and bran, which obtained great favor through the recommendation of Francis I., King of France, and which afterwards, towards the end of the eighteenth century, were introduced by the Parisian physician, Bellost, as a new article, into the modern anti-syphilitic pharmacopœia. At the commencement of that century, the mercurial salts, more particularly the sublimate, had been begun to be used. They became more universally known when Van Swieten introduced into practice a solution of this salt which bears his name. More recently, the use of mercurial preparations, and of combinations of this metal with other chemical substances, has become more extensive. In the pharmacopœias of different countries we not only find calomel, sublimate, the red and white precipitate, the Mercurius solubilis Hahnemanni, but likewise the Nitrate, Phosphate, Sulphate of Mercury, the Iodide and Cyanide of Mercury, the metallic Mercury, and the Cinnabaris of ancient renown, not to mention other preparations, such as a combination of the Cyanide of Mercury and the Iodide of Potassium. All these preparations were employed more or less against the syphilitic disease, although other drugs were likewise resorted to, more especially since the danger involved in too liberal a use of the mercurial preparations became evident at a very early period in the history of this agent.

Sec. 221.—Former Anti-syphilitics.

As early as the year 1508, only a few years after the introduction of Mercury against syphilis, the first of the so-called exotic *sudorifics*, the American lignum vitæ or Guajacum officinale, was introduced as an anti-syphilitic agent. Since most of those who were treated with Mercury seemed to suffer more from the effects of this metal than from the ravages of syphilis, Guajac, which seems to possess a sort of antidotal power against the ill effects of Mercury, soon acquired an extraordinary reputation, which lasted until, in the year 1530, the Brazilian Sarsaparilla, which was combined with Guajac as a *sweating potion*, successfully contended with Guajac for preëminence. The Smilax-China, which was introduced about the same period, created less excitement, and met with no more favor than the laurus Sassafras and the Saponaria, whereas the Guajac and Sarsaparilla, more especially the latter, still enjoy considerable repute with physicians even to this day. However much these remedies may have helped those who suffered from the effects of Mercury rather than from those of syphilis, it was soon found that they do not cure syphilis without the employment of Mercury. Nevertheless, in view of the dread which people had of Mercury, and the belief that it was the metallic character of this agent that destroyed the syphilitic virus, several physicians conceived the idea, towards the end of the seventeenth century, to substitute *Gold* for Mercury. Already, in the year 1688, Gervay Ucay, and, after him, Lecoq, Loss, and Rebentrost, sang the praises of this metal as an anti-syphilitic agent. The introduction of three new vegetable drugs, towards the middle of the eighteenth century, soon caused Gold to lose its important rank; these new drugs were: 1) the *Spurge laurel* or Daphne Mezereum, which was more particularly praised for affections of the osseous system; 2) the *American Lobelia* or the Lobelia antisyphilitica; and 3) the *Astragalus exscapus*, the two last-named of which are now so entirely ignored by physicians, that the roots are no longer offered for sale by any European druggist. *Opium*, as well as *Silver* and *Platina*, were used against syphilis towards the end of the last, and at the beginning of the present century, after the *Volatile Ammonium* (Ammonium causticum), and even *oxygen* had been used in 1774 as anti-syphilitic remedies, to be abandoned again, like the rest, in a short time, with the exception of two officinal preparations, in which they are contained as leading constituents, namely: the *soluble Mercury of Hahnemann* (sub-proto-nitratum ammoniaco-mercuriale) and *Nitri acidum*, containing a large proportion of oxygen. These two drugs are but little used by Old-School physicians, who, since Coindet's discovery of the medicinal properties of Iodine in the first twenty years of the present century, are more particularly fond of employing as anti-syphilitics the combinations of Iodine with Mercury and other substances, such as *Iodide of Mercury*, *Iodide of Potassium*, etc., in addition to which we now have the combinations of *Mercury and Kali with Bromine*, such as: the Bromide of Mercury (Mercurius bromatus), the *Bromide of Potassium* (Kali bromatum), the *Bromide of Sodium* (Natrum bromatum), etc. First employed for buboes, and afterwards, by

Martini, of Lübeck, for syphilitic ulcers in the throat, *Iodine*, on account of its dangerous effects upon the organism, was very little used internally until, in the years 1832–1836, Doctor Wallace, of Dublin, recommended the *Iodide of Potassium* as a much milder and yet equally efficacious remedy for syphilis. Ebers, of Breslau, Haselberg and Kluge, of Berlin, soon after followed his example, recommending this salt strongly for secondary and inveterate syphilis, but more particularly for affections of the bones. This agent, which probably will never cure primary forms of syphilis where *Mercurius* is not used in the first place, is abused at the present time about as much as Mercury has been formerly.

Sec. 222.—The Physiological Method.

After what we have stated in the preceding paragraphs of the different means of treatment recommended for syphilis, the reader must have seen that these different recommendations are based upon two sets of opinions diametrically opposed to each other: 1) the *specific* view, according to which syphilis depends upon a *specific virus* that has to be annihilated by *specific remedies*, and 2) the so-called *physiological view*, which teaches that the syphilitic disease can be cured by the simple restoration of the organic functions to a normal condition, and which, although first reduced to a scientific doctrine by Broussais, had already, long before his time, guided the practice of a number of physicians. The fearful accidents caused by the insensate use of Mercury, in the very first years of the syphilitic plague, caused the lignum vitæ to be received with so much satisfaction as early as the year 1508, that the employment of Mercury as an anti-syphilitic was almost abandoned, until it was resumed in 1527. Since then Mercury has been steadily adhered to. Nicolas von Blegny's attempts, in 1673, to revive the use of Guajac-decoctions were unsuccessful; Payrilhe, who in 1774 sought to substitute the volatile Ammonium for Mercury, remained without imitators; nor was Scott able, in 1796, to replace Mercury by Nitric acid. Nevertheless, the trials which were instituted with mineral acids, in 1799, had somewhat shaken the old belief in Mercury, when Ferguson published a memoir in England, in the year 1813, in which he laid before the public the magnificent results he had witnessed in Portugal, of the treatment of syphilis without Mercury. They were confirmed by Dr. Rose, who had been with him in Portugal, and likewise by a German physician, Dr. Huber. Although Henry Robertson contradicted these statements by asserting the fact, that nowhere in the world were seen so many faces disfigured by syphilis as in Portugal, nevertheless, in several military hospitals of England, experiments with this non-mercurial treatment of syphilis were instituted. It would lead us too far to indicate all the results that were obtained by means of this mode of treating the disease; suffice it to say that no English physician, in 1838, dared to advocate this method any longer, and that the Profession generally resumed the use of Mercury. Despite the English notion of the non-use of Mercury, the employment of this agent as an anti-syphilitic had been steadily and very generally continued by the French and German physicians, when, in 1813, Broussais' Physiological School, denying all idiopathic diseases, ascended the throne, and the treatment of syphilis with so-called specific remedies was especially opposed by Jourdan, who set up the antiphlogistic method as the only rational mode of treatment, and would allow the use of Mercury only in its capacity of a powerful revulsive. Since then, a number of French and German physicians, who embraced these doctrines of the Physiological School, treated all the primary forms of venereal diseases with external *local means*, such as injections in gonorrhœa, cauterization of chancres, sanguineous depletions to relieve violent pains, swellings, inflammations, until, at least in France, the more deeply penetrating physicians saw that the pathological and therapeutic doctrines of the Physiological School were absolutely untenable, *illogical*, and *unscientific*, and, in 1835, summoned a medicinal congress in Nantes for the purpose of discussing the new doctrines. The opinions of the different medical Societies in France, especially the society of Lyons, represented in this congress, went almost unanimously against the errors of the Physiological School; a *viva voce* vote likewise showed an opposition of fifty to two against the fallacies of Broussais, who has only a few partisans left, more especially in our own German fatherland. Whatever the present position of the Physiological School may be, it is certain that, at the present day, two opposite views are contending for supremacy among Old-School physicians: 1) the *specific* doctrine, according to which syphilis is to be treated with *specific* means: and 2) the *physiological* doctrine, denying the existence of this disease, and claiming, as its highest object of cure, a restoration of the normal organic functions, by the best possible use of palliatives at every proper and favorable moment. Let us now see what our own School proposes to do to overcome the enemy Syphilis.

III. THE HOMŒOPATHIC TREATMENT OF SYPHILIS.

Sec. 223.—Theoretical Views.

There was a time when a homœopathic physician, who should have undertaken to demonstrate to Hahnemann's adherents the specific idiopathicity of syphilis, and the necessity to oppose it with specific remedies, would have been deemed slightly crazed for putting himself to the trouble of advocating and defending a proposition which every homœopath believes in as religiously as he believes in the existence of his own soul. Some of our physicians still cling to this doctrine; but there are others who, influenced by the doctrines of the Physiological School, have been led to regard a chancre as a purely local affection, and who, with a show of dictatorial assumption and superior knowledge, would fain impose their opinions upon the rest of our brotherhood. Hence, the propriety of touching on this subject. That syphilis is a special disease, emanating from some specific virus, has already been shown in a previous division of this work (§§ 152–154 and §§ 167–170) with so much clearness, that it now behooves Hahnemann's opponents to refute our opinions by cogent and scientific arguments; that is, if they wish us to abandon the master's doctrines, and to change our present mode of treating syphilis. That the breaking out of the chancre is preceded by a general subjugation of the organism by the syphilitic virus, has likewise been shown in §§ 190–192, where, when speaking of the period of incubation, we have given our reasons for an *immediate absorption* of the poison at the very moment when the infection takes place. For the benefit of those who assert the total absence of all precursory symptoms previous to the breaking out of the chancre, we shall offer a few additional statements. We have stated in previous paragraphs, that we, too, have observed these precursory symptoms; what is particularly noteworthy, in reference to this matter is, that, according to the unanimous statements of Gaspard Torella, Massa, Fracastorius,

Fallopius, and other physicians who lived during that first period of the syphilitic epidemic, when the disease was much more violent than it now is, every patient who was attacked with it walked about for several months in a drooping and miserable condition, without the least local symptoms having been perceptible, until, finally, the chancre broke out in all its fury, after which the general constitutional symptoms at once moderated. This evidently shows that the appearance of the chancre is preceded by a general disharmony of the organism, that can only be removed by internal treatment. But, if evidence of this kind should not be deemed sufficient to settle the existence of preliminary symptoms with positive certainty; and if such evidence should only be accepted as proof that preliminary symptoms may *possibly* take place in the organism, would it be proper, from a mere spirit of opposition to Hahnemann, to assert with Girtauner, Hecker, Ricord, and others, that the removal of chancres by cauterizing agents is not succeeded by pernicious consequences? The time is, fortunately, no more when a faithful adherent of Hahnemann could be denounced and laughed at by a set of pretended critics among us, who were in the habit of setting up their authoritative *ipse dixit* in the place of his own teachings; though we are sorry to admit that there are good and trusty homœopaths, at the present day, who do not hesitate to cauterize the chancre at the same time as they employ internal treatment. If we consider (see § 207) that the sole reliable sign by which we recognize the total eradication of the virus from the organism is the *spontaneous* disappearance, as it were, of all external signs of syphilis, in consequence of internal specific treatment; it must be evident that a removal of the characteristic syphilitic product by purely external applications is no safe criterion for the radical cure of the disease, which, indeed, may break out again from its latent condition, either on the patient thus improperly and unreliably treated, or even upon his offspring. How much better it would be to effect the cure more tardily, but to effect it safely, without entailing upon the poor victim of a rash and unscientific treatment the danger of seeing the disease break out again, at a later period, in a much more destructive and more obstinate form.

Sec. 224.—Homœopathic Specifics.

Fortunately we possess specific remedial agents that render

all use of cauterizing agents superfluous. If one specific does not seem to reach the case, we have others that may be more specifically adapted to the symptoms. Whether *primary* or *secondary*, the therapeutic range of our remedies extends over every form and period of the syphilitic disease, *including all its characteristic modifications and metamorphoses* (see §§ 195–198 and §§ 177, 178). He who knows from experience what *Mercurius* and its different preparations are capable of effecting against the *primary* chancre; *Nitri acidum*, *Thuja*, *Cinnabaris*, against the fungoid vegetations of the chancre; *Kali jodatum*, *Aurum*, *Lycopodium*, Sarsaparilla (*Iodide of Mercury*, Ed.), and other remedies for such modified forms of the disease as have lost their infectious character—must admit that, in spite of all existing imperfections, we are much more successful in the treatment of syphilis than the Old School, with all its caustics, starvation-cures, inunction-cures, and mercurial poisonings. It is to be regretted that, as yet, we have no other specific for chancre than the mercurial preparations, which never show their curative powers in as small doses as almost any other drugs, and, even in half-grain doses of the first centesimal trituration, are still capable, by a too long continued use, of exciting artificial symptoms in the mouth, throat, and upon the skin. Even the preparations which some of our physicians have imported from the old school, such as the combinations of Mercury with Iodine, Bromine, Nitri and Phosphori acidum, have not lessened the danger involved in the use of mercurial preparations, since Mercury is the chief constituent in all these combinations. The *Nitrate of Mercury*, recommended by Trinks, is even much more dangerous than the Corrosive sublimate. As yet, few of those remedies have been proved, so that, in case aggravations should occur after their use, it is difficult to decide whether such aggravations are caused by an over-dose of the drug, or constitute natural exacerbations of the disease itself. It is true that, among the effects of the different mercurial combinations, the effects of Mercury always hold the most prominent rank, and that the preparations of Mercury with acids seem more energetic, probably on account of their great solubility. On the other hand, do we know whether some of the characteristic effects of Mercury are not neutralized in those combinations, and whether the *diagnostic* signs by which we recognize an excess of mercurial action in contradistinction to syphilitic phenomena, such as *itching*, the *milky-*

white color, and other properties of mercurial ulcers, etc., are not suspended in these newly-imported agents? Considerations like these deserve the most careful attention of our practitioners. It is more particularly to be regretted that our provings of the Iodide of Potassium are, as yet, very imperfect. For, if the mercurial preparations are best calculated to destroy the chancre-virus and its primary products; *Nitri acidum* and *Thuja* to reach the fungoid vegetations of chancre; the Iodides, on the contrary, are best adapted to that phase in the secondary period of the syphilitic disease where it seems to have undergone a radical metamorphosis, and perpetuates its products in the tissues by sending off shoots in the diseased organism, but is no longer capable of producing new parasites in other organisms by its own inherent fecundating power. This statement is not impaired by the fact, that the Iodide of Potassium has shown curative effects against products of the infectious period of syphilis; since, in spite of all the modifications which the virus may undergo, it remains *essentially the same thing;* like the caterpillar, its chrysalis and the butterfly, or the child and the man, growing out of it even to old age; all of which, in their different stages of existence, have a great many characteristics in common, and, on the other hand, have each their different individual wants.

Sec. 225.—Dose.

It is well known that a few pellets of the thirtieth potency, which Hahnemann has recommended as sufficient for the cure of chancre, are entirely inadequate to destroy this enemy. Any one who, finding even half a grain of the first centesimal trituration of Mercury insufficient, prescribes one or two grains of the same trituration, may deviate from the letter of Hahnemann, but, nevertheless, remains true to the spirit of his doctrine. This doctrine demands that the dose should be sufficiently small not to produce any unnecessary or injurious effects; but that, on the other hand, it is to be sufficiently large to effect a cure as radically and promptly as possible. A physician who, knowing that a dose of one-tenth of a grain is sufficient to effect a cure, or who, seeing that the exhibition of Mercury is followed by an evident exacerbation of the symptoms, should continue this agent in increasing doses—or go even so far, as was done even recently by one of our

Paris homœopaths, as to prescribe one hundred grains of Calomel in ten days, and to give out such a murderous proceeding as an improvement on Homœopathy—is not only no adherent of Hahnemann, but is no *rational* physician, since Hahnemann's exceedingly rational maxims demand that a physician should constantly seek to know how far a dose can be reduced without impairing the efficiency of the remedial agent in bringing about a speedy, safe, and permanent cure. Starting from the principle of effecting a safe cure with mild and perfectly safe means, one-half of a grain of the first centesimal trituration, twice a day, seems to be a sufficiently small dose to avoid all dangerous effects of the drug, and, on the other hand, sufficiently large to effect a sure cure; whereas a similar dose of the first decimal trituration not only seems unnecessarily large, but even dangerous, although it may not develop its medicinal effects at once. What is particularly worthy of notice is, that medicinal symptoms, caused by large doses of Mercury, sometimes disappear again after a second dose of the same drug, a phenomenon that has already been substantiated by Old-School experience; on which account symptoms, that really were mercurial effects, are frequently mistaken for syphilitic manifestations, for which repeated doses of Mercury are given, until the cumulative effect of the poison breaks forth with a dangerous and scarcely controllable violence. It is very strange, indeed, that such large doses of this most dangerous and most insidious of all metals, should be required for the cure of chancre, whereas *Nitri acidum*, *Thuja*, and other drugs, will cure the fungoid vegetations of chancre and other analogous symptoms in the thirtieth attenuation, provided these drugs are in specific rapport with the case. Perhaps, by giving three or six globules of the third, sixth, or twelfth attenuation of Mercury in half a tumbler of water, in tablespoonful doses, and thus treating a chancre as we would any other acute disease, we might achieve a cure still more rapidly; I confess, however, that I have never yet dared to pursue such a course. What I can affirm with positive certainty is, that if the virus has once been subdued by repeated doses of Mercury, and the chancre seems to be in a fair way of improvement, the further use of this agent may be safely discontinued, and the cure may be expected to take place without any further medication. I have seen acute recent chancres improve after three doses of Mercury—one dose in the evening, one next morning, and a third the following evening—to such an extent that I have felt authorized to discontinue the further use of the drug, after which the chancre continued to improve, and finally to cicatrize; in one case this happened in ten days. In other cases I have seen chancres get well in twenty days, from a dose of Mercury every other day. I speak, of course, of the simple and Hunterian chancre, to which Mercury seems to be more specifically adapted than to phagedænic chancre. In many cases of *elevated chancres*, if I have charge of the treatment at the outset, three or four doses of Mercury every other day, are sufficient to control the disease, after which the chancre gets well much more rapidly without any further medicine than old chancres, where the Mercury has to be given in frequently repeated doses. Moreover, as Vehsemeyer has noticed of the Sublimate, too large, and too frequent doses of Mercury may have the effect of causing a premature cicatrization of the chancre, and simply masking the disease. Here, too, it is better to progress slowly and safely, than rapidly and with danger to the patient. *Medio tutissimus ibis!*

Sec. 226.—Treatment of Complicated Syphilis.

One of those complications, that is most frequently met with when patients come to us out of allopathic hands, is the complication with mercurial symptoms, which it is of the utmost importance not to overlook, since we might otherwise be induced to continue the Mercury, and to cause great injury to the patient. We have stated before that mercurial symptoms have the peculiarity of disappearing in one place, under the effects of repeated doses of Mercury, in order to break out again at a subsequent period in some other part, and perhaps with more violence. A misapprehension on the part of the physician might lead him to continue the use of Mercury, in the supposition that the symptoms before him are syphilitic symptoms, until finally, completely bewildered, he no longer knows what course he ought to pursue. If a patient comes to us out of allopathic hands, the first thing the homœopathic physician has to do is, to inquire what remedies the patient has used. If the still existing chancres, exanthems, or other ulcers are accompanied by *itching;* or, as was the case with Hofrichter's patients (see All. hom. Zeit., vol. 35), if the symptoms manifest themselves in places where we are wont to see the effects of Mercury located instead of syphilitic phenomena, for instance, on the margin of the tongue; or if the ulcers exhibit the milky-white color of Mercury, instead of the copper color of syphilis, we may rest assured that we have a combination of syphilis and mercurial disease to deal with, and that we have to resort to other drugs than mercurial preparations. At this moment, I am treating a boy who has hereditary syphilis, and who, when he came to me from his allopathic attendant, was affected with a distinctly marked syphilitic ecthyma. The violent itching of which he complained, led me to doubt the nature of the case. In order to obtain light on the subject, I gave the boy *Sacch. lact.*, requesting the mother, when she called again, to bring all the boy's former receipts along. These showed me that the boy had not only been treated with large doses of the Iodide of Mercury, but had likewise taken strong baths of Corrosive Sublimate. I now prescribed ten grains of the *Iodide of Potassium* in four ounces of water, a dessertspoonful every four hours, and for the last ten days the case has visibly improved.

Beside the combination with mercurial symptoms, syphilis can likewise appear combined, or rather associated, with other diseases (see §§ 204 and 111–114), in which case the following rules are to be observed:

1) If, in the course of an acute or chronic syphilis, some other acute malady supervenes, such as typhus, smallpox, measles, scarlatina, etc., the course of the syphilitic disease is usually suspended for the time, and, for this reason, the other supervening disease has to be treated first, until it is either cured, or convalescence is, at any rate, far advanced. The same remark applies to non-miasmatic, acute inflammatory diseases, such as pneumonia, hepatitis, angina faucium, and other acute inflammations; these, too, have first to be removed before the treatment of syphilis can be continued. The supervention of syphilis, while an acute disease is running its course, could only take place, provided such a thing is at all possible, if an infection that had been caught shortly previous to the acute disease, should break out during the course of the latter; but even in such a case the intervening acute disease has to be seen to first, before we institute any special treatment for the syphilitic malady.

2) If an attack of acute or recently-acquired syphilis should take place during the course of a *chronic* malady, such as itch, herpes, scrofula, tubercles, etc., we first attend to the syphilis, without troubling ourselves about the chronic malady until the syphilis is cured. The same course is to be pursued, if, while we are treating some other chronic malady, a syphilitic infection that had been acquired years ago, and had remained in a *masked* condition, should suddenly break out into an active disease; in such a case we first attend to the syphilis, and, after this is cured, resume the treatment of the chronic affection.

3) If, during the presence of acute and recently-caught syphilis, a new chronic disease, like the itch for example, supervenes, we leave this latter disease unattended to, until the syphilis is cured. If the itch should be caught while we are managing an old, chronic, or constitutional syphilis, the itch is to be cured first, after which, we again direct our attention to the syphilitic disease.

THIRD CHAPTER.

PHARMACO-DYNAMIC OBSERVATIONS.

I. REMEDIES AGAINST THE DESTRUCTIVE CHANCRE-VIRUS.

Sec. 227.—Precursory Remark.

In the introduction to this work we have asked the important question, with what right we adopt a single syphilitic contagium, and yet believe that our patients are cured and protected against all further attacks from the syphilitic virus, even if they never took a single dose of Mercury, which, however, is our chief anti-syphilitic remedy, and were treated with entirely different medicines. Our readers, if they have followed us in our discussion up to this point, must have noticed that, in the third division of this work (§§ 194–198), we have shown four periods in the existence of chancre, representing four different *conditions* or *metamorphoses* of the chancre-virus, the two first of which are still possessed of the faculty of transmitting the contagion as embodied in their own forms, whereas the two latter can only perpetuate their existence by sending off *shoots* in the same tainted organism. We have

First: *Contagious* period, or *primary Syphilis:*

1. The *ulcerous* or *chancre-breeding* virus;
2. The *fungoid* or *condylomatous* virus, breeding fungoid forms.

Secondary: *Non-contagious* syphilis:

1. Development of the new off-shoots;
2. Retrogression into a masked condition, stage of involution.

Inasmuch as the original chancre-virus undergoes, in each of these periods, as we have shown above, a metamorphosis, not only according to its form, but likewise according to its pathological essence, it must seem quite natural that the remedies which, in the first of these periods, have power to *annihilate* the virus in its very being, as it were, are no longer adapted to the other period, after the essential nature of the virus has undergone a complete modification, or actual change. Hence, it is exceedingly questionable whether Mercury, which is a true *specific* for the primary chancres, is equally adapted for the protopathic or consecutive products of the fungoid period, such as mucous tubercles and figwarts, or even for chancre itself, after it has become correspondingly altered in its essential characteristics, in consequence of the fungoid metamorphosis. For the fungoid chancre, and for all the protopathic or consecutive symptoms that are specially characteristic of this modification, *Nitri acidum*, *Thuja*, and such like remedies are specifically curative agents. Hence it is, that the curative action of the *Iodides* against the primary and consecutive products of the chancre-virus is exceedingly unreliable, and even without effect; whereas they produce distinguished curative results when brought to bear upon almost any product of the *secondary*, no longer contagious syphilis. We have shown, in § 224, that the sphere of action of these specifics is not as sharply circumscribed in Nature as it seems to be in print. Mercurial preparations will afford help in *secondary* syphilis, if the secondary period sets in while primary phenomena are still existing; or if, in the secondary period, ulcers or other products break out, that seem to denote a tendency on the part of the organism to return to its *primitive* or *primary* condition of existence. This rule applies whenever the signs of the different periods are mixed up together. It would be more correct not to classify remedies in accordance with the different periods, but in accordance with the characteristic phenomena of these periods. Instead of saying: Remedies of the *primitive*, *consecutive*, *secondary syphilis*, we should classify the remedies as follows: Remedies for the *destructive* syphilis, the *fungoid* syphilis, the *off-shoots* of syphilis, and for *constitutional* syphilis. This is the classification that we shall follow. In this article, we shall first mention the remedies for the destructive or primitive form of *primary* syphilis; these remedies comprehend all the *mercurial preparations*, from which, however, we exclude *Cinnabaris*, as belonging rather among those that are more particularly useful for *fungoid vegetations*. *Mercurius vivus*, *Merc. sol.*, *Merc. præcip. rub.*, *sublimatus corrosivus*, *Merc. præcipitatus*, *Merc. nitrosus*, these being the only mercurial preparations, that are commonly used by homœopathic physicians, of which we here present a list.

Sec. 228.—Mercurius Vivus and Mercurius Solubilis Hahnemanni.

Although some practitioners have denounced Merc. vivus as absolutely useless as a remedy for syphilis, and are only willing to allow the solubilis exceptional rights in this direction—in the place of which they have sought to substitute the much more dangerous *Mercurius nitrosus*—too many splendid curative results obtained with these remedies are found recorded in the writings of our School, to justify the contempt with which some of our modern critics have seen fit to treat them. It is true that *Mercurius vivus*, if we mean to obtain thorough results from its use, has to be rubbed up for a long while, for the reason that its curative action is proportionate to the solubility of the preparation; if this rubbing is continued sufficiently long, the vivus is preferable to any other preparation of Mercury. As long as I prepared my own medicines, I have always got along with *Mercurius vivus* alone; at present, however, when I can no longer spare the time for this kind of work, I likewise use *Mercurius solubilis*. The following symptoms were cured, with scarcely a single exception, with Merc. sol., by the following observers: Ægidi, Attomyr, Baudis, Bernstein, Bigel, Buchner, Goullon, Hartlaub, Hartmann, Herrmann, Knorre, Kramer, Kreussler, Liedbeck, Cl. Müller, Rummel, Sommer, Schréter, Schrœn, Seidel, Stapf, Tietze, Thorer, Trinks, Vehsemeyer, Wesselhœft, Wolf. The principal symptoms that have been cured by these practitioners, as well as by myself, with Merc. sol., are the following:

1.) *Chancres and Mucous Tubercles.*—A) Several superficial excoriations on the glans secreting a white mucus.—Lardaceous chancre on the frænulum, almost separating it from the glans.—Lardaceous, suppurating chancre behind the corona glandis.—Two large, flat chancres behind the corona.—Scurfy, somewhat itching ulcer on the outer surface of the prepuce.—Chancre near the frænulum, of the size of a pea, accompanied by an itching ulcer on the outer surface of the prepuce.—Round, deep ulcer on the glans, with elevated, bright-red, pouting edges.—Two ulcers on the upper portion of the glans, with hard edges, which are sensitive to contact, and a pain that seems as if felt throughout the whole body.—*Hunterian Chancres* of some duration, having not yet changed to a fungoid growth, but no longer lardy, with agonizing, boring pains, from nine o'clock in the evening until three in the morning, depriving the patient of sleep.—*Simple*, and also recent *Hunterian* chancres on the glans and prepuce.—*Elevated* chancres on the prepuce.

B) A number of ulcers of different sizes, with pouting edges, profuse suppuration, and enormous swelling of the penis and prepuce.—Small ulcers in the folds of the prepuce.—Seven ulcers on the glans, prepuce, and body of the penis.—Two small, red, flat ulcers on the private parts.—Dry, coniform warts, of the size of split peas, resting upon an oval base, not bleeding, firm and undivided at their base, the smallest of them like ordinary condylomata, dotting the glans, prepuce, and body of the penis.

C) *Consensual phenomena:* Pains that permeate the whole body.—Nocturnal, boring pains.—Swelling of the prepuce.—Paraphimosis like a cartilaginous ring around the glans, with a bag-shaped swelling towards the outer side.—Painful inflammation and redness of the inner prepuce.—Ulcers on the glans and prepuce, but chiefly on the posterior surface of the glans.—Chancres, more particularly behind the corona glandis, chiefly on the frænulum.—Edges surrounded with a copper-colored areola, with somewhat rounded indentations, not very painful, but sensitive to the contact of the linen.—Ulcers that eat more rapidly downwards than they spread laterally.—*The bottom of the ulcer is hard, lardaceous, the ichor firmly adhering, corrosive, having a fetid odor, and leaving stains on the linen like molten tallow.*

2) *Consecutive buboes and ulcers* in the throat.—A) Painfulness of the inguinal glands, especially on the left side.—Hardness of the left inguinal gland, with slight redness and inflammation.—Swelling, hardness, and inflammation of the right inguinal gland, with a yellowish softness at the most elevated places, and tension and stinging in the gland when walking.—As long as the bubo has not yet outgrown the chancre, and seems to be more like a consensual

painful swelling, *Merc. sol.* may suffice against these phenomena, and disperse the swelling at the same time as it heals the chancre; if the chancre is on the point of passing into the secondary stage of its existence, and the bubo has become inflamed, *Merc. sol.* will be of no use, and *Merc. præc. rub.* or *Nitri acidum* will have to be used.

B) Ulcers in the throat.—Three syphilitic ulcers in the throat, with erysipelatous inflammation of the soft parts.—Flat ulcers in the throat, with pale redness and stinging when swallowing, itching between the acts of deglutition.—Stinging in the throat, as if the parts were excoriated, aggravated by swallowing liquids, especially cold liquids. Excoriation, swelling, and redness of the tonsils and salivary glands, with increased secretion of saliva, and painful pressure in the throat.—Evening hoarseness, with troublesome dryness of the fauces.

Dose.—Vehsemeyer: second or third decimal trituration, two or three doses daily, increasing the dose from one to five grains each.—Hartmann and Knorre: first to third trituration, two doses daily, from one half to a whole grain each.—Wolf and Seidel: sixth to twelfth attenuation; Wolf also gives the third.—Jahr: first centesimal trituration, two doses daily, of half a grain each, sometimes only every two or three days, according to circumstances.

Sec. 229.—Præcipitatus Ruber.

This preparation is distinguished from Merc. sol. and vivus by being more penetrating, and is frequently useful when the solubilis does not seem to act with sufficient force. In the case of old chancres that have not yet assumed the fungoid form, I resort to it if no improvement shows itself after having prescribed Solubilis for eight days. We possess clinical records of the curative powers of this drug by the following observers: Buchner, Haustein, Hofrichter, Cl. Müller, Rosenberg, Trinks, and Jahr. The following symptoms have been cured with it:

1) *Chancres.*—A) Chancre of the size of a bean between the glans and prepuce.—Deep ulcer, with swelling and induration of the prepuce.—Lardy chancre on the prepuce, with pouting edges and dirty lining, accompanied by syphilitic excoriation on the glans,

and enormous secretion of pus.—Chancre between the glans and prepuce, with thick lardy lining, hard edges, and spreading, both laterally and to the subjacent textures, to such an extent that the glans seems threatened with falling off.—Cup-shaped ulcers, with red, hard edges, and a lardaceous bottom.—Considerable ulcer on the glans, the bottom of which seems to become raised.—*Hunterian chancres, especially when old and neglected.*—Ulcer between the glans and prepuce, the latter being so enormously swollen and inflamed that it can no longer be drawn over the glans, together with purulent discharge between the glans and prepuce, nocturnal tearing in the penis proceeding from the ulcer.—B) Five small ulcers on the labia minora.—The whole glans is covered with ulcers, with dark-brown redness of the prepuce, that can no longer be drawn over the prepuce, and discharge of quantities of pus having a fetid odor.—C) *Consensual ailments:* Fearful swelling of the penis.—Enormous swelling and inflammation of the prepuce, with phimosis.—*Cartilaginous, violet-red induration, and swelling of the prepuce, following the removal of Hunterian chancres by cauterization.*

2) *Consecutive and secondary phenomena.*—A) Inflamed, also suppurating buboes.—B) Swelling of the tonsils, with two ulcers on the hairy scalp, of the size of a dime, having arisen from itching pimples, with lacerated edges, yellow pus, smarting and cutting; attended with cutting pain in the right side of the throat, when swallowing solid food, not when swallowing liquids, with ptyalism and phlegm in the throat; after giving *Merc. sol.*, lardaceous ulcer in the throat, which was cured by *Præcipitatus albus.* (This case, reported by Hofrichter in All. hom. Zeit., vol. 35, does not seem very clear to me. The itching vesicles, bursting when using the comb, and forming ulcers of the size of a dime, have been cured by me more than once with *Hepar sulph.;* the Hepar was given in the belief that these ulcers were mercurial symptoms; the fact that they here yielded to *Præcip. ruber* does not show that they were syphilitic ulcers. We have shown, § 225, that mercurial symptoms sometimes disappear very suddenly, for a time, when a second dose of Mercury is administered, after which they either return or are *soon* replaced by other symptoms. In the present case they were replaced by the lardaceous ulcer in the throat, which I should like to have seen in order to determine the pathological nature of this ulcer for myself; if there is *itching*, as was

the case with those ulcers on the hairy scalp, there is trouble; mercurial cutaneous affections always itch, syphilitic affections never itch, properly speaking. The "burning from the pit of the stomach to the throat, with occasional choking," is no syphilitic, but a real *mercurial symptom.* The same criticism applies to the other case reported in the same volume, page 84, where the following symptoms made their appearance subsequent to the allopathic treatment of gonorrhœa: Itching condyloma on the nates, bleeding when touched; lardy-looking, deep, lacerated, condylomatous ulcer, with uneven base, on the left margin of the tongue (one of the diagnostic signs of mercurial and syphilitic ulcers is, that the latter never occupy the margin, but always the root or dorsum of the tongue; or, if caused by direct contact with infectious matter, they may be seen at the tip of the tongue; likewise, the nocturnal tearing in the limbs points to mercurial disease rather than to syphilis. Jahr).

Hanbold recommends this preparation particularly for buboes, chancres in the throat (especially the true, *metastatic*, not secondary, but consecutive chancres on the tonsils, Jahr), and for other glandular affections; Trinks recommends it for syphilitic destructions of the tonsils, fauces, and palate, also for syphilitic exanthems (especially tubercular and pustulous, Jahr), for cutaneous ulcerations and osseous affections. More than once I have been able to verify its good effects in obstinate Hunterian chancres, and fully subscribe to Buchner's and Cl. Müller's favorable recommendations of this agent.

The dose employed by these authorities was the first trituration, repeated in the same manner as Merc. solubilis.

Sec. 230.—Sublimatus corrosivus. Merc. bijodatus. Merc. nitrosus.

These three preparations have not been used as much as other mercurial preparations; for the present, the following clinical observations can be offered in reference to their use:

1) *Sublimatus corrosivus.*—One of the most intensely-penetrating mercurial preparations, which, as Hartmann very justly remarks, is chiefly adapted to the treatment of phagedænic chancres; but which, according to Vehsemeyer's exceedingly practical observation, must not be continued too long in the treatment of

simple and Hunterian chancres, in order not to bring about a premature cicatrization of the chancre in the place of a radical cure. We have to speak, however, less approvingly of Goullon's method (see Arch. xx., 2, page 142), who likewise employs the Sublimate as a wash in cases of confluent chancre. According to our view of chancre, it should never be touched by external applications that might remove it from the surface before the root is destroyed; on the other hand, we agree with this excellent practitioner in opinion, when he advises, in case the itch and syphilis should break out simultaneously on the same individual, to first cure the syphilis with *Sublimate*, and afterwards to prescribe *Sulphur* for the itch; in a case of this kind, the Sublimate would likewise exert, incidentally, a curative effect upon the itch. Nor can we indiscriminately sanction the use of sublimate-baths in treating chronic eruptions combined with syphilis; in all such cases, the chief indication always is to cure the syphilis with internal remedies, from the centre towards the periphery, unless we wish to run the risk of masking the disease, which, although it may seem cured on its present victim, yet may be transmitted to the offspring. We are able to confirm Hofrichter's recommendation of the Sublimate for exostoses on the tibia, as well as for all similar exostoses, when caused by syphilis; we have found it serviceable in exostoses on the cranium. If this practitioner recommends the Sublimate as an external application to figwarts (see All. hom. Zeit., vol. 35, pages 68 and 85), we must energetically protest, in the name of humanity and all coming generations, against the incorrect diagnosis that leads to an identification of mucous tubercles and figwarts (see §§ 68–72, 177, 178). Among the dry figwarts, there are some that bear touching with *Thuja*, inasmuch as, after the poison has been destroyed, these excrescences are nothing else than abnormal outgrowths from the skin or mucous membranes, the form of which still testifies to the former syphilitic action in the affected parts. In the case of *moist tubercles*, or such like excrescences, external applications may drive the poison back upon internal organs, and give rise, in the most favorable cases, to a *latent* syphilitic disease that can still be communicated to the offspring. Moreover, Sublimate has cured: Small, dusky-red ulcers on the margin of the glans;—red ulcers on the breast and abdomen, of the size of lentils, breaking out after cauterization of chancres, attended with swelling of the tibiæ, and a sensation at night as if these bones would break;—deep ulcers on the corona glandis, with gonorrhœa and bubo.

2) *Mercurius bijodatus.*—This is recommended by Trinks for *inveterate syphilis* of scrofulous individuals; by Clotar Müller chiefly for *syphilidæ.* Müller has likewise used it, with excellent effect, for *ulcers* in the face, at whose bottom the bone was seen denuded, rough, dry, and blackish, of the size of a dime.

3) *Mercurius nitrosus.*—Recommended by Trinks for the most inveterate, most malignant forms of syphilis (which he, however, does not specify more particularly), and has been used by Rummel with success for sycosic excrescences, and more particularly for dry, filiform figwarts, in cases where neither *Thuja*, nor *Nitri acidum*, nor *Staphysagria* were of any avail.

4) *Mercurius phosphatus.*—Recommended by Vehsemeyer as useful in cases of primary chancres, if Merc. sol. or Sublimate are without any effect.

II. REMEDIES FOR FUNGOID SYPHILIS.

Sec. 231.—Cinnabaris.

The chief remedies belonging to this category, are: *Cinnabaris*, *Nitri acidum*, and *Thuja*. Although *Cinnabaris* is likewise of good effect in the *primitive* form of chancre, we mention it in this place, for the reason that it forms the transition from the remedies for *destructive* syphilis to those for *fungoid vegetations*. *Cinnabaris* is particularly effective, if the chancre has not yet assumed the fungoid form, but is on the point of doing so. Clotar Müller has derived benefit from Cinnabaris in cases of neglected Hunterian chancre; and has not only cured with it old and neglected chancres, with or without buboes, or chancres arising from condylomata (mucous tubercles? Jahr), but likewise figwarts accompanied by syphilitic tetter. The cases cured with Cinnabaris by Müller, Sommer, Hofrichter, Lingen, and myself, were characterized by the following symptoms:

1) *Chancres and mucous tubercles.*—A) Not very large, oozing ulcer behind the corona glandis.—Wreath-shaped ulcer on the inner

surface of the prepuce and glans, sprouting upwards.—Flat, cheesy ulcers on the corona glandis, of the size of a split pea; after the cheesy lining is wiped off, the bottom of the ulcer exhibits a red, tolerably smooth surface (mercurial ulcer? Jahr).—Horrid ulcer exactly in the middle of the dorsum of the penis; the bottom of the ulcer is raised two lines, and the edges three lines above the level of the skin.—Indurated chancre on the dorsum of the penis.—Chancrous ulcer on the cicatrix of an old issue on the upper arm. B) Four raised, lardy-looking ulcers on the border of the swollen prepuce; they discharge but little, had sprung from condylomata (mucous tubercles?), became visible after the swelling of the prepuce had subsided, and they afterwards disappeared.—Four small, elevated warts, discharging a moisture (Mucous tubercles? Jahr); they were seated on the border of the swollen prepuce, with phimosis.—Elliptic figwarts on the frænulum and the inner surface of the prepuce, ranged *seriatim* side by side.—*Mucous tubercles* on *the sexual organs, anus, and lips.*—*Elevated chancres.*—*Neglected, simple,* and *Hunterian chancres,* both fungoid and not fungoid. C) *Accompanying phenomena.*—Painless phimoses from swelling of the prepuce.—Swelling of the glans and prepuce.—The glans has a dark, blue-gray color, with swelling of the follicles.—The bottom of the ulcer seems like lard, with uneven granulations very painful to the touch.—Daily discharge of a fetid pus, having a pungent odor, oozing out from behind the prepuce.—Copious discharge of a thin, watery pus.—Secretion of a quantity of yellow, thin mucus having a putrid smell, accompanied by a pricking, burning pain in the glans.—Whitish secretion from the ulcer, having a nauseous-sweetish, pungent odor.—Discharge of a quantity of fetid, purulent mucus, with bleeding of the prepuce when an attempt is made to draw it back.—Offensive smell from the mouth, like amalgam; the whole individual has this odor, notwithstanding the greatest cleanliness.—Emaciated, hollow-eyed, cachectic appearance.

2) *Consecutive and secondary phenomena.*—Bubo in the left inguinal region, of the size of a pigeon's egg, having existed for some months, and painful only when touched.—Chancrous ulcer on the cicatrix of an old issue of the upper arm.—Herpetic spots on the extremities, and around the corners of the mouth, oval and sharply circumscribed.

Cinnabaris is, moreover, indicated in the case of patients who come under homœopathic treatment after having been treated allopathically, without, however, exhibiting traces of mercurial poisoning as plainly as was the case with Hofrichter's patients (see § 229). In cases of the latter kind, *Nitri acidum*, *Thuja*, or some other remedy has to be prescribed; even Cinnabaris would not be allowed, for the reason that nothing is more dangerous than to combat mercurial symptoms with Mercury. There is, indeed, no danger of latent syphilis being brought about by such a proceeding. The danger is that an inexperienced diagnostician may confound the subsequently reappearing mercurial with syphilitic symptoms, for which he again prescribes Mercury, until the patient falls a victim to mercurial poisoning.

Sec. 232.—Nitri Acidum.

Next to Thuja, this is a chief remedy in that stage of syphilis where the chancre-virus changes to the *condylomatous poison;* hence it is a remedy for all the protopathic products that emanate from this modified chancre-virus, and are known by the names of mucous tubercles, figwarts, etc.; in one word, for all kinds of *fungoid vegetations*, whether they grow out of chancre or manifest themselves as protopathic products. It is likewise an excellent, and indeed indispensable remedy, if mercurial poisoning and syphilis are combined together. Hence, Lobethal recommends it very properly for old chancres, for which large doses of Mercury had been taken without effect; instead of growing smaller, the chancres spread; he likewise recommends it for general syphilis after the ineffectual cures à la Dondi, Berg, Zittman, and Rust. Attomyr's recommendation of this drug for the second class of his chancres, is very proper; except that the ulcers, which he describes as clean, flesh-colored, spongy, seem to coincide with our mucous tubercles (see § 68). Buchner's painless *ulcers*, with gray, everted edges, for which this practitioner recommends *Nitri acidum*, seem somewhat tainted with Mercury. Nitri acidum is likewise very properly recommended for buboes; I know of no remedy that is more capable of dispersing an inflammatory bubo than Nitric acid, provided always that the suppurative process can yet be prevented. I am likewise able to confirm every thing that Rummel has said in favor of this agent as a remedy for psoriasis.

In the cases that have been cured by Attomyr, Buchner, Hahnemann, Hartmann, Fielitz, Horner, Hofrichter, Guylas, Langhammer, Liedbeck, Lobethal, Rosenberg, Rummel, Vehsemeyer, and myself, the following chief characteristics were present:

1) *Chancres, mucous tubercles, and figwarts.*—A) Painless, readily-bleeding ulcers, with gray, everted edges.—Flat, or even perceptibly-raised ulcers, with sharply-circumscribed, indented, painless edges.—Chancrous ulcer, surrounded with hard, cartilaginous, lardy-looking borders.—Ulcer with dark-blue, greasy bottom, and covered with a crust, from beneath which ichor oozes out. Ulcers with enormous abnormal granulations.—Lardaceous, painless ulcers on the frænulum, with elevated base and swelling of the prepuce.—Chancrous ulcers on the frænulum, with hard, lardy-looking borders, and redness and swelling of the prepuce.—Deep ulcer where the frænulum had already been eaten away, filled with pus, of the size of a pea.—Deep ulcers on the right side of the corona glandis, and on the left side near the frænulum, which had already become detached.—*Fungoid Hunterian or other chancres, or chancres threatening to change to the fungoid form;* they had been unsuccessfully treated with Mercury, and their bottom had already become red.—B) Clean, flesh-colored, almost spongy ulcers.—Several flat, elongated ulcers on the prepuce, existing simultaneously. — Cauliflower-shaped condylomata on the inner surface of the prepuce, and on the corona glandis, secreting a fetid matter.—Pedunculated condylomata, of the size of a pin's head, growing out of ulcers on the prepuce.—C) *Accessory symptoms:* The ichor from the ulcers does not adhere, is mixed with blood, more copious and thinner than gleet. — Copious, watery secretion from ulcers that have become quite flat, and whose edges are almost obliterated.—The pus, which is secreted in large quantity, is corrosive, smells like brine, and causes a furious itching (mercurial syphilis—Jahr).—Secretion of ichorous pus.—A lymphatic vessel on the penis is inflated, when proceeding from the ulcer, it looks like a raven's quill.—Hard, elongated swelling on the inner surface of the prepuce, round the ulcer.

2) *Consecutive and secondary symptoms.* — A) *Inflamed buboes,* threatening to suppurate.—B) The tonsils are red and swollen. The tonsils are enlarged, uneven, covered with purulent

vesicles of the size of a pin's head (Mercurial syphilis).—The velum palati, especially on the left side, is fiery-red, shining (Mercurial syphilis? Jahr).—Deep, shaggy ulcer on the border of the tongue (Merc. syphilis, Jahr).—C) Isolated, moist, burning pustules on the hairy scalp (Merc. syphilis, Jahr).—The face is covered with pustules, with broad red borders, and forming crusts.—Scurfy elevation on the alæ nasi, of the size of a bean, resembling a mucous tubercle.—Brown spots on the glans, of the size of lentils, scaling off.—Rather hard brown tubercles on the scrotum and perineum, of the size of peas, ulcerating.

Sec. 233.—Thuja Occidentalis.

The chief sphere of action of this remedy are the modifications of the chancre-virus that are described as *idiopathic condylomata*, *mucous tubercles*, and *sycosic excrescences*. It is more particularly the humid products of this kind, such as cauliflower-excrescences, and still more, *mucous tubercles* (see § 68), against which this remedy will prove most efficient, whereas this agent, according to Rummel's very correct observation, is of little or no use against the dry, filiform figwarts, which sometimes continue even after the virus has been entirely destroyed (see § 78). Nevertheless, it may be useful in certain old chancrous forms, and likewise in secondary ulcerations of the skin and throat, although the chancrous forms for which Attomyr recommends this agent seem to be *mucous tubercles*, rather than true chancres. Wolf, of Dresden, is quite right in recommending *Thuja* for dubious ulcers on the sexual organs, in the mouth and fauces, more particularly if it is not quite certain whether the ulcers are mercurial or syphilitic; in such cases, I have likewise used it with much success, especially among females. In the cases successfully treated with this remedy by Attomyr, Bernstein, Gentzke, Hahnemann, Hartmann, Kurtz, Lobethal, Mayrhofer, Nithack, Rosenberg, Rummel, Schelling, Trinks, Wolf of Dresden, and myself, the following symptoms were the chief indications:

1) *Chancres, Mucous Tubercles, and Figwarts.*—A) Chancres, becoming more elevated above the skin (after Nitri acidum).—Ulcers, secreting a corrosive ichor mixed with blood.—Small ulcers scattered over a hard base, lined with a whitish pus, burning and

smarting, or biting a good deal.—Several ulcers on the prepuce and glans, growing above the skin, clean-looking, but suppurating profusely.—Vegetating ulcers on the glans, prepuce, and penis. —Deep, humid furrows, covered with pus, seated in the prepuce, which is swollen all around, and surrounded with wrinkled, red borders.—Ulcers on the prepuce, discharging a profuse quantity of ichor, and raised above the skin like warts cut half through (mucous tubercles? Jahr). — B) Cauliflower excrescences. — Comb-shaped, horny excrescences on the inner surface of the prepuce.—Twelve condylomata on the margin of the glans.—A number of warts and tubercles, part ulcerated and part dry, on the scrotum, perineum, and anus, the skin of these parts being excoriated here and there.—Warts, partly hard and reddish, partly suppurating, densely covering the anus and scrotum all around.—Smooth condylomata on the perineum, scrotum, and anus; they secrete a good deal of moisture, and are covered with a purulent and viscid fluid. —A continued line of condylomata on both sides of the external labia, extending as far as the promontary of Venus.—Numerous condylomata on the thighs and swollen labia majora, with corrosive leucorrhœa.—A mulberry-shaped, shining condyloma at the anus, with a broad base; on both sides of it deep rhagades, secreting a fetid ichor, and surrounded by a brownish-yellow areola.—*Mucous tubercles on the labia, at the anus, in the corners of the mouth, on the alæ nasi, eyelids, nipples, especially in the case of women and children.*

2) *Syphilitic Erosions.*—Female gonorrhœa, with numerous erosions and profuse secretion.—*Humid erosions between the thighs and on the sides of the scrotum.*—Excoriation and bright redness on the inner side of the thighs, with intolerable burning.—*Superficial, syphilitic erosions* in the fauces, with mucous tubercles.—Suspicious redness of the palate, with occasional stinging in the throat.

Most of the condylomata alleged to have been cured by the above-mentioned observers, seem to have been mucous tubercles. It is a pity that these so-called condylomata have not been described more minutely; the mucous tubercles that are usually confounded with figwarts, or classed with the latter in the same category with condylomata generally, differ from common excrescences both pathologically and anatomically, and appear protopathically much more frequently than figwarts. This shows, however, how mischievous a mere nomenclature may become in Therapeutics; yet modern homœopaths seem to work in favor of such a change.

III. REMEDIES FOR SECONDARY SYPHILIS.

Sec. 234.—Other Substances that have been used by Various Practitioners.

Most of the remedies, that have been mentioned heretofore, have been chiefly employed in cases where mercurial syphilis was suspected; many of them might likewise be used, more frequently than has been done, for *secondary syphilis*; such as:

1) *Aurum foliatum* and *muriaticum.*—Hahnemann recommends this remedy for nocturnal bone-pains and for the ill effects of abuse of Mercury; Trinks denies the efficacy of this drug; he has given it in vain, even in large doses, for syphilitic affections of the mouth, palate, and nasal bones. Wolf, of Dresden, is satisfied that it has no effect whatever in syphilitic affections. On the other hand, Clotar Müller, one of our most competent practitioners, recommends *Aurum muriaticum* as one of the most efficient remedies for secondary ulcers on the scrotum. I have given Aurum with distinguished success for *mercurial affections* of the skull-bones; tearing bone-pains in the extremities; periosteal swellings on the forearms and tibiæ; mercurial destructions of the nasal and palatine-bones; constantly returning ulcers on the margins of the tongue; falling off of the hair; and a desponding melancholy and undefinable *prostration* of body and soul, which is one of the most dangerous symptoms of Mercury.

2) *Carbo animalis.*—This agent has been recommended by Gross, and afterwards by Gaspary, for inflamed buboes threatening to suppurate. I have not only used it with advantage in similar cases, especially for protopathic buboes, but likewise in a case of *gummatose swellings of the cellular tissue* (§§ 147, 151).

3) *Lycopodium.*—According to my observations, this is one of

our best remedies for certain herpetic affections of the throat, accompanied by *secondary exanthems*, secondary ulcers in the throat, condylomata on the sexual organs, deeply-penetrating mercurial symptoms, more particularly if, as has likewise been stated by other practitioners, the following symptoms are present: Pedunculated, dry, almost insensible condylomata on the sexual parts;—dark-gray-yellow, lardy-looking lining in the throat (or wrinkled spots) on the tonsils, palate, and velum, as far as the tongue;—lardaceous ulcers in the mouth and throat;—hoarseness and desire to cough, as in laryngeal phthisis;—loose and bleeding gums and teeth;—copper-colored eruption or tubercles and pustules in the cachectic-looking face;—tearing pains in the limbs at night and in cold weather;—disposition to lie down, melancholy, aversion to life;—mercurial debility, nervousness.

4) *Phosphori acidum.*—This agent is perhaps equally important as Nitri acidum; it has rendered me good service in mercurial syphilis, with ulceration of the lips, velum, and gums; in swelling of bones, bone-pains, and condylomata; Rosenberg has likewise cured with this remedy truly syphilitic, boil-shaped ulcers on the skin and penis, surrounded with a copper-colored border.

5) *Staphysagria.*—In accordance with Wahle's and Rummel's recommendations, I have used this remedy with good results, not only in dry, filiform, but also in soft, cock's-comb-shaped figwarts, and likewise in cases of mucous tubercles. It seems to me particularly indicated when syphilis and mercurial poisoning are combined. I have used it for two or three months in succession, in alternation with Phosphori acidum for mercurial-syphilitic bone-pains; and, in alternation with Aurum, for mercurial bodily and moral prostration.

6) *Sulphur.*—Whatever may be said in its favor, this remedy will never do the least thing against true syphilis, but may be of some use for the mercurial symptoms in this disease. Attomyr's itching chancre, if it is not a præputial herpes, cannot be any thing else than a mercurial-syphilitic ulcer, for there never is any itching in syphilitic ulcers, until mercurial symptoms begin to develop themselves in them. With these explanatory remarks, we may recommend Sulphur as useful in the following affections:

Violently-itching ulcers which in a few days already become covered with a scurf;—thick scurfs on the prepuce, from beneath which pus oozes out;—cock's-comb-shaped, soft, spongy, readily-bleeding excrescence on the corona glandis, of the size of a pigeon's egg;—moist warts and condylomata on the hard-swollen labium;—excoriation and inflammatory redness around the sexual parts, with burning, and secreting a moisture;—excoriation on the swollen prepuce, readily adhering to the linen;—copper-colored spots on the forehead;—hard, large, inflamed buboes;—scattered warts on the thigh;—chronic, mild gleet.

Sec. 235.—Remedies that are less frequently used.

According to circumstances, these may be as important as the other remedies. We have:

1) Guajacum.—In mercurial syphilis, this remedy deserves much more attention than it has enjoyed heretofore, and which I have used with good effect for: tearing and stinging in the limbs;—bone-pains with swelling;—stinging-drawing, tearing pains in the skull and nasal-bones;—itching, herpetic, ill-defined exanthems.

2) Hepar sulphuris.—Of no account in pure syphilis, but useful for the following mercurial symptoms: Falling off of the hair;—painful tubercles on the head, and nocturnal pains in the integuments of the skull;—painfulness of the nose when pressing upon it, with inflamed eyes;—eruption around the mouth;—ulcerated gums, with ptyalism;—swelling of the tonsils, hardness of the cervical glands, with stinging during deglutition, or when coughing, drawing in air, and turning the neck;—abscesses in the groin and axilla;—diarrhœic stools, composed of blood and green mucus;—inflammatory swelling of the knee, hands, fingers;—readily-bleeding ulcers, with nocturnal burning, beating, stinging;—nocturnal bone-pains, with chilliness;—prostration, nervousness.

3) Lachesis.—Truly suitable only in mercurial syphilis, although Gross has cured with it a malignant, ulcerated syphiloid, consisting of unclean, flat ulcers, of the size of peas; likewise a malignant syphilitic ulcer, spreading rapidly, and penetrating to the bone. I have cured with it syphilitic throat-affections, cuta-

neous pustules and ulcers. Hering relates a case of mercurial syphilis, with the following symptoms: Velum and fauces covered with cicatrices, and small, greenish-yellow ulcers, deeply seated in the folds, with constant titillation, exciting a cough and retching; —violent pain when swallowing food, with regurgitation of liquids by the nose;—continual spitting, coughing and hawking;—painful tubercles on the neck, and soreness of the throat, extending even to the ears, which feel as if stopped up;—badly-colored countenance, and yellowish cheeks, with red little veins;—nose pointed, with fluent discharges from it, red and swollen, and as if excoriated;—paroxysms of headache, as if the head would burst;—nocturnal bone-pains.

4) MEZEREUM.—Chiefly suitable in mercurial syphilis, with or without affections of bones; also for affections of the fauces; Hofrichter has cured: dark redness of the pharyngeal mucous membrane, worse every winter, caused by suppression of gonorrhœa and chancre, with burning dryness of the fauces and larynx down to the chest, together with huskiness of voice, and hawking up of mucus.

5) PHOSPHORUS.—I have used this remedy with more or less success for: syphilitic psoriasis in the palms of the hands, and on the soles of the feet;—old roseola syphilitica;—syphilitic psoriasis; —mercurial-syphilitic ulcers on the prepuce;—vague bone-pains and exostoses.

6) SABINA.—Hahnemann informed me, when I assisted him, in 1833 and 1834, in getting out his Chronic Diseases, that he considered *Sabina* equally important as Thuja in sycosis; I know that he had provings of this drug which have never seen the light. Hartmann recommends Sabina for *abnormal granulations*, and Cl. Müller for figwarts, with intolerable burning and itching; in such cases, large doses of Mercury had most probably been employed.

7) SARSAPARILLA.—Recommended by Trinks and others for secondary syphilis, more properly, perhaps, for *mercurial syphilis*. Rummel has used a decoction of Sarsaparilla, with good effect, for *syphilitic psoriasis;* in one case, where I gave Sarsaparilla 30 for

arthritic pains, I have seen old, dry figwarts, remaining after mercurial treatment, disappear. It has also done me good service in mercurial bone-pains, where I used it together with *Phosphorus*, *Aurum*, and *Nitri Acidum*.

Sec. 236.—More Recent Remedies that have been but little used.

1) ARGENTUM.—This remedy was proposed in 1811, as a substitute for Mercury. Its range of action is confined to mercurial affections, more particularly to *angina*. Under the internal use of *Argentum nitricum*, 3d attenuation, I have seen cock's-comb-shaped *protopathic figwarts* on the pudendum disappear in two cases; in one case, they were seated, like a silvery wreath, on the margin of the labia majora. I have found it of no use in cases of inflamed buboes; in one case, it has seemed to promote the healing of a bubo.

2) BADIAGA.—On account of the resemblance which this sea-sponge bears to Lycopodium, it may become an important remedy for secondary and perhaps consecutive products of syphilis. Rosenberg has cured with it an oblong, rather hard swelling of the left inguinal gland, of the size of a pigeon's egg, and coming on after suppression of chancre.

3.) CORALLIA RUBRA.—According to Attomyr, Corallia is chiefly indicated for *syphilitic erosions*, or superficial, lardy-looking, mostly red ulcerations. Attomyr has cured with Corallia a case of balanorrhœa, and Bernstein a flat, round ulcer on the prepuce.

4.) FERRUM IODATUM.—May become highly useful in mercurial cachexias caused by abuse of Mercury, even to ptyalism.

5.) IODINE.—Recommended by Trinks and Lobethal for mercurial cachexia, and more particularly for mercurial ptyalism.

6.) KALI HYDROJODICUM.—Recommended by Lobethal, who remarks that small doses of this agent are of no use, but that it has to be employed in gradually increased quantities of thirty to sixty grains to several ounces of water. Rosenberg prescribed one grain in six ounces of water, curing with this dose more rapidly than Lobethal. The latter recommends it for *figwarts*, *swelling of the bones*, *inflam-*

mation of the periosteum, tubercular and papulous eruptions in the face, carious ulcers, and other products of secondary syphilis. Rosenberg has cured with it idiopathic buboes. This remedy seems particularly adapted to combinations of mercurial and syphilitic symptoms, but likewise to that period of the syphilitic disease (see § 196) where the metamorphosed products of the virus are *no longer contagious* (truly secondary period.) When given in large doses for *contagious* primary symptoms, its effect is only palliative. Such results should be avoided by the physician, unless he does not mind changing the character of the disease to that of latent syphilis. Where the virus had become essentially modified by a previous use of large doses of Mercury, the *Iodide of Potassium* becomes indispensable. The chief symptoms that Lobethal and Rosenberg have cured with this remedy, are the following: Deep, lardaceous chancres, of the size of peas, with hard edges, on the inner surface of the labia majora;—buboes in both groins, of the size of pigeon-eggs;—deep, ulcerated bubo, with pouting lips;—tubercular pustules in the face, on the forehead and nose;—roseola on the chest and extremities;—broad, badly-colored gummatose ulcerations in the cellular tissue;—badly-colored, large cutaneous ulcerations;—swelling of bones;—mercurial, bloody diarrhœa, with tenesmus;—horrid nocturnal bone-pains;—falling off of the hair.

7) Platina.—Rosenberg has employed a preparation of Platina, which was probably the *Chloride of Platina and Sodium.* He cured with this preparation a bleeding, violently tearing, and stinging fungoid chancre, together with an almost painless bubo, except in the warmth when stitches, as with red-hot pins, darted through it.

I wish to direct attention to four other remedies that are but seldom, if ever, used in syphilitic affections, and which have proved very effectual in my hands; they are:

a) Arsenicum, for tubercular exanthems of secondary syphilis;

b) Fluoris acidum, for mucous tubercles, balanorrhœa, and syphilitic erosions;

c) Sepia, for syphilitic erosions, and gonorrhœa occasioned by them, especially among females;

d) Silicea, for ulcerated cutaneous affections in mercurial syphilis.

ADDENDA.

I.—To Sections 35 and 36.

Not only these two paragraphs, but upwards of two thirds of this work, had already been printed, and the whole of my manuscript had already been sent off, when, in the course of last month, I had an opportunity of making two interesting observations, that, on the one hand, seemed to confirm my views concerning the essential oneness and purely accidental, external, or phenomenal differences of the various kinds of chancre, and, on the other hand, seem to favor the views of those who hold, with Virchow and Yvaren, that syphilis is at the bottom of every thing, and that even tubercular phthisis, cardiac polypi, disorganizations of the liver, several kinds of jaundice, even scrofula, white swellings, and sarcocele, originate in syphilis. However firmly I have been resolved not to discuss points of doctrine that, owing to the absence of reliable facts, are still exceedingly problematical, yet I deem it incumbent upon me to publish these two cases.

The first is the case of a man of seventy, who consulted me in the month of August on account of a profusely-secreting soft ulcer on the prepuce, for which I prescribed *Merc. sol.*, first trituration, half a grain twice a day. However, dreading Mercury a good deal, he took, without my knowledge, two pellets of Merc. 12, and several other remedies. On the 7th of November he came again, his forehead manifestly covered with isolated, scattered syphilitic tubercles. The chancre had become cicatrized, without having shown the least hardness in its course; at the place where the chancre had been located, a tolerably large, cock's-comb-shaped figwart was seen. Last September he had had two buboes, which he had cured himself with *Nitri acidum*, on which account I gave him *Lycopodium* 30. Since then (now December 7th), the figwart and the dry, scattered tubercles on the forehead have disappeared; in their places, a cough, with purulent expectoration, has set in, which might lead others to suspect phthisis pulmonalis. Unfortunately for this diagnosis, this patient has had such a cough twice before, during the twenty-five years that I have been acquainted with him.—The other case is that of a young married woman, who consulted me in the month of May on account of a soft chancre at the lower commissure, that had been there for about a fortnight. She continued her visits for eight days, when I did not see her again until the 15th of November following. Not having perceived any improvement the first four days of my treatment, and fearing the return of her husband, who happened to be absent on a journey, she had had the chancre removed by cauterization, and had, at the same time, continued my prescription for another week. She thought herself free from all trouble, when, all at once, in the month of November, an unmistakable papulous exanthem broke out, which covered chiefly the abdomen and lower extremities, particularly the thighs.—Individuals, with old soft chancres, and simultaneously existing roseola syphilitica, have frequently applied to me for treatment, so that, notwithstanding the observations recently published by the hospital-physicians of Lyons concerning the supposed *essential* differences between the contagia giving rise respectively to the soft, Hunterian, and phagedænic chancres, I am unable to regard such a distinction as founded in fact; for, if it is certain, as I know from personal observation, that a Hunterian chancre may, according to circumstances, produce any of the other forms, and that any of these forms may superinduce the same secondary consequences, although these results may not always follow, the fact that there inheres, in all these forms, a faculty of superinducing the secondary consequences, is sufficient to induce us to regard the identity of the contagium as an established fact, and to attribute the apparent differences of forms to the influence of as yet unknown, but, at all events, *non-essential* circumstances. Who knows whether the *ulcus molle* is not derived from the Hunterian chancre, by the bare fact, that the profuse secretion of the former prevents the specific inflammation upon which the characteristic induration of the Hunterian chancre depends. It is true that, beside the Hunterian chancres, all other chancres, as we have shown in the third division, §§ 156–166, seem to have existed since the remotest period; but, in the same place, we have likewise shown that the great epidemic of the fifteenth century produced a new unitary syphilitic disease, from which not only the ancient gonorrhœa and condylomata arose in their new forms of syphilitic gonorrhœa, and syphilitic mucous tubercles, but likewise the ancient soft and phagedænic, even gangrenous chancres, modified by the new syphilitic virus.

II.—To Sections 176–178.

What I have said just now, leads me to utter a few other remarks which I should have kept suppressed, but for the fact that I met in the past week a young man who had fallen a victim to a new pathological and therapeutic theory in Homœopathy. I allude to the theory which accords an undue extension to the boundaries of Sycosis, and accepts a large number of new remedies for this disease upon purely speculative grounds. There is no doubt, whatsoever, that there are chancrous-syphilitic as well as non-chancrous syphilitic figwarts, although we may not as yet have it in our power to distinguish these two kinds from each other. If we adopt, after the example of Hahnemann, a special contagium, the so-called sycosic contagium, which is different from the contagium of chancre; and if we class, as some French homœopaths are in the habit of doing, in the category of sycosis any thing that bears the remotest anatomical analogy to sycosic excrescences, such as: common warts, steatomata, sarcomata, polypi of the nose, ears, heart, bladder, uterus; it seems to us, that this mode of generalizing is carrying the application of a theory beyond the bounds of logic and even of the most superficial pretensions to science. Either these theorizers admit, with Hahnemann, that some of these condylomata are of venereal origin, and can be communicated again by the act of coïtion; and that others cannot; or else they regard all these condylomata as elements of one and the same pathological series. If they regard only some of these condylomata as contagious, they can no more class the non-contagious excrescences in the same category with the former, than simple maculæ, vesicles, papulæ, pustules, etc., can be classed with their syphilitic analogues in the same series. If yonder theorizers regard all the above-mentioned excrescences, on the ground of their pathological resemblance, as elements of the same pathological series, they must, for consistency's sake, either regard all of them as contagious, or else as non-contagious, for the simple reason that what constitutes the pathological unity of a series, is the pathological identity of the generating cause or principle of the whole series, and consequently of each of its constituent elements. Now, if we mean to assert that steatomata and sarcomata, as well as common warts, are equally contagious as the figwarts whose contagious character is established by abundant experience, we shall find purely anatomical demonstrations utterly insufficient, and we shall have to call in aid arguments based upon the etiological, physiological, and pathological origin and behaviour of those excrescences. A confusion of this kind, introduced in our anatomical and pathological definitions, is to be deplored all the more, since, when therapeutic measures are to be governed by such erroneous theories, the selection of remedial agents is no longer regulated by positive and decisive science, but by superficial sophisms. That the anatomical structure of certain pathological products is sometimes determined by an analogous pathological activity, and, hence, may lead to the selection of the same remedial agent, cannot be denied; but that which is decisive in the selection of a remedy, is not the inanimate pathological product, but, on the one hand, the specific *generative cause*, and, on the other hand, the *physiological* and *pathological activities*, and *vital manifestations* of the disease; where these are alike, the most diversified anatomical malformations can be cured by the same remedy; but, if the causes and vital manifestations of such malformations are of a different kind, anatomical products that are ever so much alike, require the most varied remedies for their cure. Those are to be pitied who, misled by such erroneous theories, and failing to cure evidently venereal figwarts, in a hurry, with *Nitri ac.*, *Thuja*, *Staphys.*, *Phosph. ac.*, *Cinnabaris*, and *Lycopodium*, now jump at *Calcarea*, *Teucrium*, *Secale cornutum*, *Sepia*, and *Dulcamara*, for no better reason than because these last-mentioned remedies have cured steatomata, polypi, or common warts, and, in accordance with the new theory, should be powerful *anti-sycotica*. Even if, by pursuing this course, physicians do not always allow the figwarts to grow to the size of one or more inches, it is certain—we can prophesy this result most positively—that, by this means, they will most uselessly incur the loss of precious time that it may be beyond their power to repair.

JUST PUBLISHED:

A MANUAL OF PHARMACODYNAMICS.

BY RICHARD HUGHES, L.R.C.P. Edin.

London: H. Turner & Co. Bound, $3.00.

SECOND EDITION, WITH ADDITIONS.

This is the first volume of a manual of homœopathic practice for students and beginners. The second part, which we are promised shortly, will be on therapeutics.

Dr. Hughes is already favorably known to the homœopathic public and profession as a thoughtful writer, and as one of the editors of the *British Journal of Homœopathy*. His essays in our periodical literature are characterized by their eminently practical tone and by their scientific precision. It was therefore with much pleasurable expectation that we waited his promised work, and our expectations have been fully realized on its perusal.

Homœopathy has long wanted such a work as this which is now before us. Our Materia Medica, in its entirety, is cumbrous, and is yearly becoming more and more unwieldy. It is worse than that, it is disjointed and fragmentary. It is full of pearls of great value, but at present they lie at the bottom of their beds, and the diving for them is an effort, always requiring great exertion, sometimes exhausting and baffling even to the strongest swimmer. We therefore hail with no little joy and gratitude any attempt to gather or to arrange these pearls for our use. If this want has been felt by homœopaths, how much more does it appear an essential to allopathic inquirers, who have been long accustomed to generalizations?

Dr. Hughes exactly describes the state of chaos of our chief works on Materia Medica, which we have so often brought under the notice of our readers, when reviewing the several attempts hitherto made to reduce this chaos into order. These efforts to reform our Materia Medica may be described as of two kinds: the one, of which Dr. Hempel's "Materia Medica" may be regarded as the type; the other, which is well represented by the more recent "Text Book of Materia Medica" by Dr. Lippe.

The former of these books is synthetical, the latter analytical. Dr. Hempel's admirable work attempts to arrange the Homœopathic Materia Medica and Therapeutics on a physiologico-pathological basis. Dr. Lippe adheres to the arrangement of Hahnemann, and attempts to simplify it by an arbitrary blotting out of certain symptoms.

Adhering to Dr. Hughes' metaphor, we should say that Dr. Hempel's attempt is, as it were, to put each picture together again so as to form a pleasing and meaning landscape: placing the trees, the clouds, the lakes and mountains all in their natural order and position. On the other hand, Dr. Lippe cuts out a few trees, or wipes out a few clouds, and blots out a few sheets of water, but does not attempt to place any one of these essentials to a landscape in its proper position so as to form a whole. Thus the one book gives us a series of pictures conveying pleasing ideas of a rational kind, and is eminently practical. The other is more like the property room of a theatre, and presents a very dreamy amount of confused out of places, trees and clouds and pieces of water piled up, each after its own kind, without any definite or mutual relation the one to the other.

The refusal on the part of certain homœopaths to group and classify the effects of medicines, with their corresponding refusal to group and to classify the symptoms of disease, has done more to retard the true progress of homœopathy than all the opposition of its enemies.

We therefore welcome as a valuable addition to our literature, this new and rational effort to give us clear and concrete notions of each drug; to put before us its whole shape and size and habits in a readable manner.

Very readably and pleasantly, does the author of the MANUAL OF PHARMACODYNAMICS lead us through 590 pages of his well-written discourses, which, for reasons set forth on p. ix, he has given to us in the form of letters to a medical friend.—*Brit. Hom. Review.*

C. Neidhard, M. D., Diphtheria, as it prevailed in the United States from 1860 to 1867, preceded by an Historical Account of its Phenomena, its Nature, and Homœopathic Treatment. Price, bound, ... $1 75

After the publication of several able works on diphtheria by the Homœopathic Press, it might be considered superfluous to issue another work on the same subject. A superficial glance at the Index and Table of Contents will make it evident that the present work is more complete in the details of its history, symptoms, and treatment, than any of its predecessors. The author's own rich experience (having attended over six hundred cases of the disease), and his discovery of a valuable homœopathic remedy, will make it a standard work on diphtheria. It ought to be in the hands of every practitioner.

Gross', Dr. H., Comparative Materia Medica, translated and edited by Dr. Constantine Hering. Bound, . $10 00

It is needless to dwell upon the fact how much the value of this work has been enhanced by being edited by Dr. Hering, for he not only rendered the original into English scrupulously correct, but also greatly enriched it from his own inexhaustible storehouse.

Hempel, Dr. Chas. J., A New and Comprehensive System of Materia Medica and Therapeutics. Second Edition. In two volumes. Bound. Price, ... $12 00

The almost unanimous desire of the profession has induced the publisher to put forth a second edition of this work, which has been greatly improved and considerably enlarged by the addition of *new remedies*, and by a more careful elaboration of a number of the older remedies, to which a rather short space had been allotted in the first edition. In this work the subject of Homœopathic Materia Medica and Therapeutics is presented, as it should be, in connection with pathology and physiology. Homœopathic physicians will find this work a reliable and most comprehensive guide in the treatment of diseases. Students and allopathic practitioners may acquire a thorough and comparatively easy knowledge of Homœopathy by a perusal of its pages. In no work that we know of, is the subject of Homœopathy presented to the inquiring mind in the same broad and comprehensive sense as in the present one.

Marcy, Dr. E. E., and ***F. W. Hunt, M. D.,*** The Homœopathic Theory and Practice of Medicine. In two volumes. Bound. Price, ... $12 00

This work presents to the medical profession and the friends of Homœopathy a comprehensive and intelligent view of the principles and practice of our school, as it is now represented by our best writers and practitioners; it embodies, as far as our wide range of subjects permits, the latest opinions and theories of investigators of every school on pathology and collateral sciences connected with medicine; and gives to all inquirers after advanced scientific truth the opportunity to investigate our principles, and to see them tested by facts, as illustrated in the clinical experience of a large number of reliable observers.

Zehn Hauptgruende fur die Bevorzugung der Homöopathie gegen die gewöhnliche medizinische Behandlung, . . 10 cts.

www.ingramcontent.com/pod-product-compliance
Lightning Source LLC
LaVergne TN
LVHW021132110826
845150LV00005B/1005

* 9 7 8 1 4 2 5 5 5 0 1 3 4 *